MOLECULAR DIAGNOSTICS AND TREATMENT OF PANCREATIC CANCER: SYSTEMS AND NETWORK BIOLOGY APPROACHES

MOLECULAR DIAGNOSTICS AND TREATMENT OF PANCREATIC CANCER: SYSTEMS AND NETWORK BIOLOGY APPROACHES

Edited by

ASFAR S. AZMI

Amsterdam • Boston • Heidelberg • London
New York • Oxford • Paris • San Diego
San Francisco • Singapore • Sydney • Tokyo
Academic Press is an imprint of Elsevier

Academic Press is an imprint of Elsevier
32 Jamestown Road, London NW1 7BY, UK
225 Wyman Street, Waltham, MA 02451, USA
525 B Street, Suite 1800, San Diego, CA 92101-4495, USA

2014 Elsevier Inc.

Notice

British Library Cataloguing-in-Publication Data
A catalogue record for this book is available from the British Library

Library of Congress Cataloging-in-Publication Data
A catalog record for this book is available from the Library of Congress

ISBN: 978-0-12-408103-1

For information on all Academic Press publications
visit our website at elsevierdirect.com

Typeset by TNQ Books and Journals
www.tnq.co.in

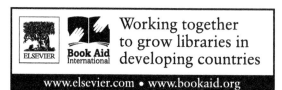

DEDICATION

This book is dedicated to my Father, Dr. Sohail Ahmad Azmi, a tireless physician who instilled in me the right values, work ethics, and scientific temperament.

CONTENTS

Preface   xiii
Acknowledgments   xv
Contributors   xvii

Section I. Current Trends and Advances in Pancreatic Cancer

1. **Epidemiology, Treatment, and Outcome of Pancreatic Cancer**   3

   Robert Grützmann

   Introduction   3
   Epidemiology and etiology of pancreatic cancer   3
   Types of pancreatic cancer   4
   Clinical presentation of pancreatic cancer   5
   Diagnosis of pancreatic cancer   5
   Treatment of pancreatic cancer   6
   Potentially curative surgical treatment   6
   Adjuvant and neoadjuvant treatment   7
   Prognosis of pancreatic cancer   8
   Outlook   8
   References   8

2. **Advances in Primary Cell Culture of Pancreatic Cancer**   11

   Niccola Funel

   Introduction   12
   Cell culture of PDAC   16
   Isolation and establishment procedure   17
   Characterization of cell cultures   26
   Morphology   26
   Genotyping   26
   Phenotyping   27
   Second level of biological models   29
   Three-dimensional cell cultures   34
   In vivo models   34
   Applications   35
   Conclusion   35
   Acknowledgments   35
   References   36

3. **Multimodal Therapies for Pancreatic Cancer**   **39**

Sara Chiblak, Kenneth E. Lipson, Amir Abdollahi

Introduction   39
Conclusion   63
References   64

4. **The Role of Notch Signaling Pathway in the Progression of Pancreatic Cancer**   **75**

Jiankun Gao, Fazlul H. Sarkar, Lucio Miele, Zhiwei Wang

Introduction   75
Notch signaling pathway   76
The role of Notch in PC   77
Notch inhibition is a novel strategy for PC treatment   83
Understanding notch signaling through systems biology   84
Conclusion   85
References   86

Section II. Gene Expression Profiling and Bioinformatics Analysis in Pancreatic Cancer

5. **Bioinformatics Analysis of Pancreas Cancer Genome in High-Throughput Genomic Technologies**   **93**

Enrique Carrillo-de Santa Pau, Francisco X. Real Alfonso Valencia

Introduction   94
Heterogeneity and quality of samples for high-throughput
    genomic technologies   95
Microarrays   96
Next-generation sequencing   101
Databases and resources   115
Conclusion and future perspectives   125
References   126

6. **Statistical Analysis of High-Dimensional Data for Pancreatic Cancer**   **133**

Haijun Gong, Tong Tong Wu, Edmund Clarke

Introduction   133
LASSO penalized cox regression   137
Doubly regularized cox regression   140

Pancreatic cancer survival analysis   144
Acknowledgments   148
References   148

7. Gene Expression Profiling in Pancreatic Cancer   151
Christian Pilarsky, Robert Grützmann

Introduction   151
Summary   164
References   165

8. Genetic Susceptibility and Risk of Pancreatic Cancer   169
Jason Hoskins, Jinping Jia, Laufey T. Amundadottir

Introduction   169
Familial risk of pancreatic cancer   170
Rare, high-risk pancreatic cancer susceptibility genes and multicancer
    syndromes   171
Common, low-risk pancreatic cancer susceptibility loci   174
Common pancreatic cancer risk loci in non-European populations   179
Pathway analyses of pancreatic cancer GWAS data sets   181
Future GWAS and gene mapping approaches   186
Websites   188
References   188

Section III. Pancreatic Cancer Proteomics

9. Proteomics in Pancreatic Cancer Translational Research   197
Sheng Pan, Ru Chen, Teresa A. Brentnall

Introduction   198
Overview of proteomics technologies   198
Proteomics study of pancreatic tissue   202
Blood biomarker discovery   205
Analysis of pancreatic juice and cyst fluid   207
Functional and hypothesis-driven proteomic studies   209
Post-translational modifications   211
Summary   213
Acknowledgment   213
References   214

10. **Proteomic Differences and Linkages between Chemoresistance and Metastasis of Pancreatic Cancer Using Knowledge-Based Pathway Analysis**   **221**

Jin-Gyun Lee, Kimberly Q. McKinney, Sun-Il Hwang

Introduction   221
Proteomic analysis at subcellular level   222
Protein identification and data compiling   224
Comparative analysis of differentially expressed proteins   225
Biological network analysis   230
Canonical pathway analysis using metacore™   233
Vimentin expression and chemoresistance   238
Conclusion   241
References   242

11. **RNAi Validation of Pancreatic Cancer Antigens Identified by Cell Surface Proteomics**   **245**

Candy N. Lee, Tao He, Ian McCaffrey, Charles E. Birse, Katherine McKinnon,
Bruno Domon, Steven M. Ruben, Paul A. Moore

Introduction   245
Summary   272
Acknowledgments   273
References   273

Section IV. Systems and Network Understanding of Pancreatic Cancer Signaling

12. **The Significance of the Feedback Loops between Kras and Ink4a in Pancreatic Cancer**   **281**

Baltazar D. Aguda

Introduction   281
Threshold of Kras activation   282
Kras effector pathways in PDAC development   285
Negative versus positive feedback loops between Kras and Ink4a   288
Ink4a against microRNAs in the control of Kras   289
Concluding remarks   291
References   293

13. **Systems Biology of Pancreatic Cancer Stem Cells**   **297**

Ginny F. Bao, Philip A. Philip, Asfar S. Azmi

Introduction   297
The complexity of pancreatic cancer   298

Why systems biology is needed for PC   302
PC therapy resistance and the role of cancer stem cells   307
Isolation and biological characterization of PC CSCs   308
Systems and pathway analysis of CSCs   310
Systems analysis of PC CSC microRNA network   314
Summary and future directions   316
Acknowledgment   318
References   318

14. Characterizing the Metabolomic Effects of Pancreatic Cancer   323

Oliver F. Bathe

Introduction   323
Conclusion   337
References   338

15. Prioritizing Diagnostic, Prognostic, and Therapeutic MicroRNAs in Pancreatic Cancer: Systems and Network Biology Approaches   345

Osama M. Alian, Shadan Ali, Ramzi M. Mohammad, Asfar S. Azmi, Fazlul H. Sarkar

An introduction and brief overview of microRNAs   345
MicroRNAs and disease priming and progression   346
Diagnostic, prognostic, and therapeutic value of miRNAs in pancreatic cancer   349
Prioritizing miRNAs from pancreatic biospecimens using pathway tools   352
Clinical targeting of miRNAs   352
Implications—new hope or wild-goose chase?   357
Conclusion   359
References   359

Section V. Systems Approaches to Pancreatic Cancer Therapeutics

16. Integration of Protein Network Activation Mapping Technology for Personalized Therapy: Implications for Pancreatic Cancer   367

Mariaelena Pierobon, Julie Wulfkuhle, Lance A. Liotta, Emanuel F. Petricoin III

Introduction   367
Defective protein signaling networks underpin tumorigenesis   368
Reverse phase protein microarrays as a tool for personalized cancer therapy   371
Pre-analytical factors influence phosphoprotein pathway activation mapping   374
Case studies in pathway activation mapping of human cancer   375
Generation of a cellular circuit diagram for patient management: a summary   377
References   379

17. Computational and Biological Evaluation of Radioiodinated Quinazolinone Prodrug for Targeting Pancreatic Cancer   385

Pavel Pospisil, Amin I. Kassis

Introduction to EMCIT concept	385
Computational evaluation	387
Sequence alignment of extracellular sulfatase	388
Biological evaluation	394
Discussion	397
Conclusions	401
References	402

18. Systems and Network Pharmacology Strategies for Pancreatic Ductal Adenocarcinoma Therapy: A Resource Review   405

Irfana Muqbil, Asfar S. Azmi, Ramzi M. Mohammad

Introduction	405
Need for revisiting the progression model of PDAC: departure from genes to network	407
Defining biological networks	408
Network pharmacology to unwind PDAC microRNA complexity	414
Network pharmacology in drug repositioning for PDAC	416
Networks in polypharmacology strategies against PDAC	418
Conclusions and future perspectives	420
References	421

Index	427

Pancreatic cancer remains a deadly disease that is receiving more and more attention nowadays. Its diagnosis is still considered a death sentence and sadly every two minutes a patient dies from the disease somewhere in the world (~300,000 annual deaths). It is quite unfortunate to note that unlike other cancers that have witnessed major progress in early diagnostics, better management and some success in the identification of molecularly targeted drugs, the field of pancreatic cancer research lags behind on all these fronts. There is an urgent need for the identification of diagnostic and prognostic markers and a dire need for effective drugs to tame the disease. A major reason for such poor progress is due to the reductionism in approaches that for the past few decades have focused on studying single or few pathways and searching for magic bullet drugs. Being a heterogeneous disease, there is a need for interdisciplinary strategies that take a holistic view at the whole system instead of individual components.

The scale of the complexity of pancreatic cancer calls for equally complex solutions and holistic computational technologies, especially systems biology, are expected to play pivotal roles in current and future research. The depth and breadth of opportunities provided by systems sciences are endless and researchers are increasingly relying on these interdisciplinary areas to enhance the understanding of this invariably terminal disease of the pancreas. Although the cross talk between different scientific disciplines has increased, a wide gap still exists between basic biologist and computational experts; the former hesitant to dwell into unchartered bioinformatics territory and the later unable to obtain opportunities to test and validate their powerful analytical tools in actual biological systems.

The literature on pancreas cancer systems biology is sparsely distributed in the web of knowledge and no previous work has satisfactorily integrated this new interdisciplinary subject area. Unlike prior works, this book brings together wide-ranging modern topics and for the first time, showcases the recent advancement in systems approaches to pancreatic cancer under one comprehensive volume. The 18 chapters presented here are from leading pancreas cancer experts who have been using many novel computational tools to get new information by reaching to previously unfathomable depths. Many of these experts are founders in their own fields. They have discussed a wide range of topics such as pancreatic cancer bioinformatics, expression analysis, and proteomics. Other topics highlight the use of systems sciences in unraveling the complexities of pancreas cancer signaling, understanding disease metabolomics, the role of microRNAs, overcoming therapy resistance, resolving the pancreatic cancer stem cell debate, understanding the cross talk between different components that make up the microenvironment, pursuing patient stratification for tailored treatments, and many more. These chapters carry more than a thousand updated references and numerous web resources and detailed illustrations. They should be very helpful for the researchers that are seriously engaged in the area of translational pancreatic cancer research. It is anticipated that this book will bridge the gap among basic researchers, clinicians, and computational biologists, all of whom have a common goal—to defeat pancreatic cancer.

Asfar S. Azmi, PhD.

ACKNOWLEDGMENTS

First of all I would like to thank Elsevier Academic Press for appreciating the value of this concept and allowing me to edit this book. Special thanks to Nisbet Graham for entertaining the idea of this volume. I am extremely grateful to the constant support provided by Catherine Van Der Laan (Cassie) and her editorial team during the various stages of this project. Her help in setting up the submission website and cover design is deeply appreciated. I would like to especially thank Professor Ramzi Mohammad, Division Head, Hamad Medical Corporation, Doha, Qatar for giving his unending support in my editorial ventures. The scholarly guidance from Professor Fazlul Sarkar (Distinguished Professor), Wayne State University is deeply acknowledged. I am highly grateful to the entire Gastrointestinal Cancer Research Team at Karmanos Cancer Institute, especially our team leader Dr Philip A. Philip for developing in me the enthusiasm to work in the area of pancreatic cancer.

CONTRIBUTORS

Amir Abdollahi
German Cancer Consortium (DKTK), Heidelberg, Germany; Molecular & Translational Radiation Oncology, Heidelberg Ion Therapy Center (HIT), Heidelberg Institute of Radiation Oncology (HIRO), University of Heidelberg Medical School and National Center for Tumor Diseases (NCT), German Cancer Research Center (DKFZ), Heidelberg, Germany

Baltazar D. Aguda
DiseasePathways LLC, Bethesda, MD, USA

Shadan Ali
Department of Oncology, Karmanos Cancer Institute, Detroit, MI, USA

Osama M. Alian
Department of Oncology, Karmanos Cancer Institute, Detroit, MI, USA

Laufey T. Amundadottir
Laboratory of Translational Genomics, Division of Cancer Epidemiology and Genetics, National Cancer Institute, National Institutes of Health, Bethesda, MD, USA

Asfar S. Azmi
Department of Pathology, Wayne State University School of Medicine, Detroit, MI, USA

Ginny F. Bao
Department of Pathology, Wayne State University School of Medicine, Detroit, MI, USA

Oliver F. Bathe
Departments of Surgery and Oncology, University of Calgary, Calgary, AB, Canada

Charles E. Birse
Department of Protein Therapeutics, Celera, Rockville, MD, USA; Celera, Alameda, CA, USA

Teresa A. Brentnall
Department of Medicine, University of Washington, Seattle, WA, USA

Ru Chen
Department of Medicine, University of Washington, Seattle, WA, USA

Sara Chiblak
German Cancer Consortium (DKTK), Heidelberg, Germany; Molecular & Translational Radiation Oncology, Heidelberg Ion Therapy Center (HIT), Heidelberg Institute of Radiation Oncology (HIRO), University of Heidelberg Medical School and National Center for Tumor Diseases (NCT), German Cancer Research Center (DKFZ), Heidelberg, Germany

Edmund Clarke
Computer Science Department, Carnegie Mellon University, Pittsburgh, PA, USA

Bruno Domon
Department of Protein Therapeutics, Celera, Rockville, MD, USA; Luxembourg Clinical Proteomics Center, CRP-Sante, Luxembourg

Niccola Funel
Department of Surgical, Molecular and Medical Pathology, University of Pisa, Pisa, Italy

Jiankun Gao
Department of Basic Medical Sciences, Sichuan College of Traditional Chinese Medicine, Mianyang, Sichuan, China

Haijun Gong
Department of Mathematics and Computer Science, Saint Louis University, St. Louis, MO, USA

Robert Grützmann
Department of General, Thoracic, and Vascular Surgery, University Hospital "Carl Gustav Carus", Dresden University of Technology, Dresden, Germany

Tao He
Department of Protein Therapeutics, Celera, Rockville, MD, USA; Pfizer, Cambridge, MA, USA

Jason Hoskins
Laboratory of Translational Genomics, Division of Cancer Epidemiology and Genetics, National Cancer Institute, National Institutes of Health, Bethesda, MD, USA

Sun-Il Hwang
Proteomics and Mass Spectrometry Research Laboratory, Carolinas HealthCare System, Charlotte, NC, USA

Jinping Jia
Laboratory of Translational Genomics, Division of Cancer Epidemiology and Genetics, National Cancer Institute, National Institutes of Health, Bethesda, MD, USA

Amin I. Kassis
Department of Radiology, Harvard Medical School, Boston, MA, USA

Jin-Gyun Lee
Proteomics and Mass Spectrometry Research Laboratory, Carolinas HealthCare System, Charlotte, NC, USA

Candy N. Lee
Department of Protein Therapeutics, Celera, Rockville, MD, USA; Pfizer, South San Francisco, CA, USA

Lance A. Liotta
Center for Applied Proteomics and Molecular Medicine, George Mason University, Manassas, VA, USA

Kenneth E. Lipson
FibroGen, Inc., San Francisco, CA, USA

Ian McCaffrey
Department of Protein Therapeutics, Celera, Rockville, MD, USA; Genentech, South San Francisco, CA, USA

Kimberly Q. McKinney
Proteomics and Mass Spectrometry Research Laboratory, Carolinas HealthCare System, Charlotte, NC, USA

Katherine McKinnon
Department of Protein Therapeutics, Celera, Rockville, MD, USA; NCI, Bethesda, MD, USA

Lucio Miele
University of Mississippi Cancer Institute, Jackson, MS, USA

Ramzi M. Mohammad
Department of Oncology, Karmanos Cancer Institute, Wayne State University, Detroit, MI, USA; Hamad Medical Corporation, Doha, Qatar

Paul A. Moore
Department of Protein Therapeutics, Celera, Rockville, MD, USA; MacroGenics Inc., Rockville, MD, USA

Irfana Muqbil
Department of Biochemistry, Faculty of Life Sciences, AMU, Aligarh, UP, India

Sheng Pan
Department of Medicine, University of Washington, Seattle, WA, USA

Emanuel F. Petricoin III
Center for Applied Proteomics and Molecular Medicine, George Mason University, Manassas, VA, USA

Philip A. Philip
Department of Oncology, Karmanos Cancer Institute, Detroit, MI, USA

Mariaelena Pierobon
Center for Applied Proteomics and Molecular Medicine, George Mason University, Manassas, VA, USA

Christian Pilarsky
Department of Visceral-, Thoracic- and Vascular Surgery, Medizinische Universität Carl Gustav Carus, TU Dresden, Dresden, Germany

Pavel Pospisil
Philip Morris International R&D, Philip Morris Products S.A., Neuchâtel, Switzerland

Francisco X. Real
Spanish National Cancer Research Center (CNIO), Madrid, Spain

Steven M. Ruben
Department of Protein Therapeutics, Celera, Rockville, MD, USA

Enrique Carrillo-de Santa Pau
Spanish National Cancer Research Center (CNIO), Madrid, Spain

Fazlul H. Sarkar
Department of Pathology and Oncology, Karmanos Cancer Institute, Wayne State University, Detroit, MI, USA

Alfonso Valencia
Spanish National Cancer Research Center (CNIO), Madrid, Spain

Zhiwei Wang
The Cyrus Tang Hematology Center, Jiangsu Institute of Hematology, the First, Affiliated Hospital, Soochow University, Suzhou, China; Department of Pathology, Beth Israel Deaconess Medical Center, Harvard Medical School, Boston, MA, USA

Tong Tong Wu
Department of Biostatistics and Computational Biology, University of Rochester, Rochester, NY, USA

Julie Wulfkuhle
Center for Applied Proteomics and Molecular Medicine, George Mason University, Manassas, VA, USA

Current Trends and Advances in Pancreatic Cancer

Epidemiology, Treatment, and Outcome of Pancreatic Cancer

Robert Grützmann

Department of General, Thoracic, and Vascular Surgery, University Hospital "Carl Gustav Carus", Dresden University of Technology, Dresden, Germany

Contents

Introduction	3
Epidemiology and Etiology of Pancreatic Cancer	3
Types of Pancreatic Cancer	4
Clinical Presentation of Pancreatic Cancer	5
Diagnosis of Pancreatic Cancer	5
Treatment of Pancreatic Cancer	6
Potentially Curative Surgical Treatment	6
Adjuvant and Neoadjuvant Treatment	7
Palliative Treatment	7
Prognosis of Pancreatic Cancer	8
Outlook	8
References	8

INTRODUCTION

Pancreatic cancer is a relatively rare cancer type, but a major cause of cancer-related death because there are quite rare histologically proven long-time survivors of pancreatic cancer. The main reasons for the worse prognosis are: late clinical presentation, aggressive biology, and failure of surgical and systemic treatment. The aim of this introductory chapter is to provide an update on the known causes, clinical presentations, and most current management strategies of pancreatic carcinoma.

EPIDEMIOLOGY AND ETIOLOGY OF PANCREATIC CANCER

Pancreatic adenocarcinoma comprises only 3% of estimated new cancer cases each year but with 44,030 new cases and 37,660 deaths expected in 2011 is the fourth most common cause of cancer mortality [1]. The annual incidence rate of pancreatic cancer is approximately 8/100,000 persons worldwide. Adenocarcinoma is the most frequent type of pancreatic cancer. Others are endocrine and cystic tumors, which have a different, mostly better, prognosis [2]. There are established risk factors for developing pancreatic cancer including chronic pancreatitis, increased age, family history, smoking, and diabetes [3]. Obesity and physical activity have been implicated in pancreatic cancer etiology.

TYPES OF PANCREATIC CANCER

Ninety-five percent of pancreatic cancers originate from the exocrine portion of the gland. A proposed mechanism for the development of invasive pancreatic adenocarcinoma is a stepwise progression through genetically and histologically well-defined noninvasive precursor lesions, called pancreatic intraepithelial neoplasias (PanINs). They are microscopic lesions in small (less than 5 mm) pancreatic ducts and are classified into three grades (PanIN 1–3). The understanding of molecular alterations in PanINs has provided rational candidates for the development of early detection biomarkers and therapeutic targets. Another precursor of invasive pancreatic carcinomas is pancreatic intraductal papillary mucinous neoplasia (IPMN). IPMNs belong to the increasingly diagnosed and treated group of cystic tumors. They progress from a benign intraductal tumor through increasing grades of dysplasia to invasive adenocarcinoma and therefore provide models of neoplastic pancreatic progression [4]. Other tumor types within the pancreas are endocrine tumors and a variety of rare pancreatic tumors like acinar cell carcinoma (Table 1.1) [5].

Table 1.1 Main Types of Pancreatic Cancer

Pancreatic Exocrine Cancers	Pancreatic Endocrine Neuroendocrine Tumor
Pancreatic ductal adenocarcinoma	Nonfunctional islet cell tumor insulinoma
Intraductal papillary mucinous neoplasia (IPMN)	Gastrinoma
Mucinous cystadenocarcinoma	Glucagonoma
Adenosquamous carcinoma	Somatostatinoma
Solid pseudopapillary tumors	Vasoactive intestinal peptide releasing tumor (VIPoma)

CLINICAL PRESENTATION OF PANCREATIC CANCER

Most cases of pancreatic cancer are diagnosed for nonspecific abdominal pain or jaundice or both. The peak incidence for pancreatic cancer is in the seventh and eighth decades of life. Men are affected slightly more often than women.

The only specific clinical sign, jaundice, develops if the tumor is growing in the pancreatic head near to the bile duct. Many patients present late with secondary symptoms related to a larger malignant tumor and/or metastatic spread with back pain (direct invasion of the celiac plexus) or malignant ascites. Unexplained weight loss is sometimes the only sign. Approximately 80% of patients have unresectable disease at the time of diagnosis due to metastatic spread or locally advanced disease.

Development of diabetes should strongly alert the physician to the possibility of pancreatic cancer. Patients over the age of 50 with late onset diabetes have an eightfold increased risk of developing pancreatic cancer within three years of the diagnosis compared to the general population [6]. Most malignant tumors develop in the pancreatic head; because of late presentation the tumors within the pancreatic tail have a lower resectability and worse prognosis.

DIAGNOSIS OF PANCREATIC CANCER

Tumor markers seemed to be ideal for early diagnosis of cancer. However, the lack of sensitivity and specificity has been a major problem in the use of most serum tumor markers for diagnosis of pancreatic cancer. In the vast majority of research studies over the past two decades, CA19-9 alone has been applied as the "gold standard" for monitoring and diagnosis of patients with pancreatic cancer [7].

The aim of imaging is to detect pancreatic cancer, to detect metastases, to evaluate the risk for malignancy, and to predict resectability. Transabdominal ultrasonography (US) serves as a basic imaging examination. In experienced hands, it is possible to predict resectability with high accuracy using US. Endoscopic ultrasonography is a useful diagnostic method, especially in small pancreatic tumors. It enables fine-needle aspiration for pathological analysis. Pancreatic cancer also can be visualized by endoscopic retrograde cholangiopancreatography (ERCP) [6]. The appearance of double duct sign (occlusion of both the pancreatic and the bile duct) is a pathognomic of a malignant pancreatic head tumor. However, ERCP has been mostly replaced by contrast enhanced multislice computed tomography (CT) and magnetic resonance cholangiopancreatography (MRCP) because they are much less invasive than ERCP. Both CT and magnetic resonance imaging with MRCP are useful for the diagnosis and characterization of pancreatic masses. Both modalities provide an accurate assessment of a tumor and its relationship with surrounding organs and vessels.

TREATMENT OF PANCREATIC CANCER

At present, surgical resection is the only curative treatment for pancreatic adenocarcinoma. For unresectable tumors and patients unwilling or not medically fit enough to undergo major pancreatic surgery, alternatives include systemic chemotherapy, chemoradiotherapy, image guided stereotactic radiosurgical systems (such as CyberKnife), surgical bypass, ablative therapies, and endoscopic biliary and gastrointestinal stenting. These are palliative procedures that can improve patients' quality of life by alleviating tumor-related symptoms like pain.

POTENTIALLY CURATIVE SURGICAL TREATMENT

The majority of pancreatic adenocarcinomas are located within the head, neck, and uncinate process of the pancreas and require a pancreaticoduodenectomy with lymphadenectomy. First described in the 1930s, it involves resection of the proximal pancreas, along with the distal stomach, duodenum, distal bile duct, and gallbladder as an en bloc specimen. It is the so-called Whipple procedure. Intestinal reconstruction is restored via a gastrojejunostomy, hepaticojejunostomy, and pancreatojejunostomy. It has been shown that the preservation of the stomach is oncologically safe, faster, and blood sparing, and therefore most of the pancreatic head resections today are performed as pylorus preserving pancreaticoduodenectomy. Pancreatic tail tumors are treated with a pancreatic left resection.

The absolute contraindications to pancreatic resection are distant metastases to the liver or the peritoneum. The age of the patient, size of the tumor, local (and even distant) lymph node metastases, and continuous invasion of the stomach or duodenum are no general contraindications to resection. Tumor involvement of the major vessels around the pancreas is no longer an absolute contraindication to curative resection, especially in venous infiltration. Encasement of the hepatic artery, superior mesenteric artery, and coeliac axis means that potentially curative surgery is unlikely but not always impossible.

A complete resection with microscopically free margin (R0) should always be intended, but cannot always be achieved. If an R0 resection can be obtained, median survival is vastly improved compared to resections with tumor positive.

Advances in surgical techniques and perioperative care made pancreatico-duodenectomy safe and feasible, but morbidity following pancreatic head resection can be as high as 50%. The most common complications are pancreatic fistula formation, delayed gastric emptying, and postpancreatectomy hemorrhage. In many specialized centers the operation has a 30-day mortality below 5%, dependent on the surgical volume of the center and the surgeon [8].

ADJUVANT AND NEOADJUVANT TREATMENT

Adjuvant treatment of pancreatic cancer is standard of care. The ESPAC-1 (European Study Group for Pancreatic Cancer) trial showed a clear advantage for adjuvant chemotherapy in patients with resected pancreatic cancer over chemoradiotherapy, which had a deleterious impact on survival [9]. Therefore, in Europe the standard of care after resection of pancreatic cancer is adjuvant chemotherapy [10]. The ESPAC-3 trial showed there was no difference between 5-flurouracil/folinic acid and gemcitabine, which is now the most commonly used chemotherapy agent [11].

The rationale for neoadjuvant therapy is to increase the incidence of R0 resections, downstage borderline resectable disease to allow resection, and reduce loco-regional recurrence. However, there are no large multicenter randomized controlled trials of neoadjuvant therapy for pancreatic cancer. Meta-analysis of the available data shows that one-third of patients with locally advanced disease without distant metastases can achieve a significant oncological response to neoadjuvant treatment, increasing the chances of achieving an R0 resection, thereby reducing local recurrence and potentially improving disease-free survival [12].

Palliative Treatment

Biliary tract or duodenal obstruction can be relieved by surgical, endoscopic, or radiological techniques. Palliative chemotherapy usually involves gemcitabine-based regimes. Efforts to improve survival outcomes with gemcitabine-based combination chemotherapy regimens have been largely disappointing, with the possible exception of the addition of the targeted agent erlotinib. The multiagent cytotoxic chemotherapy regimen FOLFIRINOX (FOL- Folinic_acid(leucovorin), F – Fluorouracil (5-FU) IRIN – Irinotecan

(Camptosar), OX – Oxaliplatin (Eloxatin)) (sequential administration of oxaliplatin immediately followed by leucovorin over 2 h, and then irinotecan, followed by a bolus dose of 5-fluorouracil, and finally, a 46-h infusion of 5-fluorouracil) has significantly improved survival compared with gemcitabine alone [13]. However, this regimen can be highly toxic and may need to be reserved for those with an excellent performance status.

PROGNOSIS OF PANCREATIC CANCER

PDA is still extremely resistant to currently available regimens, which results in poor prognosis, with only 5% of patients alive at three years. Surgery with curative intent has a five-year survival of 10–25%, and median survival of 11–18 months. Main prognostic factors include age, tumor size, nodal and margin status, and tumor grade [7]. Patients with locally advanced disease have a median survival time of 8–12 months, and patients with distant metastases have significantly worse outcomes, with a median survival time of 3–6 months [14]. Recently, a new our algorithm using computational approaches has been proposed for personalized pancreatic cancer therapy [15].

OUTLOOK

The surgical treatment of pancreatic cancer has a high quality in many specialized centers. Rather than from new surgical techniques, improvement of the treatment and prognosis of pancreatic cancer will come from new diagnostics and (molecular) targets. There has been a spurt in the application of newer technologies, particularly computational biology, which is being utilized for diagnostic and therapeutic discoveries in pancreatic cancer. Researchers and clinicians are able to model the disease and obtain information on critical weak points within the complex molecular network in pancreatic cancer. The predictive models and networks have been shown to respond to novel agents in pancreatic cell lines and xenograft models. In the clinical setting, such technologies are projected to be helpful in stratifying responsive patient populations and may also provide the blueprints for tailored therapies. Nevertheless, these computational developments are still in their infancy. Therefore, more computational research efforts should be put into the field of pancreatic cancer.

REFERENCES

[1] Poruk KE, Firpo MA, Adler DG, Mulvihill SJ. Screening for pancreatic cancer: why, how, and who? Ann Surg 2013;257(1):17–26.
[2] Yadav D, Lowenfels AB. The epidemiology of pancreatitis and pancreatic cancer. Gastroenterology 2013;144(6):1252–61.

[3] Ruckert F, Brussig T, Kuhn M, Kersting S, Bunk A, Hunger M, et al. Malignancy in chronic pancreatitis: analysis of diagnostic procedures and proposal of a clinical algorithm. Pancreatology 2013;13(3):243–9.

[4] Grutzmann R, Niedergethmann M, Pilarsky C, Kloppel G, Saeger HD. Intraductal papillary mucinous tumors of the pancreas: biology, diagnosis, and treatment. Oncologist 2010;15(12):1294–309.

[5] Ehehalt F, Saeger HD, Schmidt M, Grutzmann R. Neuroendocrine tumors of the pancreas. Oncologist 2009;14(5):456–67.

[6] Chari ST, Leibson CL, Rabe KG, Ransom J, de Andrade M, Petersen GM. Probability of pancreatic cancer following diabetes: a population-based study. Gastroenterology 2005;129(2):504–11.

[7] Distler M, Ruckert F, Hunger M, Kersting S, Pilarsky C, Saeger HD, et al. Evaluation of survival in patients after pancreatic head resection for ductal adenocarcinoma. BMC Surg 2013;13:12.

[8] Grutzmann R, Ruckert F, Hippe-Davies N, Distler M, Saeger HD. Evaluation of the International Study Group of Pancreatic Surgery definition of post-pancreatectomy hemorrhage in a high-volume center. Surgery 2012;151(4):612–20.

[9] Stocken DD, Buchler MW, Dervenis C, Bassi C, Jeekel H, Klinkenbijl JH, et al. Meta-analysis of randomised adjuvant therapy trials for pancreatic cancer. Br J Cancer 2005;92(8):1372–81.

[10] Oettle H, Post S, Neuhaus P, Gellert K, Langrehr J, Ridwelski K, et al. Adjuvant chemotherapy with gemcitabine vs observation in patients undergoing curative-intent resection of pancreatic cancer: a randomized controlled trial. JAMA 2007;297(3):267–77.

[11] Neoptolemos JP, Stocken DD, Bassi C, Ghaneh P, Cunningham D, Goldstein D, et al. Adjuvant chemotherapy with fluorouracil plus folinic acid vs gemcitabine following pancreatic cancer resection: a randomized controlled trial. JAMA 2010;304(10):1073–81.

[12] Gillen S, Schuster T, Meyer Zum Buschenfelde C, Friess H, Kleeff J. Preoperative/neoadjuvant therapy in pancreatic cancer: a systematic review and meta-analysis of response and resection percentages. PLoS Med 2010;7(4):e1000267.

[13] Conroy T, Desseigne F, Ychou M, Bouche O, Guimbaud R, Becouarn Y, et al. FOLFIRINOX versus gemcitabine for metastatic pancreatic cancer. N Engl J Med 2011;364(19):1817–25.

[14] Paulson AS, Tran Cao HS, Tempero MA, Lowy AM. Therapeutic advances in pancreatic cancer. Gastroenterology 2013;144(6):1316–26.

[15] Winter C, Kristiansen G, Kersting S, Roy J, Aust D, Knosel T, et al. Google goes cancer: improving outcome prediction for cancer patients by network-based ranking of marker genes. PLoS Comput Biol 2012;8(5):e1002511.

CHAPTER 2

Advances in Primary Cell Culture of Pancreatic Cancer

Niccola Funel

Department of Surgical, Molecular and Medical Pathology, University of Pisa, Pisa, Italy

Contents

Introduction	12
Epidemiology	12
The Molecular Genetics of PDAC	13
K-Ras	14
p53	14
p16	14
Dpc4	15
Other Genes	15
General Considerations	15
Cell Culture of PDAC	16
Cell Lines of PDAC	16
Primary Cell Cultures of PDAC	17
Isolation and Establishment Procedure	17
Pancreatic Resections for PDAC	17
The Role of Surgical Pathology Unit: Diagnosis of PDAC (Macroscopic Features)	17
Microscopic Features	20
Histological Diagnosis	22
Isolation of Tumor Tissue	23
Selection of Epithelial Cell Population	25
Culturing and Storage	25
Characterization of Cell Cultures	26
Morphology	26
Genotyping	26
Phenotyping	27
Cell Culture vs. Origin Tissue	27
Cellular Growth (Doubling Time)	28
Second Level of Biological Models	29
LMD on Primary Cell Cultures	29
Three-Dimensional Cell Cultures	34
In vivo Models	34
Applications	35
Conclusion	35
References	36

INTRODUCTION

Pancreatic cancer is a lethal disease, and despite the low incidence, it is in fact a major cause of cancer-related deaths in industrialized countries. At the time of diagnosis, 75–85% of patients present with advanced tumors and are not amenable to surgical resection with curative intent [1]. Conservative therapeutic strategies, such as chemotherapy and/or radiotherapy, have not shown to improve the prognosis of pancreatic cancer that is not operable [2]. Improvement of the surgical technique in high-volume centers has reduced the intraoperative mortality below 5%, and consequently increased the number of resections with curative intent. However, the local recurrence rate remains very high and, although in subgroups of patients there has been reported actual survival of more than 20% five years post diagnosis, the real long-term survivors are rare (<2%) [1,3]. The reasons for this aggressive nature of the disease are not fully known, but they seem to have to be sought in the particular biological structure that characterizes cancer of the pancreas. In the last two decades, scientific and technological progress in the field of molecular biology have made it possible to elucidate many of the genetic and epigenetic mechanisms underlying this disease, with the hope that they will lead to the development of better diagnostic and therapeutic modalities. Nevertheless, the lack of known risk factors and the absence of symptoms in the early stages of the disease make the implementation of strategies for primary or secondary prevention very unlikely.

Epidemiology

Pancreatic cancer has the highest incidence in industrialized countries such as the United States, Japan, and Europe, where rates are higher in the northern than the Mediterranean regions. The African and Asian countries are characterized by a low incidence (1–2 cases/10^5 habitants/year) [4]. In Italy there are regional variations; in fact, it has been reported that the incidence is around 1–2 cases/10^5 habitants/year, with an average of 8.4 new 1–2 cases/10^5 habitants/year (National Cancer Registry). Epidemiological studies have shown a constant growth in the overall incidence rate and age-standardized incidence rate until the eighties, followed by a plateau phase. The mortality rate has been shown to coincide with that of incidence [3,5]. Males are more commonly affected than females, with a ratio ranging from 1.4:1 to 2.9:1 in Brazil and France, respectively. However, in recent decades there has been an increase in the number of female patients suffering from pancreatic cancer, probably because of increased cigarette smoking in women [5]. Cigarette smoking is a clear and well-established risk factor (from two to six times higher) for pancreatic cancer, as demonstrated by some epidemiological studies. However, there is no clear evidence linking cigar or pipe smoking or chewing tobacco with the disease. The consumption of alcohol, coffee, or tea showed no clear association with the development of the disease either. In contrast, medical conditions such as chronic pancreatitis, cystic fibrosis, and diabetes do show strong correlation with the disease. Speaking of chronic pancreatitis, for example, a multicenter study conducted by Lowenfels showed a 14.4- to 16.5-fold increase in the incidence of pancreatic carcinoma compared to the general population [6], with the risk increasing even higher over the years from the onset of the disease. Individuals with hereditary chronic pancreatitis, which is characterized by an early onset, can achieve a 75% cumulative risk of developing pancreatic cancer if they have inherited the disease from the male branch of the family [7]. Although most cases of pancreatic cancer are sporadic, the disease also occurs in the context of hereditary syndromes, such as dysplastic nevus syndrome, Lynch syndrome type II (colon cancer hereditary nonpolyposis), breast-ovarian cancer syndrome, ataxia-telangiectasia, Peutz-Jeghers syndrome, and the aforementioned hereditary pancreatitis [7]. Furthermore, the possibility of an autosomal dominant inheritance of the disease in the absence of an apparent genetic disorder may have other hereditary links to it. For example, through linkage analysis, change at locus 4q32-34 has recently been identified to associate with the disease significantly, even though no specific gene has been identified responsible [8]. Overall, it is estimated that up to 10% of pancreatic cancer cases are transmitted with an autosomal dominant pattern of inheritance [7].

The Molecular Genetics of PDAC

In the last decade, with the advancement of molecular biology tools and the development of transgenic animal models, researchers have been able to identify some fundamental genetic alterations underlying the development of pancreatic cancer. Four main events are believed to be critical for the pathogenesis and/or progression of ductal adenocarcinoma:

- Activating point mutations of the *K-Ras*
- Inactivation of the tumor suppressor gene TP53
- Inactivation of the tumor suppressor gene *p16*
- Inactivation of the tumor suppressor gene *Dpc4* (deleted in pancreatic cancer 4).

K-Ras

K-*Ras* mutations are more frequent in pancreatic cancer than in any other type of human neoplasia: >80% of carcinomas of the pancreas have activating mutations in the first or second base of codon 12 [9]. The Ras family proteins have a function of transmitting growth signals within the cell: they are capable of binding GTP molecules and transform them into GDP (GTPase activity) once the signal is transmitted. Point mutations at codons 12, 13, or 61 lead to loss of the GTPase activity. As a consequence, the ras protein remains in the active state to continuously transmit growth signals. K-*Ras* mutations appear to be an early event in pancreatic carcinogenesis, as shown by numerous experimental data. In fact, the same type of mutation has been found in tumors and in the lesions associated with them [10]; also, animal models of pancreatic carcinogenesis have revealed a high incidence of ras mutations in the early stages of neoplastic transformation. Finally, K-*Ras* mutations have been identified in preneoplastic ductal lesions found in the pancreas of a patient with a family history of pancreatic cancer [11].

p53

The alterations of the *p53* tumor suppressor gene are common in human cancers. This gene encodes a nuclear protein with a short half-life. It acts as a transcription factor to exert a negative regulation of cell growth and proliferation by inducing apoptosis in the presence of genomic damage that is unrepairable. Loss of heterozygosity at the *p53* locus occurs in almost 90% of pancreatic tumors, while in 50–75% of cases there is complete loss of function of the protein due to alterations involving the inactivation of the remaining copy of the gene [12,13]. Of all the *p53* gene alterations, missense point mutations are the most frequent ones; frameshift mutations may also occur predominantly represented by intragenic microdeletions, which occur in pancreatic cancer with a frequency significantly higher (up to 30%) compared to other human cancers. The majority of *p53* mutations, with exceptions frequently represented by microdeletions and more rarely by nonsense mutations, lead to the synthesis of a mutant protein with increased half-life, which can be easily detected by immunohistochemistry staining [14,15].

p16

P16INK4a/CDKN2/MTS1 gene is located on chromosome 9p21 and encodes a protein that binds the cyclin-dependent kinase 4 (Cdk4) to prevent its interaction with cyclin D1. The cyclin D1-Cdk4 interaction regulates the transition from G1 phase to S phase of the cell cycle. In the absence of inhibition by *p16*, it leads to continuous activation and therefore uncontrolled cell growth. Three mechanisms are responsible for the loss of function of *p16* in almost all cases of carcinomas of the pancreas: (1) homozygous deletions due to loss of both alleles; (2) loss of one allele and mutation in the other allele resulting in altered function (loss of heterozygosity); and (3) methylation of cytosine nucleotides in the promoter region to suppress the expression of the gene [16].

Dpc4

Dpc4 (Smad4) is a tumor suppressor gene located on the long arm of chromosome 18 and encodes a transcription factor that participates in the cascade mediated by signal transduction-dependent growth factor TGF. It is frequently altered in pancreatic cancer. The loss of its function was observed in 50% of pancreatic carcinomas and is due to two mechanisms: (1) loss of heterozygosity; and (2) homozygous deletion. Immunohistochemistry staining allows one to obtain a very sensitive and specific assessment of the expression level of *Dpc4* [17,18]. Recently, it was shown that the loss of expression of Smad4 is associated with a poorer prognosis of carcinoma of the pancreas.

Other Genes

Alterations of other genes, mainly tumor suppressors, have also been reported in pancreatic cancer. Mutations of the gene APC (adenomatous polyposis coli) are rare in ductal adenocarcinoma but are reported more frequently in solid pseudopapillary pancreatic tumors, acinar carcinoma, and ampullary cancer [19]. DCC (deleted in colorectal cancer) is a tumor suppressor gene that encodes a protein with receptor functions involved in cell migration and apoptosis. It is located on the long arm of chromosome 18 near the gene *Dpc4*, leading to an underestimation of its involvement in the molecular pathogenesis of pancreatic cancer because the consequence of the chromosomal deletions discussed in this topic has been mainly attributed to the loss of the *Dpc4* locus. However, it has recently been shown that there are some pancreatic carcinomas in which there is a real loss to the locus DCC, while the locus *Dpc4* remains intact. BRCA2 is another tumor suppressor gene involved in the pathogenesis of some familial forms of pancreatic carcinoma [19].

General Considerations

As previously described, at the time of diagnosis pancreatic cancer appears to be an incurable disease in almost all cases, since the rate of incidence of this disease is almost coinciding with the rate of mortality. The cases that are defined as long-term survivors, disease free after five years, make up a very small cohort of patients, estimated at around 2%. This is due to the absence of early diagnosis of pancreatic cancer. The radiodiagnostic methods that are the current ones for diagnosis are not able to detect the presence of this cancer in its early stages, so at the time of diagnosis, this cancer is already in advanced stages and in some cases not operable [20]. Pancreatic surgery has made great strides in substantially reducing the operative mortality and improving morbidity of patients with unresectable tumors, but the absence of an effective drug therapy seems to be the problem [21]. Until now, the gold standard in the treatment of pancreatic cancer has been the use of gemcitabine in adjuvant setting chemotherapy in favor of other drugs such as 5-fluorouracil or platinum derivatives, both of which are less tolerable in therapy [21,22].

Our goal in the presented study was to obtain an in vitro model that closely mimics pancreatic ductal adenocarcinoma (PDAC) patients; the purpose was to measure the levels of expression of the molecular determinants involved in the metabolism of gemcitabine and relate them to the survival of patients treated with this drug in monochemotherapy [23]. To eliminate the interference of the abundant desmoplastic component, the tumor epithelial component was isolated using the laser microdissection (LMD) technology. To complete the study of expression in vivo and in vitro, primary cell cultures of pancreatic cancer have been set up [24].

The purpose of this chapter is to describe the techniques for the isolation of the epithelial component of pancreatic cancer. These methods are:

- The realization of primary cultures of PDAC
- The LMD of normal and cancerous pancreatic tissues.

The LMD and cell cultures focus on removing the "stroma", which can mask the true expression at the mRNA level of tumor cells. With microdissection you can study the molecular signature in a static manner for the reason that the tissue is locked in a precise biological moment. Cell cultures offer the opportunity to study the characteristics of the tumor in a dynamic way. Study of the molecular biology of the epithelial component of the tumor, desmoplastic excluding the component, can lead to the realization of a valid system for the study of ductal carcinoma of the pancreas.

CELL CULTURE OF PDAC

Cell Lines of PDAC

There are also many lines available for PDAC (primarily from the American Tissue Culture Collection). These biological systems can be used by researchers as a benchmark for their experiments. The main lines of PDAC used (about 20) and their characteristics were summarized by Moore [25].

Primary Cell Cultures of PDAC

The first evidence of tissue culture was done by Roux in the nineteenth century, showing its role in the basic sciences. However, it was almost 50 years later that the first tumor cell line obtained from human tissue was established [26]. The first pancreatic cell culture from a human patient was done in the 1960s [27]. This preparation was known as a primary cell culture, which can be cultivated for many passages for a long time period; these primary cell cultures were called "*Cell Line*" or "*Immortalized Cell Culture*". To isolate primary pancreatic tissues for cell culture, researchers described three most important approaches: isolation procedure, enzymatic digestion, and cell recovery from malignant fluids.

ISOLATION AND ESTABLISHMENT PROCEDURE

Pancreatic Resections for PDAC

Surgical intervention on resectable pancreas can be sorted into three types: total pancreatectomy (TP), when the entire gland is removed in a single intervention; pancreatic duodenectomy (PD), which provides for the enucleation of the head of the pancreas at the neck and the adjoining section of the duodenum; left pancreatectomy (LP), when the body and tail of the pancreas are resected. Cases where the spleen is removed surgically (in 99% of patients) are said to be left spleen-pancreatectomy. In some cases there were collected fragments of tumor tissue enucleated in the course of laparoscopy or laparotomy from patients in advanced stage of disease and therefore not operable. In the following images we can see a typical specimen of pancreatectomy (Figures 2.1 and 2.2).

The Role of Surgical Pathology Unit: Diagnosis of PDAC (Macroscopic Features)

Ductal adenocarcinoma is a malignant epithelial neoplasm composed of mucus-secreting glandular structures that show evidence of ductal differentiation. This tumor has even been called ductal adenocarcinoma or squamous cell carcinoma, pancreatic exocrine, or more simply, cancer of the pancreas. It is, together with its most common variants (nonmucinous cystic carcinoma, carcinoma with signet-ring cell carcinoma, adenosquamous carcinoma and undifferentiated), the most frequent histological type of pancreatic cancer. It represents 85–90% of all pancreatic tumors.

According to autopsy case studies, 60–70% of carcinomas of the pancreas are localized in the head of the gland, 5–10% in the body, and 10–15% in

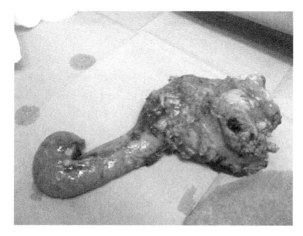

Figure 2.1 *Surgical Resection of Pancreas.* Pancreatic duodenectomy (PD). (For color version of this figure, the reader is referred to the online version of this book.)

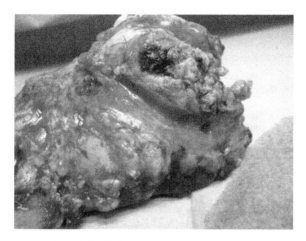

Figure 2.2 *Magnification of Head of Pancreas.* Pancreatic resection margin. (For color version of this figure, the reader is referred to the online version of this book.)

the queue in a combination of sites. The surgical series report the head of the pancreas as the most frequent site (80–90% of cases); 50% of cases are localized in the upper half of the head, close to the intrapancreatic portion of the common bile duct; and, the remaining in the region behind the ampoule Vater or, more rarely, in the uncinate process. The size of the head of the carcinoma is between 1.5 and 10 cm, with an average of between 3.5 and 4.5 cm. The tumors of the body-tail are generally larger (on average 5–7 cm), given the late onset of clinical manifestations that characterize

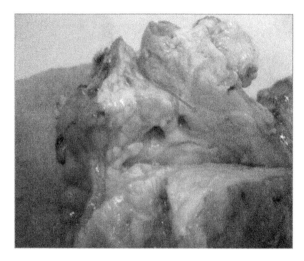

Figure 2.3 *Pancreatic Ductal Adenocarcinoma.* Macroscopic features of tumor. Desmoplastic reaction (red arrow). (For interpretation of the references to color in this figure legend, the reader is referred to the online version of this book.)

them. Macroscopically, ductal adenocarcinoma is presented as a hard mass, in ill-defined margins, with a cutting surface of whitish-yellow color that is lost imperceptibly in the surrounding parenchyma (Figure 2.3).

Hemorrhage and necrosis are rare, while there may be microcystic areas. With the exception of neoplasms originating in the uncinate process, carcinomas of the head of the pancreas are closely related to the common bile duct and the main pancreatic duct. The invasion of the wall of these ducts and growth determines stenosis and sometimes complete obstruction, with dilatation of the upstream segment of the occluded portion. The obstruction of the common bile duct leads to the development of jaundice, which is one of the most frequent clinical signs of carcinoma of the head of the pancreas; obstruction of the duct of Wirsung determines obstructive chronic pancreatitis. Involvement of the duodenum wall invasion leads to ulceration, in more advanced cases. The extrapancreatic retroperitoneal extension is often present at the time of diagnosis, with involvement of the mesenteric vessels and nerve plexus. In more advanced cases there is extension to the peritoneum, stomach, gallbladder, and retroportal tissue. This is in fact not a real anatomical structure present in the human body, but rather it is a surgical margin that separates the gland from the retroperitoneum. Histopathological evaluation of this fragment tissue is important in providing the surgeon with the success of pancreatic resection performed, since the

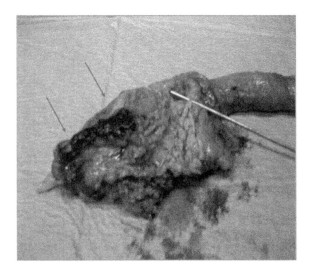

Figure 2.4 *Surgical Resection of Pancreas.* Posterior margin (green arrows) close to mesenteric vein structures (black ink). (For interpretation of the references to color in this figure legend, the reader is referred to the online version of this book.)

presence of tumor in the retroportal tissue is indicative of the presence of a residual tumor in the patient, which is indicated by the acronym of R1. In the case in which the lamina retroportal is negative, it is called pancreatic resection R0, where there is no residual tumor in the retroperitoneum of the patient (Figure 2.4). Tumors of the body-tail can infiltrate the main pancreatic duct. The extrapancreatic diffusion involves first the retroperitoneum and can thereafter extend to the spleen, stomach, adrenal gland, and peritoneum, with development of carcinomatosis [28].

Microscopic Features

From a microscopic point of view, most of the ductal adenocarcinomas are moderately or well-differentiated tumors. The well-differentiated tumors (Figure 2.5) consist of large glandular-like structures and glands of medium size, irregularly arranged in the context of a desmoplastic stroma. The latter is a typical element ductal adenocarcinoma and is responsible for the hard consistency that characterizes this malignancy. The neoplastic glands are located close to normal structures (acini, ducts, islet), and they may show a pattern of growth cribriform, micropapillary or clear mucus secretion. Mitotic activity is generally low. The moderately differentiated carcinomas are composed of glands of medium size and by tubular structures of irregular shapes and sizes and variables (Figure 2.6). Usually they completely

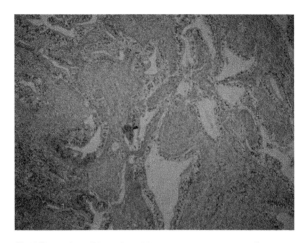

Figure 2.5 *Well-Differentiated PDAC.* H&E staining, 10× magnification. (For color version of this figure, the reader is referred to the online version of this book.)

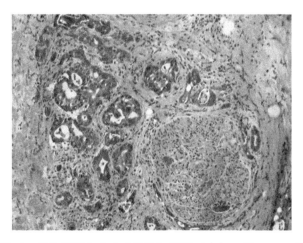

Figure 2.6 *Moderately Differentiated PDAC.* H&E staining, 10× magnification. (For color version of this figure, the reader is referred to the online version of this book.)

replace the acinar parenchyma. The cytological atypia are marked with nuclei varied in size, irregular chromatin and nucleoli, and frequent mitosis. The production of mucus is reduced.

The poorly differentiated (Figure 2.7) carcinomas are made up of small and irregular glands, as well as solid nests and cords of neoplastic cells. The stromal reaction is usually very strong, while there may be foci of necrosis and hemorrhage. The neoplastic cells are markedly atypical and do not produce mucin, although there may be individual cells containing cytoplasmic

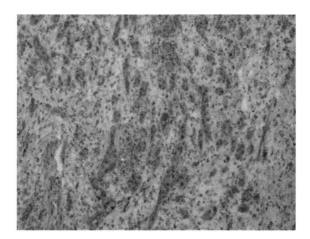

Figure 2.7 *Poorly Differentiated PDAC.* H&E staining, 10× magnification. (For color version of this figure, the reader is referred to the online version of this book.)

Table 2.1 Grading of Exocrine Pancreatic Tumor (i.e., PDAC)

Grading	Differentiation	Mitoses (10 HPF)	Nuclear atypia
1	Well	<5	Low
2	Middle	6–10	Moderate
3	Poor	>10	High

HPF, high-power field.

vacuoles. Mitotic activity is high [28]. The microscopic grading of ductal adenocarcinomas is based on the combined evaluation of histological, cytological, and mitotic activity (Table 2.1).

Histological Diagnosis

To evaluate the samples eligible for primary cell culture, we evaluated the definitive histological diagnosis of 202 patients who underwent surgery; 118 cases were classified as ductal adenocarcinoma, according to the Union for International Cancer Control (UICC) classification of 2002 and the degree of differentiation according to the criteria set by the World Health Organization (WHO).

The various degrees of differentiation and Classification of Malignant tumors (TNM) were synthesized in the following report (Table 2.2). Eighty-one carcinomas (68.64%) were from patients who underwent pancreatic resection, and 37 (31.36%) were from patients undergoing laparotomy or

Table 2.2 Relationship between Staging and TNM in PDAC Cases

TNM	Total Cases	G1/3	G2/3	G3/3
Laparoscopy (LE)	37			
pT1 N0 Mx	1	1		
pT2 N0 Mx	1	1		
pT2 N1 Mx	1	1		
pT3 N0 M1	2	1	1	
pT3 N0 Mx	12	2	4	6
pT3 N1 M1	10	8	2	
pT3 N1 Mx	54	3	29	22

Table 2.3 Cases of PDAC Sorted by Surgical Resection Type

Pathology	Total	PD	LE	LP	TP
PDAC	118	51	37	22	8
Other	84	50	6	24	4

laparoscopy (LE) (Table 2.3). The incidence of pancreatic cancer in both sexes were almost identical with a M/F ratio = 1.24 (66 males and 52 females). We used a subgroup of them [23,24] to set up the primary cell culture.

Isolation of Tumor Tissue

To set up the primary cell cultures of pancreatic adenocarcinoma, we grew only primary tumors derived from pancreatic resections total or partial as tumor biopsies of adenocarcinomas from exploratory laparotomy have never been cultured before [23,24]. The fragments of tumor tissue (Figure 2.8) cell cultures were placed in cold saline solution (4 °C) and brought under a laminar flow hood for primary cell culture preparation. For all operations we used the same synthetic medium composed as follows. RPMI 1640 supplemented with 1% L-glutamine, 1% antibiotics (ampicillin, streptomycin), and 10% fetal bovine serum. The first day the tumor is subjected to mechanical fragmentation and enzymatic digestion (collagenase type XI concentration 1 mg/mL in complete culture medium—overnight at 37 °C or for a period of time between 18 and 20 h). The second day the cellular part is harvested by centrifuging the contents of the flasks at 1200 rpm for 5 min, the supernatant is discarded, and the cell pellet is plated on two primary culture flasks. The third day finally eliminates the supernatant and adhesion of cells onto the surface of the plate occurs. Sometimes in the supernatant there is a significant component of the cell, so far as could be possible to perform

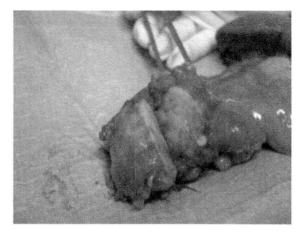

Figure 2.8 *PDAC at the Surgical Pathology Unit after Its Resection.* Sampling of tissue to start with the primary cell culture. (For color version of this figure, the reader is referred to the online version of this book.)

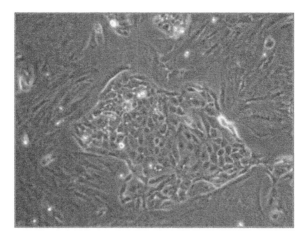

Figure 2.9 *Few Days after Culture.* Both epithelial and fibroblast cells (desmoplasia) are present in primary cell culture (magnification 20×; contrast phase microscopy). (For color version of this figure, the reader is referred to the online version of this book.)

subcultures with the same rules. Usually during the plating of the tumor at most six flasks from primary culture were established. If the procedure has been carried out correctly and there has been no contamination by bacteria or fungi, in the best cases we observed a mixed cell culture composed of fibroblasts, resulting from the tissue surrounding desmoplasia and from a fraction of epithelial tumor cells (Figure 2.9).

Selection of Epithelial Cell Population

To eliminate fibroblasts we used a solution of trypsin and EDTA (2 mL for the 25 cm^2 flasks) that is able to detach the fibroblasts prematurely compared to tumor cells. This operation is performed under a sterile hood, has a duration of about 1 min, and is reconstituted with an equal amount of complete medium used to cultivate the cells. The procedure is repeated at least every 10 days or when the growth of fibroblasts blocks the expansion of the epithelial clusters. From our observation, to totally eliminate fibroblasts from primary culture one may need a period of two to four months (Figure 2.5). After this period, the epithelial cells and fibroblasts are kept separate and grown in parallel for a short period of time (2–3 weeks), after which the fibroblasts and their culture medium are frozen for long-term preservation. After this stage the epithelial cells can be "passed" or "split" and transferred into another flask for primary cell culture. The cells are detached from the support on which they are attached forming a cell monolayer using the same solution of trypsin and EDTA used for fibroblasts extrusion, but for a longer period of time longer, about 8 min.

Culturing and Storage

After checking the detachment of the monolayer to the inverted microscope, the enzymatic action is blocked with complete medium (quantitative ratio enzyme solution/complete medium = 1:1). The cells at this moment are in suspension and are centrifuged (1200 rpm × 5 min), recovered, and resuspended in the culture medium (same solution mentioned above). This phase serves to remove the trypsin and the cells that have dissolved in the medium can be counted using a Burker chamber and seeded again with a dilution factor according the researcher's needs. In the first 10–15 passages the cells are diluted to the maximum three-fold. With the progress of life time and the increase of the steps, the dilution factor is enhanced. After the 70th passage cell cultures are passed with a dilution factor of 100.

To preserve the epithelial cells and fibroblasts, samples are cryopreserved in complete culture medium containing 10% dimethyl sulphoxide in the ratio volume/volume and 30% fetal bovine serum (FBS). This type of solution should always be freshly prepared and not exposed to direct light. The cells to be retained are suspended in 1 mL of this medium for freezing and stored in an ultrafreezer to −80 °C for a few days and then permanently transferred to liquid nitrogen at −196 °C temperature. In this way the cells can be stored even for very long periods of time. It is possible to restore frozen cells after a storage period. It is advisable not to use such cryopreserved cells beyond three years.

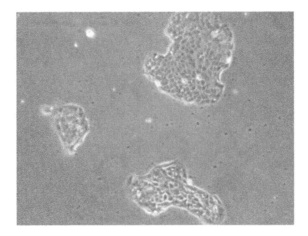

Figure 2.10 *Primary Cell Culture of PDAC.* Pure population of epithelial cells (magnification 4×; contrast phase microscopy). (For color version of this figure, the reader is referred to the online version of this book.)

CHARACTERIZATION OF CELL CULTURES

Primary cultures are important to gain molecular insights in order to understand, *in primis*, whether the primary cell cultures originate from their cognate pancreatic tumor tissues [24,28]. Since 1986, about 30 research groups have been obtaining primary cell cultures from PDAC, also showing their characteristics [29]. Here we will try to give some characterization of the primary cultures.

MORPHOLOGY

PDAC generally exhibits middle/high grade of differentiation in the tissue (Figure 2.10). Concerning cell lines their morphology is normally assessed by contrast phase microscopy. More details could be acquired by other methods such as electron microscopy and immunostaining, and histological staining is to usually find two different morphologies as reported in the following figure (Figure 2.11).

GENOTYPING

The selection of primary cell culture from the tumor, could be referred to "gain of function". As reported previously the effects of four more-frequent genetic mutations/alterations are observed in PDAC. These genes—Kras, Smad4, *p53*, and *Dpc4* [25,30,31]—are related to the preneoplastic lesion process of PDAC [32,33]. In this group of genes only one oncogene

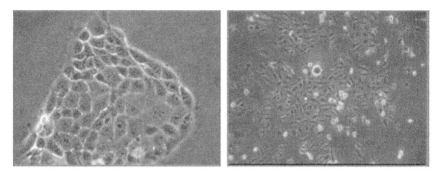

Figure 2.11 *Pure Population of Primary Cell Culture of PDAC.* Cellular growth by two different models: by cluster (left) and by single cell (right). (For color version of this figure, the reader is referred to the online version of this book.)

(i.e., Kras) has been reported. However another important oncogene is the epithelial growth factor receptor (EGFR). This resulted in alteration (gain of function) in PDAC patients who underwent surgical resection [34], in PDAC cell culture [35] and in mouse model obtained by orthotopic implant of primary cell culture of PDAC [36]. The genes cited above are used routinely in PDAC cell culture genotyping.

PHENOTYPING

The PDAC cells usually show the phenotype behaviors according to the differentiation grade of cognate origin tissues. Indeed we can find the expression of some markers related to epithelial derivation. Included in the list are: CEA, cytokeratins (i.e., Ck7, Ck8, Ck18, Ck19), EGFR, and CA 19.9 [36]. Sometimes, it could be possible to detect enhanced expression of vimentin [37].

Cell Culture vs. Origin Tissue

It should be necessary to compare the primary cell cultures and their cognate tissues to investigate whether there could be some differences in genotype and phenotype patterns. Of course, the phenotype sometimes could be different, because after many passages, the cells could shed away the antigens. Indeed, the genotypes must be close to each other, especially in the first steps of cellular growth [24]. So far *K-Ras* gene seems to be the first gene showing the pancreatic origin of primary tumor cell culture. In all cases it could be better to compare the pure population of cell vs. their origin tissues submitted to LMD. This approach could take out only epithelial cells, which represent the true target of analyses.

Cellular Growth (Doubling Time)

The doubling time (DT) of the cells directly expresses the speed of cell growth. Often this parameter is directly associated with the aggressiveness of the cell culture and then also with the tumor from which it originates. The DT expresses the interval of time associated with the duplication of cell starting number. To obtain this measure (hours are the conventional unit), it should be necessary to perform a triplicate experiment, counting the variation of cell number in front of the time. One of these formulas was reported in [29]. However, we would like to introduce a new approach to evaluate this parameter. According to the criteria described above, we would like to define the speed of growth as follows:

The function is:

$$f(x) = \text{Cellular Growth}$$

$$f(x) = \frac{(N_{t1} - N_{t0})}{(T_{t1} - T_{t0})} \tag{2.1}$$

where (N) represents the number of cells, (T) represents the time. $t1$ and $t0$ are two different moment of cellular growth (CG). So far we can express the Eqn (2.1) as "delta" of number of cells out of time.

$$f(x) = \frac{\Delta N}{\Delta T} \tag{2.2}$$

To have the variation of time could be easy, because this represents the time of experimentation, but how is it possible to measure the variation of cell number? From each cellular division we obtain two new cells, but the cell number gains one more cell only. This concept is showed in Figure 2.12.

We can consider that the number of cells increases by one unit after each cellular division. The "delta N", the number of new cells, is equal to the number of cellular divisions (D).

$$(t_1 - t_0) \Rightarrow \Delta N = D$$
$$f(x) = \frac{D}{\Delta T} \tag{2.3}$$

$$f(x) \, N_{t0} = \frac{D_{t1}}{\Delta T_{t1 - t0}} \tag{2.4}$$

In conclusion we can express the "DT" as:

$$DT_{(t1 - t0)} = \frac{D_{t1}}{N_{t0}} = 2$$

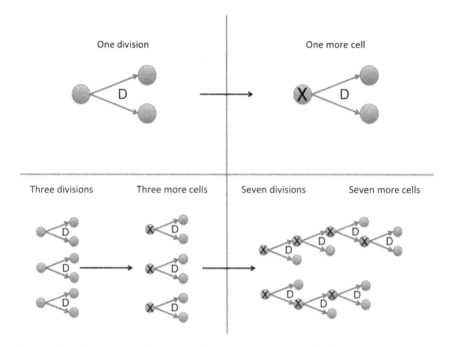

Figure 2.12 *The Scheme Shows the Theory According to Which We Have One Additional Cell After Each Division.* The number of additional cells is equal to the number of total divisions. (For color version of this figure, the reader is referred to the online version of this book.)

The calculation of the DT is important in order to count the final number for each interval of time, which is presented as Funel's equation.

SECOND LEVEL OF BIOLOGICAL MODELS

LMD on Primary Cell Cultures

LMD is a technique that has been developed over the last decade and has had great success in the molecular study of tumors. The method is defined by the third generation as this appears to be a development of the two methods specified previously that microdissected samples with two different procedures. It is worth mentioning that in all the techniques of microdissection, a laser beam is controlled by the operator who is able to directly select the affected area on the histological preparation. In the first generation the levy of the material was carried out directly on the histological preparation fixed to the slide by affixing to a solid support containing a synthetic resin that is able to withdraw the tissue following the activation of the laser beam. In the second generation, the method changed radically as the histological sample was fixed on a membrane, which was then microdissected by laser beam, which also had the task of "catapulting" the specimen within the desired container. This technique is also known as laser microdissection and pressure catapulting, manufactured by PALM Microlaser Technologies, Bernried, Germany. Between the first and the second generation techniques, three substantial differences emerged: The laser beam that was initially directed from above is directed from below in microdissection of the second generation. The chemical support containing the resin used to capture the histological preparation is replaced by a film PET (Poly-Ethylene Terephthalate), which exclusively serves as a support for the microdissection of the sample. Finally, the recovery of the material no longer occurs due to a chemical reaction, but allows the mechanical action, the fact of "catapult" [38].

The latest generation of laser microdissectors uses two approaches described previously, with a third additional approach. The laser beam strikes the specimen from above (as in the first instrument generation) and the sample is fixed on a support film (as in the second instrument generation), but the collection of the microdissected material occurs by gravity due to the fact that the sample is reversed. The advantages of this application are the following: (1) the laser beam is collinear to the optical path of the microscope, then the operator can physically follow the microdissection; (2) the collection of the material by gravity is much easier compared to other systems of previous generations.

In the study of pancreatic cancer this aspect is most important because this method allows one to select a population of pure cancer cells enucleated from the peritumoral tissue (Figure 2.13). The LMD, as we have described above, is a preparative method, since it guarantees the recovery of distinct cell populations. Through this technique it is possible to study, in the pancreas, the non–neoplastic parenchyma, separating it from infiltrating carcinomatous component [39]. By this procedure it is possible to separate and study different cell populations present in the same tissue sample. For this reason, quantitative PCR appears to be by far the most used technique, that is frequently used in combination with the LMD in the pancreatic cancer studies [40,41], in chronic pancreatitis and preneoplastic lesions [42], since the expression levels of RNA of specific molecular determinants can be compared in different cell types present within a sample [23,24,28]. Furthermore, the LMD technique is applicable also to primary cell culture through two different modalities. In the former it is possible to cut the fixed

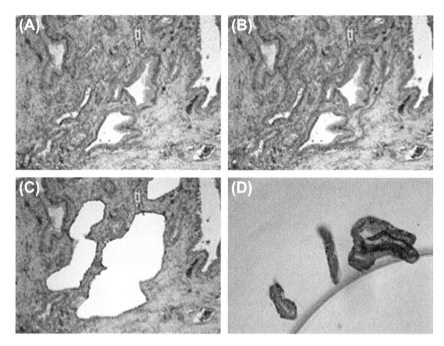

Figure 2.13 *Laser Microdissection of PDAC Tissue.* The figure shows the four most important phases of procedure: (A) Identification of Area; (B) Selection of Areas of interest; (C) Cutting: (D)Harvested fragment of Tissue. Magnification 10×; Hematoxylin staining. (For color version of this figure, the reader is referred to the online version of this book.)

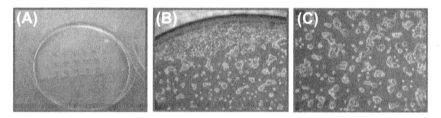

Figure 2.14 *Preparation of Primary Cell Culture for LMD.* (A) Cells seeding in appropriate chamber and condition to allow the best cell adhesion on PET membrane; original magnification; (B) Primary cell culture on PET membrane. Contrast phase light microscopy, magnification 4×; (C) Magnification 10×. (For color version of this figure, the reader is referred to the online version of this book.)

primary cells (Figures 2.14 and 2.15); in the latter it is possible to separate the live cells, during their cultivation (Figures 2.16 and 2.17) [43].

The goal of both LMD and primary cell cultures is to keep out a pure population of epithelial cells not only in PDAC but in all carcinomas. This

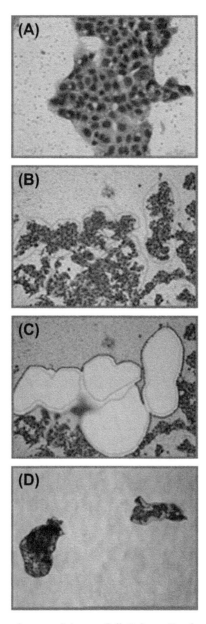

Figure 2.15 *LMD Procedure on Primary Cell Culture Fixed on PET Membrane and Stained with Hematoxylin Only; Magnification 20×.* (A) Identification and (B) Selection of interest areas; (C) Cutting; (D) Pooled samples. (For color version of this figure, the reader is referred to the online version of this book.)

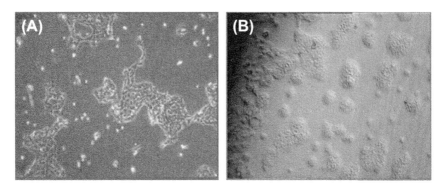

Figure 2.16 *Images of Primary Cell Cultures from Two Different Conditions.* (A) Normal cultivation of plastic support; (B) Cultivation on IDIDI support (Leica, Munchen, Germany) and direct light microscopy observation; magnification 4×. (For color version of this figure, the reader is referred to the online version of this book.)

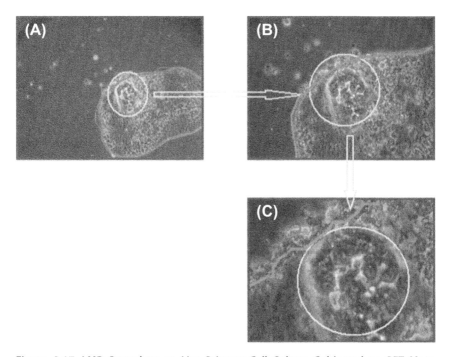

Figure 2.17 *LMD Procedure on Live Primary Cell Culture Cultivated on PET Membrane.* Microdissected areas showing living cells at different magnifications (A) 4×; (B) 10×; (C) 20×. (For color version of this figure, the reader is referred to the online version of this book.)

procedure allows the study of the true part of carcinoma that represents the real target of different therapeutic approaches.

THREE-DIMENSIONAL CELL CULTURES

Three-dimensional (3-D) culture of tumor cells was introduced as early as the 1970s. Initially, investigations focused on the morphology of and interactions between tumor cells [44]. Various PDAC cell lines were tested for their ability to grow as spheroids in 3-D culture [45,46]. Among these, the widely used Panc-1, which carries both KRAS and *p53* mutations, was shown to form aggregates under appropriate culture conditions [45]. It became apparent that 3-D cultures are generally more resistant to chemo- and radiotherapy than their 2-D counterparts [47,48], however three-dimensional in vitro tumor cell models allowing for fast and standardized drug screening are not routinely employed. Based on these observations, a new hypothesis relating chemoresistance to the microenvironment, i.e., the stroma and extracellular matrix, was proposed. This novel concept, called cell adhesion mediated drug resistance (CAM-DR), was proposed for bone marrow–derived malignancies [49], but has not been applied to solid tumors, including PDAC [50]. In this study, we characterize a 3-D tumor model in which the PDAC acquires a more stroma-rich phenotype, which simulates more closely the in vivo situation and provides evidence for the CAM-DR concept. However, the 3-D model is not referred to as spheroid only to describe their chemoresistant effects [51]. Some authors used this term to indicate the matrigel-embedded cell culture of PDAC. This model could be also important to study the modulation of growth factors (i.e., TGF-β) involved in the growth of cells and their chemoresistance [52]. Indeed, another 3-D model is represented by the integration of cell lines and primary cell culture of PDAC with different polymeric scaffold [53]. So far microenvironmental conditions regulate tumorigenesis [54,55], and biomimetic model systems are necessary to study how cancer is dependent on these conditions.

IN VIVO MODELS

It is also possible to obtain in vivo models of pancreatic cancer using cell lines [56] and primary cultures of PDAC [36]. This, for a number of features previously mentioned, could be a better preclinical model for drug testing. In the orthotopic murine model obtained using primary cultures, morphological, pathological, and molecular profiles entirely similar to those found in cognate human tissues [36] have been observed. For this reason, these types of models may be better than those obtained from cell lines in which there is no trace of the original tissue.

APPLICATIONS

Realizing that PDAC primary cell cultures could allow multiple applications in oncology, the five most important levels for primary cell culture applications are: (1) 2-D cell culture, (2) 3-D Gel matix-embedded, (3) spheroids (3-D mixed cell cultures), (4) 3-D scaffold embedding cell culture, and (5) in vivo models. The goal for each model is to test the efficacy of therapeutic approaches against PDAC. The more complicated preclinical models (i.e., in vivo systems) return better results in terms of clinical applications.

CONCLUSION

All experimental preclinical models that we have described here aim to highlight the morphological, molecular, and genetic features of PDAC in vitro and in vivo. The possibility to select pure cell populations using cell cultures and LMD allows us to have experimental models that closely mimic human PDAC. All of these models have room for improvement and are expected to become more advanced in the coming years. This will impact the development of new experimental therapies based on the molecular characteristics in vitro and in vivo. Collectively, the primary models can become the major research tools to understand and fight the drug resistance of this devastating disease.

ACKNOWLEDGMENTS

I would like to thank the following colleagues: Prof. Ugo Boggi, General and Transplants Surgery, University of Pisa, Italy; Prof. Daniela Campani, Surgical Pathology, University of Pisa, Italy; Prof. Marco Del Chiaro, General Surgery, CLINTEC Karolinska, Sweden; Prof. Irene Esposito, Surgical Pathology, Munich University, Germany; Dr Elisa Giovannetti, Cancer Center Amsterdam, VU University, Amsterdam, The Netherlands; Dr Luca Emanuele Pollina, Surgical Pathology, University of Pisa, Italy; Prof. Franco Mosca, General and Transplants Surgery, University of Pisa, Italy; and, Dr Claudio Ricci, Laboratory of Immunology, University of Verona, Italy. The author would like to thank also Fondazione Umberto Veronesi, Milano, Italy. The author was awarded the research grant "Young Investigator Program Year 2013".

REFERENCES

[1] Gudjonsson B. Cancer of the pancreas. 50 years of surgery. Cancer 1987;60:2284–303.

[2] Cullinan SA, Moertel CG, Fleming TR, Rubin JR, Krook JE, Everson LK, et al. A comparison of three chemotherapeutic regimens in the treatment of advanced pancreatic and gastric carcinoma. Fluorouracil vs fluorouracil and doxorubicin vs fluorouracil, doxorubicin, and mitomycin. JAMA 1985;253:2061–7.

[3] Greenlee RT, Murray T, Bolden S, Wingo PA. Cancer statistics. CA Cancer J Clin 2000;50:7–33.

[4] Warshaw AL, Fernandez-del Castillo C. Pancreatic carcinoma. N Engl J Med 1992;326:455–65.

[5] Lowenfels AB, Maisonneuve P, Boyle P. In: Howard J, Idezuki Y, Ihse I, Prinz R, editors. Epidemiology of pancreatic cancer. Surgical diseases of the pancreas. Baltimore: Williams & Wilkins; 1998. pp. 433–7.

[6] Lowenfels AB, Maisonneuve P, Cavallini G, Ammann RW, Lankisch PG, Andersen JR, et al. Pancreatitis and the risk of pancreatic cancer. International Pancreatitis Study Group. N Engl J Med 1993;328:1433–7.

[7] Lowenfels AB, Maisonneuve P, DiMagno EP, Elitsur Y, Gates Jr LK, Perrault J, et al. Hereditary pancreatitis and the risk of pancreatic cancer. International Hereditary Pancreatitis Study Group. J Natl Cancer Inst 1997;89:442–6.

[8] Eberle MA, Pfutzer R, Pogue-Geile KL, Bronner MP, Crispin D, Kimmey MB, et al. A new susceptibility locus for autosomal dominant pancreatic cancer maps to chromosome 4q32-34. Am J Hum Genet 2002;70:1044–8.

[9] Almoguera C, Shibata D, Forrester K, Martin J, Arnheim N, Perucho M. Most human carcinomas of the exocrine pancreas contain mutant c-K-ras genes. Cell 1988;53: 549–54.

[10] Lemoine NR, Jain S, Hughes CM, Staddon SL, Maillet B, Hall PA, et al. Ki-ras oncogene activation in preinvasive pancreatic cancer. Gastroenterology 1992;102:230–6.

[11] Di Giuseppe JA, Hruban RH, Offerhaus GJ, Clement MJ, van den Berg FM, Cameron JL, et al. Detection of K-ras mutations in mucinous pancreatic duct hyperplasia from a patient with a family history of pancreatic carcinoma. Am J Pathol 1994;144:889–95.

[12] Di Giuseppe JA, Hruban RH, Goodman SN, Polak M, van den Berg FM, Allison DC, et al. Overexpression of p53 protein in adenocarcinoma of the pancreas. Am J Clin Pathol 1994;101:684–8.

[13] Casey G, Yamanaka Y, Friess H, Kobrin MS, Lopez ME, Buchler M, et al. p53 mutations are common in pancreatic cancer and are absent in chronic pancreatitis. Cancer Lett 1993;69:151–60.

[14] Campani D, Boggi U, Cecchetti D, Esposito I, Ceccarelli F, D'Antonio L, et al. p53 overexpression in lymph node metastases predicts clinical outcome in ductal pancreatic cancer. Pancreas 1999;19:26–32.

[15] Campani D, Esposito I, Boggi U, Cecchetti D, Menicagli M, De Negri F, et al. Bcl-2 expression in pancreas development and pancreatic cancer progression. J Pathol 2001;194:444–50.

[16] Caldas C, Hahn SA, da Costa LT, Redston MS, Schutte M, Seymour AB, et al. Frequent somatic mutations and homozygous deletions of the p16 (MTS1) gene in pancreatic adenocarcinoma. Nat Genet 1994;8:27–32.

[17] Wilentz RE, Iacobuzio-Donahue CA, Argani P, MCCarthy DM, Yeo CJ, Kern SE, et al. Loss of expression of Dpc4 in pancreatic intraepithelial neoplasia: evidence that Dpc4 inactivation occurs late in neoplastic progression. Cancer Res 2000;60:2002–6.

[18] Wilentz RE, Su GH, Dai JL, Sparks AB, Argani P, Sohn TA, et al. Immunohistochemical labeling for dpc4 mirrors genetic status in pancreatic adenocarcinomas: a new marker of DPC4 inactivation. Am J Pathol 2000;156:37–43.

[19] Goggins M, Schutte M, Lu J, Moskaluk CA, Weinstein CL, Petersen GM, et al. Germ-line BRCA2 gene mutations in patients with apparently sporadic pancreatic carcinomas. Cancer Res 1996;56:5360–4.

[20] Siegel R, Naishadham D, Jemal A. Cancer statistics, 2012. CA Cancer J Clin 2012;62: 10–29.

[21] Burris III HA, Moore MJ, Andersen J, Green MR, Rothenberg ML, Modiano MR, et al. Improvements in survival and clinical benefit with gemcitabine as a first-line therapy for patients with advanced pancreas cancer: a randomized trial. J Clin Oncol 1997;15:2403–13.

[22] Rosenberg L. Pancreatic cancer: a review of emerging therapies. Drugs 2000;59: 1072–3.

[23] Giovannetti E, Del Tacca M, Mey V, Funel N, Nannizzi S, Ricci S, et al. Transcription analysis of human equilibrative nucleoside transporter-1 predicts survival in pancreas cancer patients treated with gemcitabine. Cancer Res 2006;66:3928–35.

[24] Funel N, Giovannetti E, Del Chiaro M, Mey V, Pollina LE, Nannizzi S, et al. Laser microdissection and primary cell cultures improve pharmacogenetic analysis in pancreatic adenocarcinoma. Lab Invest 2008;88:773–84.

[25] Moore PS, Sipos B, Orlandini S, Sorio C, Real FX, Lemoine NR, et al. Genetic profile of 22 pancreatic carcinoma cell lines. Analysis of K-ras, p53, p16 and DPC4/Smad4. Virchows Arch 2001;439:798–802.

[26] Gey GO, Coffmann Wd, Kubicek MT. Tissue culture studies of the proliferative capacity of cervical carcinoma and normal epithelium. Cancer Res 1952;12:264–5.

[27] Dobrynin YV. Establishment and characteristics of cell strains from some epithelial tumors of human origin. J Natl Cancer Inst 1963;31:1173–95.

[28] Giovannetti E, Funel N, Peters GJ, Del Chiaro M, Erozenci LA, Vasile E, et al. MicroRNA-21 in pancreatic cancer: correlation with clinical outcome and pharmacologic aspects underlying its role in the modulation of gemcitabine activity. Cancer Res 2010;70:4528–38.

[29] Ruckert F, Pilarsky C, Grutzmann R. *Establishment of primary cell lines in pancreatic cancer. Pancreatic cancer–molecular mechanism and targets.* Intech; 2012.

[30] Bardeesy N, De Pinho RA. Pancreatic cancer biology and genetics. Nat Rev Cancer 2002;2:897–909.

[31] Krautz C, Ruckert F, Seager HD, Pilarsky C, Grutzmann R. An update on molecular research of pancreatic adenocarcinoma. Anticancer Agents Med Chem 2011;11: 411–7.

[32] Moskaluk CA, Hruban RH, Kern SE. p16 and K-ras gene mutations in the intraductal precursors of human pancreatic adenocarcinoma. Cancer Res 1997;57:2140–3.

[33] Luttges J, Schlehe B, Menke MA, Vogel I, Henne BD, Kloppel G. The K-ras mutation pattern in pancreatic ductal adenocarcinomas usually is identical to that in associated normal, hyperplastic, and metaplastic ductal epithelium. Cancer 1999;85:1703–10.

[34] Funel N, Vasile E, Del Chiaro M, Boggi U, Falcone A, Campani D, et al. Correlation of basal EGFR expression with pancreatic cancer grading but not with clinical outcome after gemcitabine-based treatment. Ann Oncol 2011;22:482–4.

[35] Funel N, Giovannetti E, Pollina LE, del Chiaro M, Mosca F, Boggi U, et al. Critical role of laser microdissection for genetic, epigenetic and proteomic analyses in pancreatic cancer. Expert Rev Mol Diagn 2011;11:695–701.

[36] Avan A, Caretti V, Funel N, Galvani E, Maftouh M, Honeywell RJ, et al. Crizotinib inhibits metabolic inactivation of gemcitabine in c-Met-driven pancreatic carcinoma. Cancer Res 2013;3:6745–56.

[37] Chifenti B, Morelli M, Zavaglia M, Coviello DA, Guerneri S, Santucci A, et al. Establishment and characterization of 4 new pancreatic cancer cell lines: evidence of different tumor phenotypes. Pancreas 2009;28:184–96.

[38] Burgemaister R, Gagnus R, Haar B, Schutze K, Sauer U. High quality RNA retrieved from samples by using LMPC (laser microdissection and pressure catapulting) technology. Pathol Res Pract 2003;199:431–6.

[39] Fukushima N, Koopman J, Sato N, Prasad N, Carvalho R, Leach SD, et al. Gene expression alterations in the non-neoplastic parenchyma adjacent to infiltrating pancreatic ductal adenocarcinoma. Mod Pathol 2005;18:779–87.

[40] Crnogorac-Jurcevic T, Efthimiou E, Nielsen T, Loader J, Terris B, Stamp G, et al. Expression profiling of microdissected adenocarcinoma. Oncogene 2002;21:4587–94.

[41] Kettere K, Rao S, Friess H, Weiss J, Buchler MW, Korc M. Reverse transcription analysis of laser-captured cells points to potential paracrine and autocrine action neurotrophins in pancreatic cancer. Clin Cancer Res 2003;9:5127–36.

[42] Heinmoller E, Bockholt A, Werther M, Ziemer M, Muller A, Ghadimi BM, et al. Laser microdissection of small tissue samples–application to chronic pancreatitis tissues. Pathol Res Pract 2003;199:363–71.

[43] Funel N, Campani D, Del Chiaro M, Pollina L, Baron M, Boggi U, et al. Live cell capturing (LCC) and pancreatic cancer cell culture: a new methodological approach. EHPA Congress Proc 2007;9:3–43.

[44] Mueller-Klieser W. Multicellular spheroids. A review on cellular aggregates in cancer research. J Cancer Res Clin Oncol 1987;113:101–22.

[45] Sipos B, Moser S, Kalthoff H, Torok V, Löhr M, Klöppel G. A comprehensive characterization of pancreatic ductal carcinoma cell lines: towards the establishment of an in vitro research platform. Virchows Arch 2003;442:444–52.

[46] Gutierrez-Barrera AM, Menter DG, Abbruzzese JL, Reddy SA. Establishment of three-dimensional cultures of human pancreatic duct epithelial cells. Biochem Biophys Res Commun 2007;358:698–703.

[47] Olive PL, Durand RE. Drug and radiation resistance in spheroids: cell contact and kinetics. Cancer Metastasis Rev 1994;13:121–38.

[48] Horning JL, Sahoo SK, Vijayaraghavalu S, Dimitrijevic S, Vasir JK, Jain TK, Panda AK, et al. 3-D tumor model for in vitro evaluation of anticancer drugs. Mol Pharm 2008;5:849–62.

[49] Hazlehurst LA, Landowski TH, Dalton WS. Role of the tumor microenvironment in mediating de novo resistance to drugs and physiological mediators of cell death. Oncogene 2003;22:7396–402.

[50] Kleeff J, Beckhove P, Esposito I, Herzig S, Huber PE, Löhr JM, et al. Pancreatic cancer microenvironment. Int J Cancer 2007;12:699–705.

[51] Longati P, Jia X, Eimer J, Wagman A, Witt MR, Rehnmark S, et al. 3D pancreatic carcinoma spheroids induce a matrix-rich, chemoresistant phenotype offering a better model for drug testing. BMC Cancer 2013;13:95–108.

[52] Sempere LF, Gunn JR, Korc M. A novel 3-dimensional culture system uncovers growth stimulatory actions by TGFβ in pancreatic cancer cells. Cancer Biol Ther 2011;12: 198–207.

[53] Fischbach C, Chen R, Matsumoto T, Schmelzle T, Brugge JS, Polverini PJ, et al. Engineering tumors with 3D scaffolds. Nat Methods 2007;4:860–85.

[54] Bissell MJ, Radisky D. Putting tumours in context. Nat Rev Cancer 2001;1:46–54.

[55] Hanahan D, Weinberg RA. The hallmarks of cancer. Cell 2000;100:57–70.

[56] Frampton AE, Castellano L, Colombo T, Giovannetti E, Krell J, Jacob J, et al. MicroRNAs co-operatively inhibit a network of tumor suppressor genes to promote pancreatic tumor growth and progression. Gastroenterology 2014;146:268–77.

CHAPTER 3

Multimodal Therapies for Pancreatic Cancer

Sara Chiblak[1,2], Kenneth E. Lipson[3], Amir Abdollahi[1,2]

[1]German Cancer Consortium (DKTK), Heidelberg, Germany, [2]Molecular & Translational Radiation Oncology, Heidelberg Ion Therapy Center (HIT), Heidelberg Institute of Radiation Oncology (HIRO), University of Heidelberg Medical School and National Center for Tumor Diseases (NCT), German Cancer Research Center (DKFZ), Heidelberg, Germany, [3]FibroGen, Inc., San Francisco, CA, USA

Contents

Introduction	39
Diagnosis, Grading, and Treatment Strategies of Pancreatic Cancer	40
Resectable Pancreatic Cancer	40
Borderline Resectable Pancreatic Cancer	47
Locally Advanced Unresectable Pancreas Cancer	48
Metastatic Disease	52
Novel Molecular Targeted Therapies	54
Next Generation Radiation Oncology	62
Conclusion	63
References	64

INTRODUCTION

Pancreatic ductal adenocarcinoma (PDAC) comprises the fourth most common cause of cancer lethality in Western countries with a less than 5% reported five year survival [1,2]. General increases in the life expectancy of citizens in industrialized countries primarily lead to an elevation in reported cases of PDAC [3,4] with an annual incidence rate similar to its death rate. PDAC is characterized by late diagnosis, aggressive local invasion, early systemic dissemination, and resistance to chemo- and radiotherapy [5]. Despite advances in surgical techniques and therapeutic regimens in the past 30 years, no substantial improvement in the survival of PDAC patients has been noted. We aim to provide an overview on the current status and major challenges of local and systemic treatments for PDAC. Further, novel rationales behind the development of promising next-generation therapy strategies for pancreatic cancer are explored.

Molecular Diagnostics and Treatment of Pancreatic Cancer

Diagnosis, Grading, and Treatment Strategies of Pancreatic Cancer

Following diagnosis of PDAC, planning the patient's treatment regimen is optimally based on the results of diagnostic and imaging tests, and in consultation with experienced multidisciplinary professionals, preferably in high-volume care centers. Variations in clinical evaluation and local management of pancreatic tumors exist among medical institutions in Europe and the United States. Nevertheless, general guidelines have been established for selection of the best treatment options for different subentities of pancreatic cancer (http://www.nccn.org). These involve proper assessment of tumor stage at the time of diagnosis, particularly with respect to discrimination between resectable, locally advanced or metastatic, unresectable disease. Accordingly, the assignment of stage-specific treatment strategy could be appropriately designed (Figure 3.1).

Resectable Pancreatic Cancer

Only approximately one-fifth to one-sixth of patients diagnosed with PDAC are currently eligible for surgical resections, most of which display marginal clinical benefit and postoperative disease recurrences either locally (50–80%), peritoneally (25%), and/or in the liver (50%) [6,7]. Identification

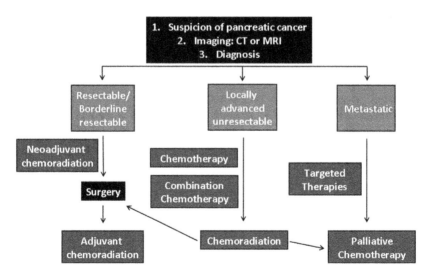

Figure 3.1 *Current Therapy Options in Management of Pancreatic Cancer.* The schematic shows the three key entities and different possible treatment approaches. (For color version of this figure, the reader is referred to the online version of this book.)

of patients with resectable disease constitutes an initial challenge in the adequate management of pancreatic cancer. Classification of the resection state of cancer patients is highly dependent on preoperative radiographic imaging such as abdominal computed tomography (CT) and magnetic resonance imaging (MRI), as well as on endoscopic ultrasound-guided fine-needle biopsy, minimally invasive laparoscopy, and serum CA 19-9 levels [8]. Abdominal CT imaging (optimized for pancreas) is the preferred method at most centers as the diagnostic tool for defining resectability [6,8]. Based on CT assessment, tumors are considered resectable when three major criteria are achieved: (1) localized intrapancreatic disease; (2) no involvement of, or extension into, the celiac axis or superior mesenteric artery (SMA), and (3) patent confluence of the superior mesenteric-portal vein (SMPV) [9].

Minimally invasive laparoscopic distal pancreatectomy (LDP) and laparoscopic pancreaticoduodenectomy (LPD) were originally introduced in the mid-1990s [10]. Studies of LDP have thereafter primarily focused on evaluating clinical outcome in patients with low-grade lesions rather than PDAC. Despite decreased blood loss, shortened hospitalization, and reduced complications, as recorded by a meta-analysis comparing LDP to open surgery, mortality rates observed for both operations were similar [11]. Improvements made later in laparoscopic devices and incorporation of robotic platforms optimized the speed, mobility, precision, and aptitude of these minimally invasive surgeries [10,12,13] as concluded by a comprehensive study of robotic-assisted LDP [14]. However, decisive conclusions on the efficacy of LDP have been impeded by the particular nature and position of the pancreas, as well as its proximity to vascular structures and the insufficiency of available data outcomes.

Postoperative Adjuvant Therapy

Improved local tumor control and increased overall survival were reported in patients with gastrointestinal (GI) malignancies (pancreatic-rectal-stomach) exposed to chemoradiation succeeding their surgery [15–17]. This improved outcome might be attributed to potency of chemoradiation in targeting microscopic lesions within the primary tumor area, or in decreasing the possibility of recurrence in regional lymph nodes [8]. Up to approximately 90% success rate in controlling local disease has been reported in a population of pancreatic cancer patients after accurate diagnosis and multidisciplinary treatment consisting of surgery and chemoradiation [18].

To date, no standard adjuvant treatment has been unambiguously accepted for treatment of pancreatic cancer, in part due to the lack of sufficiently powered randomized trials and heterogeneity of in therapy protocols. An overview of some key clinical studies is provided in Table 3.1. While chemotherapy is considered the standard treatment in Europe, centers in the United States provide chemotherapy alone, chemoradiotherapy, or chemotherapy followed by chemoradiotherapy [19]. The efficacy of 5-fluorouracil (5-FU) and 5-FU-based chemoradiation after surgical resection of pancreas tumor was evaluated in an initial clinical trial that was first reported in 1985 and was led by the Gastro-Intestinal Tumor Study Group (GITSG) [20,21]. As compared to the observation group (surgery alone), patients who received the adjuvant external beam radiotherapy (EBRT, 40 Gy) delivered in split course and chemotherapy (500 mg/m^2 5-FU), displayed significantly longer median survival times (20 vs. 11 months) and two-year survival (43% vs. 19%). However, this study was terminated due to the poor accrual of enrolled candidates (43 patients in eight years). Treatment of 30 additional patients in an expanded trial yielded a median

Table 3.1 Randomized Trials of Adjuvant Therapy for Resectable Pancreatic Cancer Patients

Trial	Year	Patients	Assigned Treatment	Overall Survival (months)	p-value
GITSG	1985	43	5-FU chemoradiation	21	0.035
			Observation (surgery alone)	10.9	
GITSG expanded	1985	30	5-FU chemoradiation	18	n/a
EORTC-40891	1999	114	5-FU chemoradiation	17.1	0.09
			Observation (surgery alone)	12.6	
ESPAC-1	2004	289	5-FU/Leucovorin chemotherapy	20.1	0.009
			No chemotherapy	15.5	0.05
			5-FU chemoradiation	15.9	
			No chemoradiation	17.9	
RTOG-9704	2006	388	Gemcitabine→5-FU chemoradiation→ Gemcitabine	20.6	0.033
			5-FU→5-FU chemoradiation→5-FU	16.9	
CONKO-001	2007	354	Gemcitabine chemotherapy	22.1	0.06
			Observation (surgery alone)	20.2	
ESPAC-3	2010	1088	Gemcitabine chemotherapy	23.6	0.39
			5-FU/Folate chemotherapy	23.0	

survival of 18 months and a two-year survival of 46%, thus confirming the findings of the initial GITSG trial.

In 1999, a second trial was reported by the European Organization for Research and Treatment of Cancer (EORTC-40891) investigating pancreatic head and peri-ampullary cancer [22]. Patients were randomized to receive either 40 Gy EBRT in a split dose with 5-FU or no treatment (observation arm) after surgery. The median survival was 19 months for observation vs. 24.5 months in the chemoradiation group ($p = 0.2$). Due to the ambiguity of data from both trials, the European Study Group for Pancreatic Cancer (ESPAC-1) initiated a randomized multicenter clinical trial investigating the effectiveness of chemoradiotherapy and chemotherapy after pancreas cancer resection [23]. Patients were randomly allocated into four treatment groups: chemotherapy (425 mg/m^2 5-FU, 20 mg/m^2 leucovorin); chemoradiotherapy (40–60 Gy EBRT split course, 425 mg/m^2 5-FU, 20 mg/m^2 leucovorin); chemoradiotherapy followed by chemotherapy; or no further treatment. This study reported beneficial effects of adjuvant 5-FU-based chemotherapy as compared to surgery alone. However, addition of radiotherapy was associated with inferior survival as compared to surgery alone or adjuvant chemotherapy arms. The outcome of the ESPAC-1 trial is controversially debated in the community. In particular, the rationale behind different radiotherapy schemes administered in these trials, i.e., split-course radiotherapy, was conceived in the 1970s. In analogy to the EORTC-40891, for example, patients were treated for two weeks with 5×2 Gy fractions, then the progression of tumor was assessed, and eventually after an interval of two weeks, the treatment was repeated to a total dose of 40 Gy. Another example would have been two courses of 20 Gy in 10 fractions each followed by a three to four week rest period. Depending on the response and the patient's clinical status, another 10–20 Gy in 5–10 fractions was administered as a final boost. Moreover, irradiation was administered sometimes with only two fields (anterior-posterior and posterior-anterior). Likewise, 5-FU-based chemotherapy was started, e.g., prior to radiotherapy as bolus or at 25 mg/kg per 24 h (at max. daily dose of 1500 mg). This is in contrast to continuous administration of 5-FU or gemcitabine-based chemotherapy delivered with modern radiotherapy techniques, i.e., four or more fields, allowing, e.g., integrated boost concepts using IMRT or additional dose escalation with IORT in doses of 45–54 Gy. Therefore, the relatively high local tumor recurrence rates constituting 62% of all recurrences (as compared to the more common pattern of distant recurrences observed in this disease), and the excess mortality observed primarily in the second year, suggest a potential role for late radiation toxicity in surrounding normal organs, such as kidney damage, and suboptimal doses prescribed to the tumor region among possible mechanisms discussed for the poor outcome of the radiotherapy arm in ESPAC-1 trial [24]. In conclusion, the low quality of radiation administered at different centers in the ESPAC-1 clearly indicates the need for randomized prospective trials using modern radiotherapy techniques to ultimately evaluate the role of this therapeutic modality in the adjuvant treatment of PDAC.

The Radiation Therapy Oncology Group (RTOG-9704) investigated the efficacy of gemcitabine ($1000\,mg/m^2$/week) or 5-FU ($250\,mg/m^2$/day) chemotherapy administered before and after 5-FU-based chemoradiation ($50.4\,Gy$ EBRT) in 388 patients with pancreatic head cancers [25]. Evaluation of data revealed prolonged overall survival in patients treated with gemcitabine (20.6 months median survival) as compared to 5-FU (16.9 months median survival). In contrast to the European ESPAC trials, the RTOG investigators have shown that failure in adhering to the specified radiation therapy protocols was associated with decreased survival in RTOG-9704 [26].

Additional evidence for the beneficial effects of adjuvant chemoradiation in PDAC is further provided by two large volume U.S. centers, Johns Hopkins University and the Mayo Clinic, which together investigated more than 1200 patients. They found an improved overall survival (OS) after 5-FU-based adjuvant chemoradiation ($50.4\,Gy$ EBRT) as compared to surgical resection alone (median survival 21.1 vs. 15.5 months, $p < 0.001$) [27]. Their data indicate sustained benefits of chemoradiation with improved two- and five-year OS rates as compared to surgery alone (44.7% vs. 34.6%; 22.3% vs. 16.1%, $p < 0.001$).

Encouraging five-year survival rate (55%) was obtained by an adjuvant interferon-based chemoradiation phase II trial performed at the Virginia Mason University and followed up by the American College of Surgeons Oncology Group (ACOSOG) [28,29]. However, these data were not confirmed by the randomized phase III trial led by the University of Heidelberg [30]. In this study, patients were treated after surgery with cisplatin, interferon alpha2b, 5-FU, and radiotherapy followed by two cycles of 5-FU monotherapy (arm A) or with six cycles of 5-FU monotherapy (arm B). Median survival for the patients who received at least one dose of the study medication was 32.1 months in the combination arm A and 28.5 months in 5-FU alone arm B ($p = 0.49$). Patients treated with the combination therapy more frequently experienced grade III/IV toxicities as compared to the 5-FU alone arm (85% vs. 15%). Nonetheless, this study demonstrates that management of operable PDAC patients with surgery and chemotherapy and/or chemoradiotherapy has improved over time as the relatively high median survival in both arms suggest. Currently, a phase III trial conducted by the RTOG-0848 is joining American and European efforts (EORTC) in evaluating efficacy of postoperative erlotinib treatment after five months of gemcitabine-based chemoradiation [7].

Toward further development in the direction of chemotherapy alone in the adjuvant setting, the ESPAC-3 trial compared the influence of gemcitabine to that of 5-FU/folate–based adjuvant chemotherapies [31]. Although no differences in median survival were observed for both treatment modalities (23.6 vs. 23 months), better tolerance to gemcitabine (revealed by fewer adverse effects) was detected in corresponding patients. In a randomized trial initiated in Germany and Austria by the Charité Onkologie Clinical Studies in GI Cancer-001 (CONKO-001), patients treated with gemcitabine also revealed significantly longer median disease-free survival (13.4 months) as compared to the surgery alone group (6.9 months) [32]. Consequently, based on these studies postoperative chemotherapy has become standard in treatment of operable PDAC in Europe. Later on, the Japanese Study Group of Adjuvant Therapy for Pancreatic Cancer conducted a randomized phase III trial comparing gemcitabine with surgery, but only in 118 patients with resectable disease [33]. Treatment with gemcitabine ($1000 \, mg/m^2$) contributed to prolonged disease-free survival as compared to surgery alone (11.4 vs. 5 months).

Preoperative Neoadjuvant Therapy

Several rationales favor the implementation of radiochemotherapy prior to surgery in a "neoadjuvant" setting [7,8]. First, surgery itself is associated with increased risk of morbidity and mortality, which may consequently result in delayed/canceled postoperative adjuvant treatment. Therefore, preoperative chemo- or radiotherapy may ensure full dose delivery, unlike for adjuvant treatment. Second, development of metastatic disease during the time frame of neoadjuvant therapy would select patients with advanced systemic disease that might benefit less from more aggressive local regimens including surgery. Third, improved delivery of chemotherapeutic agents may be possible by the still intact blood supply prior to surgery. Fourth, disrupted perfusion caused by the interruption of the tumor's blood flow after initial surgery reduces oxygen levels within tumors, rendering cells resistant to radio- as well as chemotherapy. Fifth, reduced adverse and toxic effects have been reported in patients with GI malignancies exposed to preoperative treatment regimens, as shown by a German Rectal Cancer Study [34].

Successive phase II clinical trials testing the efficacy of neoadjuvant therapy have been initiated at MD Anderson Cancer Center [35–39]. In 1992, efficacy of 5-FU (300 mg/m²/day) and irradiation (50.4 Gy, in certain cases intraoperative radiation therapy (IORT)) was tested in 28 patients with cytologic or histologic proof of localized adenocarcinoma of the pancreas head [35]. Four to five weeks of neoadjuvant chemoradiation provided a window for metastatic development in approximately 40% of enrolled patients, as displayed by pathological restaging. The remaining patients were treated with 5-FU (300 mg/m²/day) and irradiated with rapid fractionation (30 Gy in 2 weeks, i.e., 10 daily fractions of 3 Gy, ±10–15 Gy intraoperative radiotherapy (IORT) in 74% of patients) [36]. Around 40% of subjects displayed a pathologic partial response to treatment (>50% non-viable tumor cells). Both irradiation modalities (standard 50.4 Gy [35] vs. rapid [36]) yielded similar local tumor control. Median survivals recorded were 18 and 25 months for standard and rapid chemoradiation regimens, respectively. This study concluded that favorable locoregional control may require a combination of preoperative 5-FU/rapid fractionation chemoradiation, surgery, and IORT [36]. Investigation of the influence of paclitaxel (60 mg/m²) in combination with rapid fractionation (30 Gy EBRT), conducted later on resectable pancreas cancer, showed no advantage of this neoadjuvant therapy over 5-FU-based chemoradiation [37]. Of note, paclitaxel-based neoadjuvant chemoradiation demonstrated a higher relative toxicity (nausea, dehydration, vomiting) as compared to conventional 5-FU-based regimens. Subsequently, two phase II trials, including 86 and 90 resectable pancreatic cancer patients, evaluated preoperative chemoradiation using gemcitabine alone (400 mg/m²) or in combination with cisplatin (30 mg/m²) and radiotherapy (30 Gy in 10 fractions), respectively [38,39]. Patients treated with gemcitabine displayed better pathological findings, i.e., higher rates of microscopic tumor clearance (R0 resection) and longer overall survival than those treated with 5-FU– or paclitaxel-based neoadjuvant treatments. Addition of cisplatin with gemcitabine had no obvious improvement on patient outcome as compared to gemcitabine alone [39]. In conclusion, the MD Anderson data clearly suggest favorable outcomes for primarily operable patients using a neoadjuvant gemcitabine-based hypofractionated (30 Gy in 10 fractions ± IORT) radiochemotherapy regimen.

Borderline Resectable Pancreatic Cancer

In clinical practice, definition of resectability of PDAC is often made by multidisciplinary boards consisting of specialist surgeons and radiologists. Nevertheless, an operable tumor may turn out to be not resectable and vice versa during the preoperative laparoscopy or later surgery. Considering these uncertainties, the final decision on operability is made by surgeons and could tremendously vary between different centers, depending on their expertise. Based on CT assessment, and in the absence of metastatic disease, two definitions of borderline resectable have been introduced by the MD Anderson Cancer Center (MDACC) [40] and the National Comprehensive Cancer Network (NCCN) [41]. The NCCN describes borderline resectable pancreatic head cancer as "tumor abutment of the superior mesenteric artery (SMA), severe unilateral superior mesenteric vein (SMV) or portal vein (PV) impingement, gastroduodenal artery (GDA) encasement up to its origin from the hepatic artery, or colon and mesocolon invasion" [41]. Likewise, borderline resectable tumors are defined at MD Anderson by tumors with "encasement of a short segment of the hepatic artery, without evidence of tumor extension to the celiac axis, that is amenable to resection and reconstruction; abutment of the SMA involving ≤180° of the circumference of the artery; or short-segment occlusion of the SMV, PV, or SMPV confluence with a suitable option for vascular reconstruction available because of a normal SMV below and normal PV above the area of tumor involvement" [40].

One therapy strategy for this category of PDAC involves induction chemotherapy followed by chemoradiation and restaging prior to surgery [7]. Katz et al. recently reported the outcome of a trial including borderline resectable patients treated with either chemotherapy, chemoradiation, or both [42]. Out of the 125 patients who completed neoadjuvant therapy, partial response (PR, >50% reduction of viable tumor cells) was observed in 56%, 79 patients were eligible for surgery after restaging, and 94% underwent a margin-negative pancreatectomy. Data revealed that neoadjuvant therapy succeeded by surgery prolonged median survival by 27 months as compared to those patients who could not undergo surgical resection (40 vs. 13 months, $p < 0.001$). A pilot study, led by the Alliance for Clinical Trials in Oncology, National Cancer Institute (NCI), is currently testing the feasibility of FOLFIRINOX (5-FU, leucovorin, oxaliplatin, and irinotecan) and 5-FU-based chemoradiation for patients with borderline resectable disease [7].

Locally Advanced Unresectable Pancreas Cancer

Patients with surgically unresectable disease and with no sign of metastatic spread comprise around 15–20% of pancreatic cancer patients. Until recently these patients were treated similar to those with advanced metastatic disease. However, a growing body of data indicated a higher median survival (~1 year) in these patients as compared to patients with metastatic lesions [38,40] suggesting that they may benefit from a more intensified therapy. Treatment options optimally selected for these patients are still to be established. Chemoradiation in addition to chemotherapy comprise the foundation of treatment for locally advanced unresectable pancreatic cancer (LAPC) disease. Various clinical studies have been initiated to investigate clinical outcome in this relatively new category of pancreatic cancer patients (Table 3.2).

Table 3.2 Randomized Trials of Therapy for Advanced Pancreatic Cancer Patients

Trial	Year	Patients	Assigned Treatment	Overall Survival (months)
GITSG	1981	194	5-FU + moderate dose radiation	10
			5-FU + high dose radiation	10
			High dose radiation	5.5
GITSG follow-up	1988	43	5-FU chemoradiation → Strepto-zocin/Mitomycin/5-FU	9.5
			Streptozocin/Mitomycin/5-FU chemotherapy	7.5
ECOG	1985	191	5-FU chemoradiation	8.3
			5-FU chemotherapy	8.2
Taiwan study	2003	34	Gemcitabine chemoradiation	14.5
			5-FU chemoradiation	6.7
GERCOR	2007	181	Chemotherapy → Chemoradiation	15
			Chemotherapy	11.7
MDACC	2007	323	Gemcitabine chemotherapy → Gemcitabine chemoradiation	11.9
			Gemcitabine chemoradiation	8.5
FFCD/SFRO	2008	119	Gemcitabine chemotherapy → Gemcitabine chemotherapy	13
			5-FU/Cisplatin chemoradiation → Gemcitabine chemotherapy	8.6
ECOG	2011	74	Gemcitabine chemoradiation	11.1
			Gemcitabine chemotherapy	9.2

5-FU-Based Clinical Studies

The earliest clinical trial investigating 194 LAPC patients was conducted in 1981 by the GITSG [43]. Three study groups were randomized and assigned to either high dose irradiation (60 Gy in split course), moderate dose irradiation (40 Gy in split course) with 5-FU chemotherapy or to high dose with 5-FU. The median survival and one-year survival were 5.5 months and 10% for radiotherapy vs. 10 months and 40% for combined chemoradiation. No difference in OS was observed between the two chemoradiation arms [43]. In a prospective follow-up GITSG trial, the overall survival efficacy of multidrug chemotherapy alone (streptozocin, mitomycin, and 5-FU (SMF)) or continued after chemoradiation (5-FU) was evaluated in LAPC patients [44]. Patients allocated to the chemotherapy/chemoradiotherapy treatment protocol had an improved median survival (42 weeks) as compared to chemotherapy alone (32 weeks). Chemotherapy succeeding 5-FU-based chemoradiation yielded increased toxicities in patients with no evidence of improved benefit. In contrast to the GITSG trial, efficiency of 5-FU-based chemoradiation over chemotherapy alone was not demonstrated by an Eastern Cooperative Oncology Group (ECOG) trial [45]. Similar clinical outcome (median survival between 8.2 and 8.3 months) was obtained upon treatment of patients with 5-FU chemotherapy (600 mg/m²/day) or 5-FU chemoradiation (600 mg/m²/day, 40 Gy).

Gemcitabine-Based Clinical Trials

Recognition of gemcitabine's radiosensitizing properties in multiple phase I trials triggered its introduction into chemoradiation regimens for LAPC [46–50]. The Cancer and Leukemia Group B (CALGB) 89805 phase II clinical study evaluated the efficacy of gemcitabine (40 mg/m²/day) administered twice weekly with upper abdominal irradiation (50.4 Gy), directly followed by five cycles weekly gemcitabine (1000 mg/m², three weeks on, one week off per cycle) [51]. The high rate of local control (~87%) was not translated into a substantial improvement of overall survival (OS) (median survival 8.5 months). This might have been in part due to the considerable toxicity of this protocol with 58% and 21% of patients experiencing grade III and IV hematologic toxicities (leukocytopenia and neutropenia) and 31% and 10% of patients displaying grade III and IV gastrointestinal toxicities, respectively. In a phase I study initiated later by the University of Michigan, the maximum tolerated dose (MTD) for radiotherapy was determined at the fixed dose of gemcitabine (1000 mg/m² on days 1, 8, and 15 of a 28-day cycle) concurrent to radiotherapy [48]. The dose-limiting toxicity (DTL) was identified at 42 Gy in 2.8-Gy fractions. Out of six patients treated at DTL one experienced grade 4 vomiting, one patient developed duodenal ulceration, and two patients developed late gastrointestinal toxicity that required surgical management. Therefore, 36 Gy in 2.4 Gy fractions were recommended to be safely administrated for further phase II evaluation. Accordingly, a phase II clinical trial was conducted using this 36 Gy in 3 weeks and full dose gemcitabine schedule in patients with non-metastatic pancreatic cancer; one-year survival rates were 73% for all, 94% for resectable, 76% for borderline resectable, and 47% for unresectable patients [52]. Further developments moved toward lowering the gemcitabine dose (to reduce toxicity) while increasing the radiotherapy dose that has been progressively more frequently administered with better techniques to reduce toxicity and to improve the therapeutic window in order to achieve local tumor control in LAPC. For example, ECOG conducted a trial validating the impact of 50.4 Gy radiotherapy administered at 1.8 Gy fractions combined with concurrent reduced dose gemcitabine GEM $(600\,mg/m^2$ week 1–5) followed by four weeks break, followed by full dose maintenance gemcitabine $(1000\,mg/m^2$ for three of four weeks). This radio-chemotherapy scheme showed an acceptable toxicity profile and was superior to full dose gemcitabine alone with median survival of 11.1 vs. 9.2 months, $p < 0.01$ [53].

Capecitabine-Based Clinical Trials

Capecitabine has gained attention as an orally administered radiosensitizing agent to substitute for 5-FU-based regimens from studies on various malignancies including advanced pancreas cancers [54–56]. In a phase II trial, treatment of 42 pancreatic cancer patients (advanced or metastatic) with capecitabine $(2500\,mg/m^2/day)$ resulted in significantly beneficial effects on tumor-related symptoms [57]. Combining other drugs with capecitabine, such as bevacizumab and cisplatin, along with radiation therapy was also shown to be well tolerated by LAPC patients [58,59].

Gemcitabine-Based Combination Chemotherapy

Gemcitabine and FU: Apart from gemcitabine as a sole chemotherapeutic drug in LAPC treatment, several other studies have evaluated additional combinations to be delivered with, or in comparison to, gemcitabine. For example, a small study in Taiwan assigned 34 LAPC patients to receive either 5-FU-based $(500\,mg/m^2/day)$ or gemcitabine-based $(600\,mg/m^2/day)$ chemoradiation (50.4–61.2 Gy) [60]. Both treatments were similarly tolerated, however, the gemcitabine-based therapy was more effective as compared to 5-FU chemoradiation, with median survival of 14.5 vs. 6.7 months. A phase III trial was later conducted by the Fédération Franco-phone de Cancérologie Digestive (FFCD) and the Société Francophone de Radiothérapie Oncologique (SFRO) [61]. The two treatment arms of this study involved either induction chemoradiotherapy (CHRT) with concomitant 5-FU ($300\,mg/m^2/day$), cisplatin ($20\,mg/m^2/day$), and radiation ($60\,Gy$), or induction gemcitabine chemotherapy ($1000\,mg/m^2/week$). Maintenance gemcitabine succeeded both treatment regimens until signs of disease progression or adverse toxic effects were detected. Patients undergoing the intensive CHRT suffered more from toxicity, thus reporting a shorter median survival (8.6 months) as compared to chemotherapy alone (13 months). On the other hand, the Groupe Coopérateur Multidisciplinaire en Oncologie (GERCOR) has adopted other therapeutic strategies and compared survival of LAPC patients enrolled onto prospective phase II and III studies. In their trial, 181 patients randomly received gemcitabine-based chemotherapy either alone or in combination with 5-FU or oxaliplatin. This was followed by treatment with 5-FU-based chemoradiation or continuation with chemotherapy alone. Of note, chemotherapy and chemoradiation significantly increased survival as compared to chemotherapy alone (15 vs. 11.7 months) [62]. This finding was confirmed by a separate study in which 323 patients received either initial chemoradiotherapy (30 Gy in 10 fraction (85%) combined with 5-FU (41%), gemcitabine (39%), or capecitabine (20%)) or 2.5 months of gemcitabine-based induction therapy followed by chemoradiotherapy. As observed in the first trial, induction gemcitabine treatment preceding chemoradiotherapy improved patients' median OS as compared to chemoradiotherapy alone (11.9 vs. 8.5 months) [63].

Gemcitabine and capecitabine (GemCap): Capecitabine and gemcitabine combination regimens have also shown promising outcomes on advanced and metastatic pancreatic cancer patients in phase I/II clinical studies [64,65]. Based on these promising findings, three major phase III clinical studies have been initiated to further evaluate the efficacy of GemCap combinations on clinical outcome [66–68]. In the first trial led by the Swiss Group for Clinical Cancer Research and the Central European Cooperative Oncology Group (319 patients), GemCap combination failed to improve overall survival as compared to gemcitabine alone (8.4 vs. 7.2 months) [66]. In a recent phase III trial including meta-data, GemCap combinations significantly prolonged median overall survival compared to the gemcitabine alone group (7.4 vs. 6 months) [68].

In conclusion, LAPC patients seem to benefit from an intensified local therapy. In these populations resectability is achieved in approximately one-third of patients with median survival almost equal to those with primary resectable disease [69,70]. Therefore, efficient local control and effective maintenance regimens beyond classical chemotherapy may further improve the management of LAPC.

Metastatic Disease

Unfortunately, metastatic spread is detected in 60–70% of pancreatic cancer patients. A median survival of only six months from time of diagnosis is reported for patients with metastatic disease [71]. Control of symptoms, psychological support, and aid in decision-making fall into the context of palliative care (the standard approach) for this category of patients [71,72]. Numerous morbidities usually accompany advanced pancreatic disease such as pain, cachexia (body weight loss), hyperbilirubinuria (jaundice, icterus, due to blockade of bile duct), bowel obstruction, as well as increased risk of thromboembolic complications [71,73].

In an attempt to improve outcome for patients diagnosed with advanced pancreatic disease, several trials have been initiated using gemcitabine as a backbone. Drugs such as oxaliplatin [74,75], cisplatin [76,77], irinotecan [78], exatecan [79], and pemetrexed [80] have all shown limited improvement when combined with gemcitabine. Therefore, development of novel treatment protocols is highly crucial for improving clinical outcome in patients with metastatic pancreatic cancer.

Establishment of FOLFIRINOX treatment: Conroy and colleagues were first to introduce a combination of infusional 5-FU, irinotecan, and oxaliplatin into the therapy of metastatic pancreatic cancer [81]. Promising data observed in phase I trials prompted the initiation of single-arm phase II studies in metastatic pancreatic and colorectal cancer patients [82,83]. Eligibility criteria for enrollment of patients included good World Health Organization performance status (0 or 1), an age below 70 years old, levels of total bilirubin 1.5 times or less than the normal upper limit, as well as resectability. Cases that met these conditions involved 11 LAPC and 35 metastatic patients. FOLFIRINOX treatment resulted in median overall survival of 9.5 months in metastatic patients and 15.7 months in LAPC cases. No cases of toxicity-related deaths were reported.

The promising results of these studies encouraged conducting a phase III PRODIGE 4/ACCORD 11 study. The major aim of this French randomized trial was to compare the efficacy of FOLFIRINOX vs.

gemcitabine in metastatic pancreatic cancer patients [81]. The data indicated a 31.6% response rate for FOLFIRINOX combination as compared to 9.4% for gemcitabine alone. Although no significant difference was shown between the treatments on the median duration of response, FOLFIRINOX displayed 70.2% disease control rate as compared to only 50.9% for gemcitabine. Significantly longer progression-free (PFS) and overall (OS) survivals were also reported for FOLFIRINOX in contrast to gemcitabine (PFS: 5.4 vs. 3.3 months, OS: 11.1 vs. 6.8 months). One-year survival rates recorded for FOLFIRINOX and gemcitabine were 48.4% and 20.6%, respectively. As anticipated, FOLFIRINOX delivery was associated with higher toxicities than gemcitabine (Grade III/IV neutropenia: 45.7% vs. 21%; febrile neutropenia: 5.4% vs. 1.2%; thrombocytopenia: 9.1% vs. 3.6%; diarrhea: 11.4% vs. 1.2%; and peripheral neuropathy: 9% vs. 0%). Nevertheless, FOLFIRINOX regimen proved superior over gemcitabine in improving outcome of metastatic pancreatic cancer patients with a good performance status.

Promising data from this study paved the way for additional clinical trials. A clinical benefit of FOLFIRINOX was also reported by a multi-institutional study enrolling a total of 61 patients (median age of 58 years, 31% LAPC) [84]. Similar to the French trial, no toxicity-related fatalities were recorded. Approximately one-fifth of patients suffered from grade III/IV neutropenia including 5% febrile neutropenia. Out of the 40 evaluated cases, 25% had an overall response and 47% had a stable disease rate. Subsequent to FOLFIRINOX therapy, all borderline resectable as well as 4/19 LAPC cases were eligible for surgical resection. Including patients with poor performance status (higher than 1) in a U.S. multi-institutional study yielded a median overall survival of only 7.2 months, arguing against FOLFIRINOX as a standard of care due to its limitation to patients with only good performance [85]. Numerous other clinical studies are currently in progress to evaluate clinical advantages of FOLFIRINOX over gemcitabine-based therapy arms [85].

Activity of FOLFIRINOX treatment in combination with chemoradiotherapy on LAPC has also been recently described in various studies [85,86]. A clinical trial was initiated at the Massachusetts General Hospital in Boston to test the efficacy of this combination regimen on 22 LAPC patients. Irradiation following chemotherapy was performed on 20 patients. The overall response rate was 27.3%, and the median progression-free survival (PFS) was 11.7 months. Five patients exposed to this combination became resectable and underwent a R0 resection [87]. Despite some encouraging data of FOLFIRINOX, the value of this relatively toxic regimen in treatment of patients with limited survival expectation is still not well elaborated.

A New Chemotherapeutic: nab-paclitaxel

The extensive hypovascularity of stroma surrounding pancreas tumor cells is thought to hinder proper delivery of cytotoxic drugs that are administered to the systemic circulation. Therefore finding methodologies to increase accessibility of cytotoxic drugs to tumor cells is considered highly desirable. The original formulation of paclitaxel (Taxol®) utilized cremophor and oil-based solvents and that resulted in significant systemic toxicities in patients. Therefore, a modified albumin-bound formulation named nab-paclitaxel (Abraxane®) was developed using nanoparticle technology. The phase I clinical trial of nab-paclitaxel showed that it was better tolerated than the original formulation [88]. The exact mechanism of action of nab-paclitaxel is not yet fully elucidated but is thought to involve improved tumor uptake. Coadministration of nab-paclitaxel with gemcitabine into a genetically engineered mouse model of pancreatic cancer strikingly resulted in tumor regression, increased intratumoral gemcitabine levels, as well as reduced levels of the primary gemcitabine metabolizing enzyme cytidine deaminase [89]. Neesse and colleagues have recently shown that chemical inhibition of cytidine deaminase resulted in increased gemcitabine concentration within the tumor of the KPC mouse model, but that was insufficient to enhance tumor cell apoptosis or to alter the growth of the pancreatic tumors [90]. Together, these observations suggest that the tumor regression observed upon treatment of mice with nab-paclitaxel and gemcitabine did not result from the enhanced delivery of gemcitabine. Improved clinical outcome was observed in a phase I/II clinical trial of nab-paclitaxel and gemcitabine in metastatic patients [91]. Several other trials evaluating nab-paclitaxel with other combinations are currently in progress, and their outcomes will likely be reported over the next several years. Based on improvement of overall survival and progression-free survival (by 1.8 months for each) in a phase III clinical trial [92] the U.S. FDA approved nab-paclitaxel for treatment of pancreatic cancer on September 6, 2013.

Novel Molecular Targeted Therapies

Better comprehension of cellular and molecular mechanisms governing the resistant phenotype of this devastating disease is urgently needed. Dissecting critical players of aberrant tumor cell behavior (genetic modifications, signaling cascades) as well as altered extracellular communication (tumor stroma) is indispensable as they can be amendable to targeted therapy (Figure 3.2).

Prostaglandin synthase: Elevated levels of cyclooxygenase-2 (COX-2), crucial for prostaglandin synthesis, have been detected in pancreatic precursor lesions as well as PDAC [93,94]. Aberrant COX-2 overexpression usually predicts for a poor prognosis in pancreatic cancer [95]. Preclinical studies have reported resistance in tumor development within COX-2– deficient mice, while overexpression of COX-2 in various transgenic mouse models promotes angiogenesis, dysplasia, and tumorigenesis [94]. A phase II trial, enrolling 42 cytologically or histologically confirmed PDAC patients, tested the effect of the COX-2 inhibitor celecoxib when delivered in combination with gemcitabine (GECO) [96]. As compared to the gemcitabine-alone group, 62% of patients treated with GECO had stable disease and 71% showed total disease control. This combination was also less toxic than gemcitabine alone. Further clinical investigation is thus warranted.

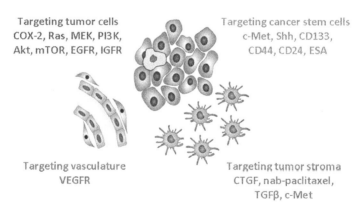

Targeting tumor cells
COX-2, Ras, MEK, PI3K,
Akt, mTOR, EGFR, IGFR

Targeting cancer stem cells
c-Met, Shh, CD133,
CD44, CD24, ESA

Targeting vasculature
VEGFR

Targeting tumor stroma
CTGF, nab-paclitaxel,
TGFβ, c-Met

Figure 3.2 *Molecular Targets for Pancreas Cancer.* Inhibitors of (1) critical tumor cell effectors, e.g., cyclooxygenase-2 (COX-2), Ras, mitogen-activated protein kinases (MEK), phosphatidylinositol 3-kinases (PI3K), Akt, mammalian target of rapamycin (mTOR), epidermal growth factor receptor (EGFR), and insulin-like growth factor receptor (IGFR); (2) tumor stroma, e.g., connective tissue growth factor (CTGF), transforming growth factor beta (TGFβ), hepatocyte growth factor receptor (c-Met), and albumin-conjugated paclitaxel (Abraxane); (3) tumor endothelium, e.g., vascular endothelial growth factor receptor (VEGFR); and (4) cancer stem cell markers, e.g., c-Met, Sonic hedgehog (Shh), CD133, CD44, CD24, and epithelial-specific antigen (ESA). *Adapted from Ref. [119].* (For color version of this figure, the reader is referred to the online version of this book.)

Ras synthesis and downstream signaling: GTPases of the Ras superfamily act as binary switches controlling multiple signaling pathways in eukaryotic cells. They exist in an inactive guanosine diphosphate (GDP)-bound "off" state and an active guanosine triphosphate GTP-bound "on" state. Stimulation of a vast array of upstream receptors by ligand binding, e.g., binding of ligand to the epidermal growth factor tyrosine kinase receptor (EGFR), elicits a signaling cascade activating adaptor molecules, which in turn switch Ras between both of its states. SOS-1 and SOS-2 are guanine nucleotide exchange factors (GEFs) known to be crucial activators of Ras via the replacement of a GDP by a GTP moiety [97,98]. They act downstream from GRB2, which binds to the autophosphorylated tail of EGFR [99]. Activation of Ras is terminated by another set of adaptor proteins called Ras-GTPase activating proteins (Ras-GAP). These soluble cytosolic proteins increase the rate of intrinsic GTPase activity of normal Ras proteins [100]. Upon hydrolysis of GTP, Ras-GTP shifts back to its inactive Ras-GDP state, thus terminating all Ras-stimulated signaling [101,102].

Mutationally activated Ras proteins share a potent ability to transform cells, and their activation is mostly correlated with cancer development. Activating mutations in the K-Ras proto-oncogene are the earliest genetic alterations associated with pancreatic cancer development [103,104]. Therefore, aberrant Ras signaling is thought to play a crucial role in initiating pancreatic carcinogenesis [105].

Inhibition of farnesyl protein transferase (FPT), a critical enzyme of Ras protein synthesis, was thought to demolish aberrant protein activity in pancreatic tumors. Examples of FPT inhibitors include lonafarnib (SCH66336) and tipifarnib (BMS-214662) inhibitors. Unfortunately, in a randomized phase III trial (688 advanced pancreatic cancer patients) treatment with gemcitabine and tipifarnib had no clinical advantage over gemcitabine and placebo combination [106]. Both treatment arms yielded overall survival of around 185 days.

These disappointing findings suggested that inhibitors that target crucial downstream effectors of K-Ras signaling such as the mitogen-activated protein kinases 1/2 (MEK1/2) might be a more effective intervention point for tumors with activated Ras. Therapeutic efficacy of several MEK inhibitors GSK1120212 (trametinib), MSC1936369B, and AZD6244 (selumetinib) was successfully validated in vitro [107]. This led to initiation of a series of phase II clinical trials evaluating MEK inhibitors in combination with gemcitabine or EGFR inhibitors [108].

A second critical Ras downstream signaling pathway involves the phosphatidylinositol 3-kinases (PI3K)/Akt/mammalian target of rapamycin (mTOR) regulating growth, proliferation, and survival of cells [109]. Activation of the PI3K/Akt/mTOR pathway has been associated with carcinogenesis, and therefore its inhibition reflects an attractive therapeutic option. PI3K inhibitor BKM120 and PI3K/mTOR inhibitor BEZ235 are currently being tested in combination with MEK inhibitors in phase I trials of solid tumors with K-Ras, N-Ras, or B-Raf mutations. Abrogation of Akt/mTOR signaling using MK-2206 (allosteric Akt inhibitor) alone or in combination with c-Met or EGFR inhibitors are currently under investigation [91]. Use of RX-0201 antisense oligonucleotides selectively inhibiting Akt is also thought to be therapeutically promising as indicated in preclinical setting [110]. Combination of RX-0201 with gemcitabine is currently being evaluated in a phase II trial for metastatic pancreatic cancer patients. Inhibitors of mTOR such as RAD001 (everolimus) have also been investigated in a phase II study. Treatment of 33 metastatic PDAC patients, who were refractory to gemcitabine, with RAD001 was of minor benefit [111]. Based on these findings, two smaller studies enrolling patients with advanced disease examined the efficacy of temsirolimus (study A) and everolimus combined with EGFR inhibitor erlotinib (study B). Unfortunately both studies displayed no objective responses or disease stability [112].

Epidermal growth factor receptor (EGFR): Four main members belong to the human epidermal growth factor receptor family: EGFR, Her-2/Neu, Her-3, and Her-4. Aberrant EGFR signaling was reported in pancreatic cancer to causally contribute to its therapy-refractoriness [113]. Therefore, EGFR inhibitors were evaluated in PDAC. Erlotinib is a small molecule inhibitor of EGFR kinase that prevents its autophosphorylation and consequently inhibits its downstream signaling. A randomized phase III trial was conducted at the National Cancer Institute of Canada to compare gemcitabine treatment alone to gemcitabine combined with erlotinib in patients with advanced pancreatic disease [114]. The combination regimen led to a slight but statistically significant improvement of median OS and one-year survival as compared to gemcitabine alone (6.24 months and 23% vs. 5.91 months and 17%, respectively). In a separate phase III German trial, led by the Arbeitsgemeinschaft Internistische Onkologie (AIO), first-line treatment with gemcitabine plus erlotinib was compared to therapy with capecitabine plus erlotinib, demonstrating similar survival benefit in both arms (6.6 vs. 6.9 months) [115].

Cetuximab is a monoclonal antibody that inhibits EGFR signaling by binding to the extracellular domain of the receptor. Therapeutic efficacy of cetuximab in combination with gemcitabine was compared to gemcitabine alone in advanced pancreatic disease by Southwest Oncology Group–directed intergroup Phase III trial (SWOG-S0205) [116]. In line with erlotinib data, combined modality treatment showed a trend toward improved OS of 6.3 months in cetuximab + gemcitabine vs. 5.9 months in gemcitabine alone, but it did not reach statistical significance. The time to treatment failure was significantly, but only two weeks, longer in combination vs. gemcitabine monotherapy ($p = 0.006$). In another randomized phase II study, the effect of trimodal therapy consisting of gemcitabine, intensity-modulated radiation therapy (IMRT) and cetuximab was investigated in LAPC patients [117]. The initial treatment consisted of concurrent gemcitabine weekly (300 mg/m^2), and cetuximab weekly (loading dose 400 mg/m^2 day 1, concomitant with RT 250 mg/m^2). After trimodal therapy, patients in arm A received gemcitabine weekly (1000 mg/m^2) over four weeks, and patients in study arm B received gemcitabine weekly (1000 mg/m^2) over four weeks and cetuximab (250 mg/m^2) weekly over 12 weeks. IMRT was delivered using an integrated boost concept (54 Gy to the gross tumor volume (GTV), 45 Gy to the clinical tumor volume (CTV)) over five weeks. One- and two-year survival was 61% and 20%, respectively, and median survival was 15 months. After trimodal therapy 40/68 patients were amenable for secondary, potentially curative resection, i.e., with no local tumor progression or appearance of metastatic lesions. Fourteen patients could be resected. These encouraging data suggest further exploration of multimodal regimens in the LAPC patients using advanced radiotherapy, and targeted agents are warranted [118].

Vascular endothelial growth factor receptor (VEGFR): Tumors are dependent on their vasculature to provide nutrients and remove wastes and have therefore developed mechanisms to promote angiogenesis, including increased expression of VEGFs. VEGF binding to VEGFR2 on endothelial cells induces their proliferation, motility, and survival, thereby promoting angiogenesis. The result in many tumors is increased vascularity that facilitates tumor growth and metastasis [119–121].

Bevacizumab, a humanized monoclonal antibody targeting VEGF-A, was investigated in combination with gemcitabine and erlotinib in a phase III trial enrolling metastatic patients. Adding bevacizumab to gemcitabine-erlotinib significantly improved PFS as compared to placebo, however, did not significantly improve OS (7.1 vs. 6.0 months) [122]. Similarly, combination of bevacizumab with gemcitabine and capecitabine demonstrated no clinical benefit in a phase II study of advanced pancreatic cancer [123]. Failure of other VEGF signaling pathway inhibitors in combination with various gemcitabine-based regimens to improve survival of advanced pancreatic patients was also reported in multiple studies [122–126].

In addition to a scarcity of blood vessels in PDAC tumors, high interstitial pressure appears to contribute to poor tumor perfusion. This poor tumor perfusion impairs delivery of chemotherapeutic agents to the tumor. One of the mechanisms contributing to high interstitial pressure is elevated expression of hyaluronic acid. In genetically engineered mouse models of PDAC, tumor perfusion and delivery of chemotherapeutic agents to tumors was improved by administration of a pegylated hyaluronidase (PEGPH20). This resulted in objective tumor responses and increased survival of the mice [127,128]. A phase II clinical trial is now in progress to test the activity of a pegylated hyaluronidase in combination with nab-paclitaxel and gemcitabine.

Insulin-like growth factor receptor (IGF-1R): The relevance of the IGF signaling pathway in pancreatic cancer has been previously described. Elevated levels of IGF-1R was associated with increased tumorigenicity and metastasis in transgenic mouse models of pancreas cancer [129]. Moreover, inhibition of IGF-1R by siRNA resulted in reduced tumor growth of various gastrointestinal malignancies [130,131]. Therefore, targeting the IGF signaling axis appeared to represent a promising therapeutic approach. Several IGF-1R inhibitors are currently being investigated for clinical benefit. In preclinical studies, the AMG-479 monoclonal antibody (specifically raised against IGF-1R) reduced downstream Akt signaling favoring proapoptotic and antiproliferative stimuli [132]. Although patients treated with a combination of AMG-479 and gemcitabine displayed slight improvement over gemcitabine in a randomized phase II trial, AMG-479 failed to achieve its efficacy in a phase III study [108]. Cixutumumab, a second IGF-1R inhibitor, also demonstrated no improved clinical outcome in combination with gemcitabine or erlotinib as reported by a recent phase II trial [108].

Targeting pancreas tumor stroma: Another characteristic of PDAC is the presence of "desmoplasia", defined as proliferation of fibrotic tissue with an altered extracellular matrix (ECM) conducive to tumor growth and metastasis [133]. Pancreatic cancer cells produce many extracellular matrix (ECM) proteins themselves. However, tumor cell activation of pancreas stellate cells (PSC) within the tumor stroma comprises the predominant pattern of ECM deposition in PDAC. This paracrine activation is mediated by a series of enriched growth factors notably transforming growth factor β (TGFβ), hepatocyte growth factor (HGF), IGF-1, and EGF. Moreover, autocrine signaling via TGFβ1 and connective tissue growth factor (CTGF) maintain sustained activation of PSCs [133–135]. Therefore, these factors appear to represent attractive therapeutic targets for treatment of pancreatic cancer.

CTGF is upregulated in many pancreatic cancers. CTGF overexpression in Panc1 cells was previously reported to induce proliferation of cells in a dose-dependent fashion [136,137]. It also led to increased migration and invasiveness of the CTGF-overexpressing Panc-1 cells in vitro [136,137]. Moreover, elevated CTGF levels increased pancreas tumor cell growth in soft agar and decreased their apoptosis [138,139]. Robust selection of cells overexpressing CTGF was associated with enhanced tumor growth, as observed in subcutaneous and orthotopic pancreas models [138]. Blocking of CTGF using FG-3019, a human anti-CTGF antibody, inhibited tumor growth generated by subcutaneous injection of CTGF-overexpressing MIA PaCa-2 cells in a xenograft model [139]. Treatment of mice with FG-3019, alone or in combination with gemcitabine, also reduced tumor burden and metastasis in an orthotopic Panc1 tumor model [136]; [139]. In addition, FG-3019 in combination with gemcitabine promoted apoptosis of pancreatic carcinoma cells in a genetically engineered mouse model of PDAC, thereby inhibiting tumor growth and metastasis, and improving survival [128].

Inhibition of CTGF using FG-3019 in combination with gemcitabine and erlotinib has been tested in a phase I/II trial on locally advanced and metastatic pancreatic cancer patients [140]. Results, reported at the American Society of Clinical Oncology (ASCO) meeting, showed that the antibody was well tolerated up to the highest doses tested (45 mg/kg every two weeks or 22.5 mg/kg weekly), in combination with gemcitabine and erlotinib. No adverse events were attributed to antibody administration. The median overall survival of the 75 subjects in the study was 9.1 months. No subjects in the two lowest dose cohorts (3 and 10 mg/kg every two weeks) survived for one year. However, at higher doses, one-year survival increased in a dose-dependent manner and reached a plateau at about 30%. Examining overall survival as a function of baseline plasma CTGF levels and exposure to FG-3019 (based on trough level after the first dose) suggested that clinical outcome correlates with both. Subjects with the lowest baseline CTGF and the highest exposure to FG-3019 exhibited a median overall survival of greater than 11 months, compared to less than four months for subjects with the highest baseline CTGF levels and the lowest antibody exposure [140].

CTGF promotes the activity of TGFβ by enhancing mitogenic and chemotactic activity of connective tissue cells and their synthesis of ECM proteins collagen and fibronectin [141,142]. Among various TGFβ inhibitors, efficacy of trabedersen (antisense oligodeoxynucleotide inhibiting TGFβ2) monotherapy was evaluated in 61 patients with refractory solid tumors, out of which 37 were diagnosed with pancreatic cancers [143,144]. In phase I of the study, Oettle and colleagues described excellent tolerance of the drug when administered at the dose of 140 mg/m^2/day, a dose adopted in phase II of the study. Patients receiving trabedersen at the recommended dose displayed highly satisfactory clinical outcome with a reported 13.4 months median overall survival. Another randomized trial testing the impact of specific TGFβ1 receptor inhibitor LY2157299 in combination with gemcitabine is currently ongoing [108].

The receptor for hepatocyte growth factor (HGF), c–Met, and HGF are essential for normal mammalian development and play a crucial role in branching morphogenesis [145]. Multiple studies have shown an overexpression of c–Met in pancreatic cancer. Binding of HGF to c–Met initiates a signaling cascade favoring pancreatic tumor cell motility, invasion, and metastasis [146]. Cabozantinib, a novel potent dual c–Met/VEGFR-2 inhibitor, was accepted by the FDA at the end of 2012 for treatment of patients with medullary thyroid carcinoma [147]. Preclinical data have shown the drug's ability to regress tumor vasculature, hypoxia, and apoptosis as well as to decrease aggressiveness of pancreatic tumors [147–149]. Metastatic spread of intracardiac-injected pancreatic cancer cells was also prevented after two weeks of cabozantinib delivery in mice [149]. Moreover, cabozantinib reduced viability and induced apoptosis of gemcitabine-resistant pancreas cell lines [147]. Based on these striking findings, various phase II trials including metastatic pancreatic cancer patients are currently investigating its clinical benefit.

Evidence for self-renewing cells within solid tumors, referred to as cancer stem cells (CSC), has been described for many cancers [150–152]. Li and colleagues were the first to relate CSC to pancreatic cancer progression [153]. In their work, isolation of pancreatic CSC was guided by enrichment for the previously assigned CSC markers CD44, CD24, and epithelial-specific antigen (ESA). CD44+ CD24+ ESA+ pancreatic CSC demonstrated typical stemness features such as self-renewal, generation of differentiated progeny, and activation of developmental signaling pathways such as sonic hedgehog (Shh) [153]. Systemic inhibition of Shh by IPI926 inhibitor resulted in a significant depletion of pancreas tumor stroma in a transgenic mouse model. This was accompanied by an enhanced vascularity and concentration for coadministered gemcitabine [154]. A clinical trial investigating efficacy of IPI926 has recently been terminated due to an observed inferiority to gemcitabine therapy arm on LAPC patients [108]. A subpopulation of pancreas cells with high c-Met expression also displayed stem cell–like properties. In contrast to c-Met negative, cells with high c-Met levels had better sphere formation capabilities and exhibited higher tumor uptake in nude mice. Therefore, further evaluation of c-Met as a cancer stem cell marker is of extreme importance [149]. Cabozantinib treatment downregulated expression of c-Met and several other stem cell markers (CD133, SOX-2) in primary spheroid cultures, thus emphasizing the importance of further clinical investigation [147].

Next Generation Radiation Oncology

Introduction of particle therapy into the clinic provides a novel option to improve sensitivity of cancer to radiotherapy [155]. However, biological and molecular rationales favoring particle over conventional radiotherapy are not yet fully explored.

In vitro experimentation elucidated possible mechanisms for the observed superiority of high linear energy transfer (LET) particles, e.g., carbon over conventional photon. Precise dose localization, increased relative biological effect, reduced oxygen enhancement ratio, decreased cell cycle–dependent radiosensitivity, and induced complex DNA damage are among the thus far validated advantages provided by heavy ions [156]. Strong correlation with radiobiological effects of heavy ions has been previously shown in pancreas cells [157]. Unlike photon radiotherapy, carbon ions induced more DNA damage and reduced the clonogenic survival of pancreas cancer as well as cancer stem-like cells [156]. High LET particles also enhanced cellular death in human pancreatic cancers with different genetic status. Additionally, high LET strongly correlated with G2/M arrest in pancreas cancer cell lines [157]. Advantageous killing of heavy ions was not only restricted to pancreas tumors cells. For instance apoptosis induction, autophagy, and cellular senescence are among postulated mechanisms underlying enhanced glioma cell kill by carbon irradiation [158,159].

Pancreas cells are highly aggressive and show a great potential for traversing from primary tumor site into a metastatic niche. This renders pancreatic cancers among the most therapeutically resistant tumors. Migration and invasiveness of various pancreas cell lines such as MIA-PaCa-2, BxPC3, and AsPC-1 have been previously shown to be reduced by carbon radiotherapy [160].

Apart from tumor cells, carbon radiotherapy also influenced endothelial cells [161] and enhanced antiangiogenic effects in lung [162] and colorectal cancer models [163]. The introduction of raster scanning carbon ion radiotherapy constitutes a landmark technological development in high precision radiotherapy. Efficacy of chemoradiation using gemcitabine in combination with raster scanning carbon ion on pancreas cancer cells in vitro was recently described [164]. Additional preclinical experimentation will increase our understanding of heavy ion radiotherapy. Nevertheless, current in vitro and preliminary in vivo data demonstrate a firm basis for further investigating the efficacy of heavy ion therapy alone or in combination with chemotherapy in highly resistant pancreatic cancer patients.

Initial promising data on the safety of short-course carbon ion radiotherapy in patients with resectable pancreatic cancer were shown in a Japanese clinical phase I/II study [165]. Dose escalation was performed at 5% increments from 30 to 36.8 GyE administered in eight fractions over two weeks prior to surgery. The reported five-year survival rates for all 26 patients receiving carbon radiotherapy and those who underwent surgery post radiotherapy were 42% and 52%, respectively. These very promising data need to be validated in randomized prospective trials.

CONCLUSION

Pancreatic cancer is among the most therapeutically resistant tumors. For the relatively small fraction of operable tumors, the surgical resection has evolved substantially by reducing mortality and morbidity, in particular at specialized centers with high patient volumes. In this chapter, evidence is provided for beneficial effects of adjuvant chemotherapy as well as preoperative (neoadjuvant) radiochemotherapy. Based on the promising phase I/II data, the value of modern radiotherapy techniques, such as IMRT, IORT, and particle radiotherapy with carbon ions has to be evaluated in randomized trials. Nonetheless, the maintenance chemotherapy is still suboptimal, and considering the low overall survival, the impact of antiangiogenic, tumor stroma, immune-, and other targeted therapies in tertiary prevention of tumor metastasis and local recurrence need further exploration. Failure of a plethora of targeted agents observed in advanced metastatic PDAC might not necessarily translate when the switch of micro- to macrometastatic tumors is targeted. Intensified multimodal therapies are warranted in locally advanced PDAC. Approximately one-third of LAPC patients become resectable after multimodal therapies and perform similarly to primary operable patients. After a long series of setbacks with iteration of a plethora of gemcitabine-containing chemotherapy combinations, the clinical approval of albumin-conjugated-taxol (nab-Paclitaxel) landmarks a novel era in the management of metastatic PDAC. Further studies are needed to evaluate the impact of eradicating tumor bulks, e.g., via radiotherapy or surgery in oligometastatic PDAC.

REFERENCES

[1] Siegel R, Naishadham D, Jemal A. Cancer statistics, 2012. CA Cancer J Clin 2012;62:10–29.

[2] Malvezzi M, Bertuccio P, Levi F, La Vecchia C, Negri E. European cancer mortality predictions for the year 2013. Ann Oncol 2013;24:792–800.

[3] Gudjonsson B. Cancer of the pancreas. 50 years of surgery. Cancer 1987;60:2284–303.

[4] Parker GA, Postlethwait RW. The continuing problem of carcinoma of the pancreas. J Surg Oncol 1985;28:36–8.

[5] Stathis A, Moore MJ. Advanced pancreatic carcinoma: current treatment and future challenges. Nat Rev Clin Oncol 2010;7:163–72.

[6] Wayne JD, Abdalla EK, Wolff RA, Crane CH, Pisters PW, Evans DB. Localized adenocarcinoma of the pancreas: the rationale for preoperative chemoradiation. Oncologist 2002;7:34–45.

[7] Paulson AS, Tran Cao HS, Tempero MA, Lowy AM. Therapeutic advances in pancreatic cancer. Gastroenterology 2013;144:1316–26.

[8] Crane CH, Varadhachary G, Pisters PW, Evans DB, Wolff RA. Future chemoradiation strategies in pancreatic cancer. Semin Oncol 2007;34:335–46.

[9] Fuhrman GM, Charnsangavej C, Abbruzzese JL, Cleary KR, Martin RG, Fenoglio CJ, et al. Thin-section contrast-enhanced computed tomography accurately predicts the resectability of malignant pancreatic neoplasms. Am J Surg 1994;167:104–11. discussion 111–103.

[10] Gagner M, Pomp A. Laparoscopic pylorus-preserving pancreatoduodenectomy. Surg Endosc 1994;8:408–10.

[11] Venkat R, Edil BH, Schulick RD, Lidor AO, Makary MA, Wolfgang CL. Laparoscopic distal pancreatectomy is associated with significantly less overall morbidity compared to the open technique: a systematic review and meta-analysis. Ann Surg 2012;255:1048–59.

[12] Gagner M, Begin E, Hurteau R, Pomp A. Robotic interactive laparoscopic cholecystectomy. Lancet 1994;343:596–7.

[13] Cuschieri A. Laparoscopic surgery of the pancreas. J R Coll Surg Edinb 1994;39: 178–84.

[14] Winer J, Can MF, Bartlett DL, Zeh HJ, Zureikat AH. The current state of robotic-assisted pancreatic surgery. Nat Rev Gastroenterol Hepatol 2012;9:468–76.

[15] Douglass HO. Further evidence of effective adjuvant combined radiation and chemotherapy following curative resection of pancreatic cancer. Cancer 1987;59:2006–10.

[16] Krook JE, Moertel CG, Gunderson LL, Wieand HS, Collins RT, Beart RW, et al. Effective surgical adjuvant therapy for high-risk rectal carcinoma. N Engl J Med 1991;324:709–15.

[17] Macdonald JS, Smalley SR, Benedetti J, Hundahl SA, Estes NC, Stemmermann GN, et al. Chemoradiotherapy after surgery compared with surgery alone for adenocarcinoma of the stomach or gastroesophageal junction. N Engl J Med 2001;345:725–30.

[18] Breslin TM, Hess KR, Harbison DB, Jean ME, Cleary KR, Dackiw AP, et al. Neoadjuvant chemoradiotherapy for adenocarcinoma of the pancreas: treatment variables and survival duration. Ann Surg Oncol 2001;8:123–32.

[19] Goodman KA, Hajj C. Role of radiation therapy in the management of pancreatic cancer. J Surg Oncol 2013;107:86–96.

[20] Kalser MH, Ellenberg SS. Pancreatic cancer. Adjuvant combined radiation and chemotherapy following curative resection. Arch Surg 1985;120:899–903.

[21] Woolley PV, Nauta R, Smith FP, Lindblad AS, Petrelli N, Herrera L, et al. Radiationtherapy and fluorouracil with or without semustine for the treatment of patients with surgical adjuvant adenocarcinoma of the rectum. J Clin Oncol 1992;10:549–57.

[22] Klinkenbijl JH, Jeekel J, Sahmoud T, van Pel R, Couvreur ML, Veenhof CH, et al. Adjuvant radiotherapy and 5-fluorouracil after curative resection of cancer of the pancreas and periampullary region: phase III trial of the EORTC gastrointestinal tract cancer cooperative group. Ann Surg 1999;230:776–82. discussion 782–774.

[23] Neoptolemos JP, Stocken DD, Friess H, Bassi C, Dunn JA, Hickey H, et al. A randomized trial of chemoradiotherapy and chemotherapy after resection of pancreatic cancer. N Engl J Med 2004;350:1200–10.

[24] Morris SL, Beasley M, Leslie M. Chemotherapy for pancreatic cancer. N Engl J Med 2004;350:2713–5. author reply 2713–2715.

[25] Regine WF, Winter KA, Abrams R, Safran H, Hoffman JP, Konski A, et al. Fluorouracilbased chemoradiation with either gemcitabine or fluorouracil chemotherapy after resection of pancreatic adenocarcinoma: 5-year analysis of the U.S. Intergroup/RTOG 9704 phase III trial. Ann Surg Oncol 2011;18:1319–26.

[26] Abrams RA, Winter KA, Regine WF, Safran H, Hoffman JP, Lustig R, et al. Failure to adhere to protocol specified radiation therapy guidelines was associated with decreased survival in RTOG 9704–a phase III trial of adjuvant chemotherapy and chemoradiotherapy for patients with resected adenocarcinoma of the pancreas. Int J Radiat Oncol Biol Phys 2012;82:809–16.

[27] Hsu CC, Herman JM, Corsini MM, Winter JM, Callister MD, Haddock MG, et al. Adjuvant chemoradiation for pancreatic adenocarcinoma: the Johns Hopkins Hospital-Mayo Clinic collaborative study. Ann Surg Oncol 2010;17:981–90.

[28] Picozzi VJ, Kozarek RA, Traverso LW. Interferon-based adjuvant chemoradiation therapy after pancreaticoduodenectomy for pancreatic adenocarcinoma. Am J Surg 2003;185:476–80.

[29] Picozzi VJ, Abrams RA, Decker PA, Traverso W, O'Reilly EM, Greeno E, et al. Multicenter phase II trial of adjuvant therapy for resected pancreatic cancer using cisplatin, 5-fluorouracil, and interferon-alpha-2b-based chemoradiation: ACOSOG Trial Z05031. Ann Oncol 2011;22:348–54.

[30] Schmidt J, Abel U, Debus J, Harig S, Hoffmann K, Herrmann T, et al. Open-label, multicenter, randomized phase III trial of adjuvant chemoradiation plus interferon Alpha-2b versus fluorouracil and folinic acid for patients with resected pancreatic adenocarcinoma. J Clin Oncol 2012;30:4077–83.

[31] Neoptolemos JP, Stocken DD, Bassi C, Ghaneh P, Cunningham D, Goldstein D, et al. Adjuvant chemotherapy with fluorouracil plus folinic acid vs gemcitabine following pancreatic cancer resection: a randomized controlled trial. JAMA 2010;304:1073–81.

[32] Oettle H, Post S, Neuhaus P, Gellert K, Langrehr J, Ridwelski K, et al. Adjuvant chemotherapy with gemcitabine vs observation in patients undergoing curative-intent resection of pancreatic cancer: a randomized controlled trial. JAMA 2007;297:267–77.

[33] Ueno H, Kosuge T, Matsuyama Y, Yamamoto J, Nakao A, Egawa S, et al. A randomised phase III trial comparing gemcitabine with surgery-only in patients with resected pancreatic cancer: Japanese Study Group of Adjuvant Therapy for Pancreatic Cancer. Br J Cancer 2009;101:908–15.

[34] Sauer R, Becker H, Hohenberger W, Rodel C, Wittekind C, Fietkau R, et al. Preoperative versus postoperative chemoradiotherapy for rectal cancer. N Engl J Med 2004;351:1731–40.

[35] Evans DB, Rich TA, Byrd DR, Cleary KR, Connelly JH, Levin B, et al. Preoperative chemoradiation and pancreaticoduodenectomy for adenocarcinoma of the pancreas. Arch Surg 1992;127:1335–9.

[36] Pisters PW, Abbruzzese JL, Janjan NA, Cleary KR, Charnsangavej C, Goswitz MS, et al. Rapid-fractionation preoperative chemoradiation, pancreaticoduodenectomy, and intraoperative radiation therapy for resectable pancreatic adenocarcinoma. J Clin Oncol 1998;16:3843–50.

[37] Pisters PW, Wolff RA, Janjan NA, Cleary KR, Charnsangavej C, Crane CN, et al. Preoperative paclitaxel and concurrent rapid-fractionation radiation for resectable pancreatic adenocarcinoma: toxicities, histologic response rates, and event-free outcome. J Clin Oncol 2002;20:2537–44.

[38] Evans DB, Varadhachary GR, Crane CH, Sun CC, Lee JE, Pisters PW, et al. Preoperative gemcitabine-based chemoradiation for patients with resectable adenocarcinoma of the pancreatic head. J Clin Oncol 2008;26:3496–502.

[39] Varadhachary GR, Wolff RA, Crane CH, Sun CC, Lee JE, Pisters PW, et al. Preoperative gemcitabine and cisplatin followed by gemcitabine-based chemoradiation for resectable adenocarcinoma of the pancreatic head. J Clin Oncol 2008;26:3487–95.

[40] Varadhachary GR, Tamm EP, Abbruzzese JL, Xiong HQ, Crane CH, Wang H, et al. Borderline resectable pancreatic cancer: definitions, management, and role of preoperative therapy. Ann Surg Oncol 2006;13:1035–46.

[41] Callery MP, Chang KJ, Fishman EK, Talamonti MS, William Traverso L, Linehan DC. Pretreatment assessment of resectable and borderline resectable pancreatic cancer: expert consensus statement. Ann Surg Oncol 2009;16:1727–33.

[42] Katz MH, Pisters PW, Evans DB, Sun CC, Lee JE, Fleming JB, et al. Borderline resectable pancreatic cancer: the importance of this emerging stage of disease. J Am Coll Surg 2008;206:833–46. discussion 846–838.

[43] Moertel CG, Frytak S, Hahn RG, O'Connell MJ, Reitemeier RJ, Rubin J, et al. Therapy of locally unresectable pancreatic carcinoma: a randomized comparison of high dose (6000 rads) radiation alone, moderate dose radiation (4000 rads + 5-fluorouracil), and high dose radiation + 5-fluorouracil: the Gastrointestinal Tumor Study Group. Cancer 1981;48:1705–10.

[44] Douglass HO. Treatment of locally unresectable carcinoma of the pancreas – comparison of combined-modality therapy (chemotherapy plus radiotherapy) to chemotherapy alone. J Natl Cancer Inst 1988;80:751–5.

[45] Klaassen DJ, MacIntyre JM, Catton GE, Engstrom PF, Moertel CG. Treatment of locally unresectable cancer of the stomach and pancreas: a randomized comparison of 5-fluorouracil alone with radiation plus concurrent and maintenance 5-fluorouracil–an Eastern Cooperative Oncology Group study. J Clin Oncol 1985;3:373–8.

[46] Wolff RA, Evans DB, Gravel DM, Lenzi R, Pisters PW, Lee JE, et al. Phase I trial of gemcitabine combined with radiation for the treatment of locally advanced pancreatic adenocarcinoma. Clin Cancer Res 2001;7:2246–53.

[47] Pipas JM, Mitchell SE, Barth Jr RJ, Vera-Gimon R, Rathmann J, Meyer LP, et al. Phase I study of twice-weekly gemcitabine and concomitant external-beam radiotherapy in patients with adenocarcinoma of the pancreas. Int J Radiat Oncol Biol Phys 2001;50:1317–22.

[48] McGinn CJ, Zalupski MM, Shureiqi I, Robertson JM, Eckhauser FE, Smith DC, et al. Phase I trial of radiation dose escalation with concurrent weekly full-dose gemcitabine in patients with advanced pancreatic cancer. J Clin Oncol 2001; 19:4202–8.

[49] Blackstock AW, Bernard SA, Richards F, Eagle KS, Case LD, Poole ME, et al. Phase I trial of twice-weekly gemcitabine and concurrent radiation in patients with advanced pancreatic cancer. J Clin Oncol 1999;17:2208–12.

[50] Crane CH, Wolff RA, Abbruzzese JL, Evans DB, Milas L, Mason K, et al. Combining gemcitabine with radiation in pancreatic cancer: understanding important variables influencing the therapeutic index. Semin Oncol 2001;28:25–33.

[51] Blackstock AW, Tepper JE, Niedwiecki D, Hollis DR, Mayer RJ, Tempero MA. Cancer and leukemia group B (CALGB) 89805: phase II chemoradiation trial using gemcitabine in patients with locoregional adenocarcinoma of the pancreas. Int J Gastrointest Cancer 2003;34:107–16.

[52] Small Jr W, Berlin J, Freedman GM, Lawrence T, Talamonti MS, Mulcahy MF, et al. Full-dose gemcitabine with concurrent radiation therapy in patients with nonmeta-static pancreatic cancer: a multicenter phase II trial. J Clin Oncol 2008;26:942–7.

[53] Loehrer Sr PJ, Feng Y, Cardenes H, Wagner L, Brell JM, Cella D, et al. Gemcitabine alone versus gemcitabine plus radiotherapy in patients with locally advanced pancre-atic cancer: an Eastern Cooperative Oncology Group trial. J Clin Oncol 2011;29: 4105–12.

[54] Twelves C, Wong A, Nowacki MP, Abt M, Burris 3rd H, Carrato A, et al. Capecitabine as adjuvant treatment for stage III colon cancer. N Engl J Med 2005;352:2696–704.

[55] Hofheinz RD, Wenz F, Post S, Matzdorff A, Laechelt S, Hartmann JT, et al. Chemora-diotherapy with capecitabine versus fluorouracil for locally advanced rectal cancer: a randomised, multicentre, non-inferiority, phase 3 trial. Lancet Oncol 2012;13:579–88.

[56] Dunst J, Reese T, Sutter T, Zuhlke H, Hinke A, Kolling-Schlebusch K, et al. Phase I trial evaluating the concurrent combination of radiotherapy and capecitabine in rectal cancer. J Clin Oncol 2002;20:3983–91.

[57] Cartwright TH, Cohn A, Varkey JA, Chen YM, Szatrowski TP, Cox JV, et al. Phase II study of oral capecitabine in patients with advanced or metastatic pancreatic cancer. J Clin Oncol 2002;20:160–4.

[58] Crane CH, Ellis LM, Abbruzzese JL, Amos C, Xiong HQ, Ho L, et al. Phase I trial evaluating the safety of bevacizumab with concurrent radiotherapy and capecitabine in locally advanced pancreatic cancer. J Clin Oncol 2006;24:1145–51.

[59] Schneider BJ, Ben-Josef E, McGinn CJ, Chang AE, Colletti LM, Normolle DP, et al. Capecitabine and radiation therapy preceded and followed by combination chemo-therapy in advanced pancreatic cancer. Int J Radiat Oncol Biol Phys 2005;63:1325–30.

[60] Li CP, Chao Y, Chi KH, Chan WK, Teng HC, Lee RC, et al. Concurrent chemoradio-therapy treatment of locally advanced pancreatic cancer: gemcitabine versus 5-fluorouracil, a randomized controlled study. Int J Radiat Oncol Biol Phys 2003;57:98–104.

[61] Chauffert B, Mornex F, Bonnetain F, Rougier P, Mariette C, Bouche O, et al. Phase III trial comparing intensive induction chemoradiotherapy (60 Gy, infusional 5-FU and intermittent cisplatin) followed by maintenance gemcitabine with gemcitabine alone for locally advanced unresectable pancreatic cancer. Definitive results of the 2000–01 FFCD/SFRO study. Ann Oncol 2008;19:1592–9.

[62] Huguet F, Andre T, Hammel P, Artru P, Balosso J, Selle F, et al. Impact of chemora-diotherapy after disease control with chemotherapy in locally advanced pancreatic adenocarcinoma in GERCOR phase II and III studies. J Clin Oncol 2007;25:326–31.

[63] Krishnan S, Rana V, Janjan NA, Varadhachary GR, Abbruzzese JL, Das P, et al. Induc-tion chemotherapy selects patients with locally advanced, unresectable pancreatic cancer for optimal benefit from consolidative chemoradiation therapy. Cancer 2007;110:47–55.

[64] Hess V, Salzberg M, Borner M, Morant R, Roth AD, Ludwig C, et al. Combining capecitabine and gemcitabine in patients with advanced pancreatic carcinoma: a phase I/II trial. J Clin Oncol 2003;21:66–8.

[65] Scheithauer W, Schull B, Ulrich-Pur H, Schmid K, Raderer M, Haider K, et al. Biweekly high-dose gemcitabine alone or in combination with capecitabine in patients with metastatic pancreatic adenocarcinoma: a randomized phase II trial. Ann Oncol 2003;14:97–104.

[66] Herrmann R, Bodoky G, Ruhstaller T, Glimelius B, Bajetta E, Schuller J, et al. Gemcitabine plus capecitabine compared with gemcitabine alone in advanced pancreatic cancer: a randomized, multicenter, phase III trial of the Swiss Group for Clinical Cancer Research and the Central European Cooperative Oncology Group. J Clin Oncol 2007;25:2212–7.

[67] Bernhard J, Dietrich D, Scheithauer W, Gerber D, Bodoky G, Ruhstaller T, et al. Clinical benefit and quality of life in patients with advanced pancreatic cancer receiving gemcitabine plus capecitabine versus gemcitabine alone: a randomized multicenter phase III clinical trial–SAKK 44/00-CECOG/PAN.1.3.001. J Clin Oncol 2008;26:3695–701.

[68] Cunningham D, Chau I, Stocken DD, Valle JW, Smith D, Steward W, et al. Phase III randomized comparison of gemcitabine versus gemcitabine plus capecitabine in patients with advanced pancreatic cancer. J Clin Oncol 2009;27:5513–8.

[69] Gillen S, Schuster T, Meyer Zum Buschenfelde C, Friess H, Kleeff J. Preoperative/neoadjuvant therapy in pancreatic cancer: a systematic review and meta-analysis of response and resection percentages. PLoS Med 2010;7:e1000267.

[70] Habermehl D, Kessel K, Welzel T, Hof H, Abdollahi A, Bergmann F, et al. Neoadjuvant chemoradiation with gemcitabine for locally advanced pancreatic cancer. Radiat Oncol 2012;7:28.

[71] Hidalgo M. Pancreatic cancer. N Engl J Med 2010;362:1605–17.

[72] Temel JS, Greer JA, Muzikansky A, Gallagher ER, Admane S, Jackson VA, et al. Early palliative care for patients with metastatic non-small-cell lung cancer. N Engl J Med 2010;363:733–42.

[73] Mandala M, Reni M, Cascinu S, Barni S, Floriani I, Cereda S, et al. Venous thromboembolism predicts poor prognosis in irresectable pancreatic cancer patients. Ann Oncol 2007;18:1660–5.

[74] Louvet C, Labianca R, Hammel P, Lledo G, Zampino MG, Andre T, et al. Gemcitabine in combination with oxaliplatin compared with gemcitabine alone in locally advanced or metastatic pancreatic cancer: results of a GERCOR and GISCAD phase III trial. J Clin Oncol 2005;23:3509–16.

[75] Poplin E, Feng Y, Berlin J, Rothenberg ML, Hochster H, Mitchell E, et al. Phase III, randomized study of gemcitabine and oxaliplatin versus gemcitabine (fixed-dose rate infusion) compared with gemcitabine (30-minute infusion) in patients with pancreatic carcinoma E6201: a trial of the Eastern Cooperative Oncology Group. J Clin Oncol 2009;27:3778–85.

[76] Colucci G, Giuliani F, Gebbia V, Biglietto M, Rabitti P, Uomo G, et al. Gemcitabine alone or with cisplatin for the treatment of patients with locally advanced and/or metastatic pancreatic carcinoma: a prospective, randomized phase III study of the Gruppo Oncologia dell'Italia Meridionale. Cancer 2002;94:902–10.

[77] Heinemann V, Quietzsch D, Gieseler F, Gonnermann M, Schonekas H, Rost A, et al. Randomized phase III trial of gemcitabine plus cisplatin compared with gemcitabine alone in advanced pancreatic cancer. J Clin Oncol 2006;24:3946–52.

[78] Rocha Lima CM, Green MR, Rotche R, Miller Jr WH, Jeffrey GM, Cisar LA, et al. Irinotecan plus gemcitabine results in no survival advantage compared with gemcitabine monotherapy in patients with locally advanced or metastatic pancreatic cancer despite increased tumor response rate. J Clin Oncol 2004;22:3776–83.

[79] Abou-Alfa GK, Letourneau R, Harker G, Modiano M, Hurwitz H, Tchekmedyian NS, et al. Randomized phase III study of exatecan and gemcitabine compared with gemcitabine alone in untreated advanced pancreatic cancer. J Clin Oncol 2006; 24:4441–7.

[80] Oettle H, Richards D, Ramanathan RK, van Laethem JL, Peeters M, Fuchs M, et al. A phase III trial of pemetrexed plus gemcitabine versus gemcitabine in patients with unresectable or metastatic pancreatic cancer. Ann Oncol 2005;16:1639–45.

[81] Conroy T, Desseigne F, Ychou M, Bouche O, Guimbaud R, Becouarn Y, et al. FOL-FIRINOX versus gemcitabine for metastatic pancreatic cancer. N Engl J Med 2011;364:1817–25.

[82] Ychou M, Viret F, Kramar A, Desseigne F, Mitry E, Guimbaud R, et al. Tritherapy with fluorouracil/leucovorin, irinotecan and oxaliplatin (FOLFIRINOX): a phase II study in colorectal cancer patients with non-resectable liver metastases. Cancer Chemother Pharmacol 2008;62:195–201.

[83] Conroy T, Paillot B, Francois E, Bugat R, Jacob JH, Stein U, et al. Irinotecan plus oxaliplatin and leucovorin-modulated fluorouracil in advanced pancreatic cancer–a Groupe Tumeurs Digestives of the Federation Nationale des Centres de Lutte Contre le Cancer study. J Clin Oncol 2005;23:1228–36.

[84] Peddi PF, Lubner S, McWilliams R, Tan BR, Picus J, Sorscher SM, et al. Multi-institutional experience with FOLFIRINOX in pancreatic adenocarcinoma. JOP 2012;13:497–501.

[85] Conroy T, Gavoille C, Samalin E, Ychou M, Ducreux M. The role of the FOLFIRI-NOX regimen for advanced pancreatic cancer. Curr Oncol Rep 2013;15:182–9.

[86] Hosein PJ, Macintyre J, Kawamura C, Maldonado JC, Ernani V, Loaiza-Bonilla A, et al. A retrospective study of neoadjuvant FOLFIRINOX in unresectable or border-line-resectable locally advanced pancreatic adenocarcinoma. BMC Cancer 2012; 12:199.

[87] Faris JE, Blaszkowsky LS, McDermott S, Guimaraes AR, Szymonifka J, Huynh MA, et al. FOLFIRINOX in locally advanced pancreatic cancer: the Massachusetts General Hospital Cancer Center experience. Oncologist 2013;18:543–8.

[88] Ibrahim NK, Desai N, Legha S, Soon-Shiong P, Theriault RL, Rivera E, et al. Phase I and pharmacokinetic study of ABI-007, a Cremophor-free, protein-stabilized, nanoparticle formulation of paclitaxel. Clin Cancer Res 2002;8:1038–44.

[89] Frese KK, Neesse A, Cook N, Bapiro TE, Lolkema MP, Jodrell DI, et al. nab-Paclitaxel potentiates gemcitabine activity by reducing cytidine deaminase levels in a mouse model of pancreatic cancer. Cancer Discov 2012;2:260–9.

[90] Neesse A, Frese KK, Bapiro TE, Nakagawa T, Sternlicht MD, Seeley TW, et al. CTGF antagonism with mAb FG-3019 enhances chemotherapy response without increasing drug delivery in murine ductal pancreas cancer. Proc Natl Acad Sci USA 2013;110:12325–30.

[91] Kotowski A, Ma WW. Emerging therapies in pancreas cancer. J Gastrointest Oncol 2011;2:93–103.

[92] Von Hoff DD, Ervin T, Arena FP, Chiorean EG, Infante J, Moore M, et al. Increased survival in pancreatic cancer with nab-paclitaxel plus gemcitabine. N Engl J Med 2013;369(18):1691–703.

[93] Maitra A, Ashfaq R, Gunn CR, Rahman A, Yeo CJ, Sohn TA, et al. Cyclooxygenase 2 expression in pancreatic adenocarcinoma and pancreatic intraepithelial neoplasia: an immunohistochemical analysis with automated cellular imaging. Am J Clin Pathol 2002;118:194–201.

[94] Muller-Decker K, Furstenberger G, Annan N, Kucher D, Pohl-Arnold A, Steinbauer B, et al. Preinvasive duct-derived neoplasms in pancreas of keratin 5-promoter cyclo-oxygenase-2 transgenic mice. Gastroenterology 2006;130:2165–78.

[95] Juuti A, Louhimo J, Nordling S, Ristimaki A, Haglund C. Cyclooxygenase-2 expression correlates with poor prognosis in pancreatic cancer. J Clin Pathol 2006;59:382–6.

[96] Ferrari V, Valcamonico F, Amoroso V, Simoncini E, Vassalli L, Marpicati P, et al. Gemcitabine plus celecoxib (GECO) in advanced pancreatic cancer: a phase II trial. Cancer Chemother Pharmacol 2006;57:185–90.

[97] Liebmann C. Regulation of MAP kinase activity by peptide receptor signalling pathway: paradigms of multiplicity. Cell Signal 2001;13:777–85.

[98] Ghobrial IM, Adjei AA. Inhibitors of the ras oncogene as therapeutic targets. Hematol Oncol Clin North Am 2002;16:1065–88.

[99] Lowenstein EJ, Daly RJ, Batzer AG, Li W, Margolis B, Lammers R, et al. The SH2 and SH3 domain-containing protein GRB2 links receptor tyrosine kinases to ras signaling. Cell 1992;70:431–42.

[100] McCormick F. Signal transduction. How receptors turn Ras on. Nature 1993;363:15–6.

[101] Bar-Sagi D, Hall A. Ras and Rho GTPases: a family reunion. Cell 2000;103:227–38.

[102] Downward J. Targeting RAS signalling pathways in cancer therapy. Nat Rev Cancer 2003;3:11–22.

[103] Klimstra DS, Longnecker DS. K-ras mutations in pancreatic ductal proliferative lesions. Am J Clin Pathol 1994;145:1547–50.

[104] Hruban RH, Adsay NV, Albores-Saavedra J, Compton C, Garrett ES, Goodman SN, et al. Pancreatic intraepithelial neoplasia: a new nomenclature and classification system for pancreatic duct lesions. Am J Surg Pathol 2001;25:579–86.

[105] Bardeesy N, DePinho RA. Pancreatic cancer biology and genetics. Nat Rev Cancer 2002;2:897–909.

[106] Van Cutsem E, van de Velde H, Karasek P, Oettle H, Vervenne WL, Szawlowski A, et al. Phase III trial of gemcitabine plus tipifarnib compared with gemcitabine plus placebo in advanced pancreatic cancer. J Clin Oncol 2004;22:1430–8.

[107] Poulikakos PI, Solit DB. Resistance to MEK inhibitors: should we co-target upstream? Sci Signal 2011;4:pe16.

[108] Michl P, Gress TM. Current concepts and novel targets in advanced pancreatic cancer. Gut 2013;62:317–26.

[109] Vivanco I, Sawyers CL. The phosphatidylinositol 3-Kinase AKT pathway in human cancer. Nat Rev Cancer 2002;2:489–501.

[110] Yoon H, Kim DJ, Ahn EH, Gellert GC, Shay JW, Ahn CH, et al. Antitumor activity of a novel antisense oligonucleotide against Akt1. J Cell Biochem 2009;108:832–8.

[111] Wolpin BM, Hezel AF, Abrams T, Blaszkowsky LS, Meyerhardt JA, Chan JA, et al. Oral mTOR inhibitor everolimus in patients with gemcitabine-refractory metastatic pancreatic cancer. J Clin Oncol 2009;27:193–8.

[112] Javle MM, Shroff RT, Xiong H, Varadhachary GA, Fogelman D, Reddy SA, et al. Inhibition of the mammalian target of rapamycin (mTOR) in advanced pancreatic cancer: results of two phase II studies. BMC Cancer 2010;10:368.

[113] Papageorgio C, Perry MC. Epidermal growth factor receptor-targeted therapy for pancreatic cancer. Cancer Invest 2007;25:647–57.

[114] Moore MJ, Goldstein D, Hamm J, Figer A, Hecht JR, Gallinger S, et al. Erlotinib plus gemcitabine compared with gemcitabine alone in patients with advanced pancreatic cancer: a phase III trial of the National Cancer Institute of Canada Clinical Trials Group. J Clin Oncol 2007;25:1960–6.

[115] Boeck S, Vehling-Kaiser U, Waldschmidt D, Kettner E, Marten A, Winkelmann C, et al. Erlotinib 150 mg daily plus chemotherapy in advanced pancreatic cancer: an interim safety analysis of a multicenter, randomized, cross-over phase III trial of the 'Arbeitsgemeinschaft Internistische Onkologie'. Anticancer Drugs 2010;21:94–100.

[116] Philip PA, Benedetti J, Corless CL, Wong R, O'Reilly EM, Flynn PJ, et al. Phase III study comparing gemcitabine plus cetuximab versus gemcitabine in patients with advanced pancreatic adenocarcinoma: Southwest Oncology Group-directed intergroup trial S0205. J Clin Oncol 2010;28:3605–10.

[117] Krempien R, Muenter MW, Huber PE, Nill S, Friess H, Timke C, et al. Randomized phase II–study evaluating EGFR targeting therapy with cetuximab in combination with radiotherapy and chemotherapy for patients with locally advanced pancreatic cancer–PARC: study protocol [ISRCTN56652283]. BMC Cancer 2005;5:131.

[118] Munter M, Timke C, Abdollahi A, Friess H, Jaeger D, Heeger S, et al. Final results of a phase II trial [PARC-Study ISRCTN56652283] for patients with primary inoperable locally advanced pancreatic cancer combining intensity modulated radiotherapy (IMRT) with cetuximab and gemcitabine. J Clin Oncol 2008;26.

[119] Abdollahi A, Folkman J. Evading tumor evasion: current concepts and perspectives of anti-angiogenic cancer therapy. Drug Resist Updat 2010;13:16–28.

[120] Abdollahi A, Hlatky L, Huber PE. Endostatin: the logic of antiangiogenic therapy. Drug Resist Updat 2005;8:59–74.

[121] Abdollahi A, Schwager C, Kleeff J, Esposito I, Domhan S, Peschke P, et al. Transcriptional network governing the angiogenic switch in human pancreatic cancer. Proc Natl Acad Sci USA 2007;104:12890–5.

[122] Van Cutsem E, Vervenne WL, Bennouna J, Humblet Y, Gill S, Van Laethem JL, et al. Phase III trial of bevacizumab in combination with gemcitabine and erlotinib in patients with metastatic pancreatic cancer. J Clin Oncol 2009;27:2231–7.

[123] Javle M, Yu J, Garrett C, Pande A, Kuvshinoff B, Litwin A, et al. Bevacizumab combined with gemcitabine and capecitabine for advanced pancreatic cancer: a phase II study. Br J Cancer 2009;100:1842–5.

[124] Fogelman D, Jafari M, Varadhachary GR, Xiong H, Bullock S, Ozer H, et al. Bevacizumab plus gemcitabine and oxaliplatin as first-line therapy for metastatic or locally advanced pancreatic cancer: a phase II trial. Cancer Chemother Pharmacol 2011;68:1431–8.

[125] Spano JP, Chodkiewicz C, Maurel J, Wong R, Wasan H, Barone C, et al. Efficacy of gemcitabine plus axitinib compared with gemcitabine alone in patients with advanced pancreatic cancer: an open-label randomised phase II study. Lancet 2008;371:2101–8.

[126] Kindler HL, Ioka T, Richel DJ, Bennouna J, Letourneau R, Okusaka T, et al. Axitinib plus gemcitabine versus placebo plus gemcitabine in patients with advanced pancreatic adenocarcinoma: a double-blind randomised phase 3 study. Lancet Oncol 2011;12:256–62.

[127] Jacobetz MA, Chan DS, Neesse A, Bapiro TE, Cook N, Frese KK, et al. Hyaluronan impairs vascular function and drug delivery in a mouse model of pancreatic cancer. Gut 2013;62:112–20.

[128] Provenzano PP, Cuevas C, Chang AE, Goel VK, Von Hoff DD, Hingorani SR. Enzymatic targeting of the stroma ablates physical barriers to treatment of pancreatic ductal adenocarcinoma. Cancer Cell 2012;21:418–29.

[129] Lopez T, Hanahan D. Elevated levels of IGF-1 receptor convey invasive and metastatic capability in a mouse model of pancreatic islet tumorigenesis. Cancer Cell 2002; 1:339–53.

[130] Wang Y, Adachi Y, Imsumran A, Yamamoto H, Piao W, Li H, et al. Targeting for insulin-like growth factor-I receptor with short hairpin RNA for human digestive/ gastrointestinal cancers. J Gastroenterol 2010;45:159–70.

[131] Tomizawa M, Shinozaki F, Sugiyama T, Yamamoto S, Sueishi M, Yoshida T. Insulinlike growth factor-I receptor in proliferation and motility of pancreatic cancer. World J Gastroenterol 2010;16:1854–8.

[132] Beltran PJ, Mitchell P, Chung YA, Cajulis E, Lu J, Belmontes B, et al. AMG 479, a fully human anti-insulin-like growth factor receptor type I monoclonal antibody, inhibits the growth and survival of pancreatic carcinoma cells. Mol Cancer Ther 2009;8:1095–105.

[133] Mahadevan D, Von Hoff DD. Tumor-stroma interactions in pancreatic ductal adenocarcinoma. Mol Cancer Ther 2007;6:1186–97.

[134] Bachem MG, Schunemann M, Ramadani M, Siech M, Beger H, Buck A, et al. Pancreatic carcinoma cells induce fibrosis by stimulating proliferation and matrix synthesis of stellate cells. Gastroenterology 2005;128:907–21.

[135] Omary MB, Lugea A, Lowe AW, Pandol SJ. The pancreatic stellate cell: a star on the rise in pancreatic diseases. J Clin Invest 2007;117:50–9.

[136] Aikawa T, Gunn J, Spong SM, Klaus SJ, Korc M. Connective tissue growth factor-specific antibody attenuates tumor growth, metastasis, and angiogenesis in an orthotopic mouse model of pancreatic cancer. Mol Cancer Ther 2006;5:1108–16.

[137] Bai YC, Kang Q, Luo Q, Wu DQ, Ye WX, Lin XM, et al. Role of connective tissue growth factor (CTGF) in proliferation and migration of pancreatic cancer cells. Zhonghua Zhong Liu Za Zhi 2011;33:732–6.

[138] Bennewith KL, Huang X, Ham CM, Graves EE, Erler JT, Kambham N, et al. The role of tumor cell-derived connective tissue growth factor (CTGF/CCN2) in pancreatic tumor growth. Cancer Res 2009;69:775–84.

[139] Dornhofer N, Spong S, Bennewith K, Salim A, Klaus S, Kambham N, et al. Connective tissue growth factor-specific monoclonal antibody therapy inhibits pancreatic tumor growth and metastasis. Cancer Res 2006;66:5816–27.

[140] Dimou AT, Syrigos KN, Saif MW. Novel agents in the management of pancreatic adenocarcinoma: phase I studies. Highlights from the "2011 ASCO Gastrointestinal Cancers Symposium". San Francisco, CA, USA. January 20–22, 2011. JOP 2011; 12:114–6.

[141] Ryseck RP, Macdonald-Bravo H, Mattei MG, Bravo R. Structure, mapping, and expression of fisp-12, a growth factor-inducible gene encoding a secreted cysteine-rich protein. Cell Growth Differ 1991;2:225–33.

[142] Battegay EJ, Raines EW, Seifert RA, Bowen-Pope DF, Ross R. TGF-beta induces bimodal proliferation of connective tissue cells via complex control of an autocrine PDGF loop. Cell 1990;63:515–24.

[143] Jaschinski F, Rothhammer T, Jachimczak P, Seitz C, Schneider A, Schlingensiepen KH. The antisense oligonucleotide trabedersen (AP 12009) for the targeted inhibition of TGF-beta2. Curr Pharm Biotechnol 2011;12:2203–13.

[144] Ramfidis VS, Strimpakos AS, Syrigos KN, Saif MW. Clinical studies in the second line setting of advanced pancreatic cancer: are we making any progress? JOP 2012;13:358–60.

[145] Gherardi E, Birchmeier W, Birchmeier C, Vande Woude G. Targeting MET in cancer: rationale and progress. Nat Rev Cancer 2012;12:89–103.

[146] Ebert M, Yokoyama M, Friess H, Buchler MW, Korc M. Coexpression of the c-met proto-oncogene and hepatocyte growth factor in human pancreatic cancer. Cancer Res 1994;54:5775–8.

[147] Hage C, Rausch V, Giese N, Giese T, Schonsiegel F, Labsch S, et al. The novel c-Met inhibitor cabozantinib overcomes gemcitabine resistance and stem cell signaling in pancreatic cancer. Cell Death Dis 2013;4:e627.

[148] You WK, Sennino B, Williamson CW, Falcon B, Hashizume H, Yao LC, et al. VEGF and c-Met blockade amplify angiogenesis inhibition in pancreatic islet cancer. Cancer Res 2011;71:4758–68.

[149] Li C, Wu JJ, Hynes M, Dosch J, Sarkar B, Welling TH, et al. c-Met is a marker of pancreatic cancer stem cells and therapeutic target. Gastroenterology 2011;141:2218–27. e2215.

[150] Reya T, Morrison SJ, Clarke MF, Weissman IL. Stem cells, cancer, and cancer stem cells. Nature 2001;414:105–11.

[151] Al-Hajj M, Wicha MS, Benito-Hernandez A, Morrison SJ, Clarke MF. Prospective identification of tumorigenic breast cancer cells. Proc Natl Acad Sci USA 2003;100:3983–8.

[152] Singh SK, Hawkins C, Clarke ID, Squire JA, Bayani J, Hide T, et al. Identification of human brain tumour initiating cells. Nature 2004;432:396–401.

[153] Li C, Heidt DG, Dalerba P, Burant CF, Zhang L, Adsay V, et al. Identification of pancreatic cancer stem cells. Cancer Res 2007;67:1030–7.

[154] Olive KP, Jacobetz MA, Davidson CJ, Gopinathan A, McIntyre D, Honess D, et al. Inhibition of Hedgehog signaling enhances delivery of chemotherapy in a mouse model of pancreatic cancer. Science 2009;324:1457–61.

[155] Castro JR, Saunders WM, Tobias CA, Chen GT, Curtis S, Lyman JT, et al. Treatment of cancer with heavy charged particles. Int J Radiat Oncol Biol Phys 1982;8:2191–8.

[156] Oonishi K, Cui X, Hirakawa H, Fujimori A, Kamijo T, Yamada S, et al. Different effects of carbon ion beams and X-rays on clonogenic survival and DNA repair in human pancreatic cancer stem-like cells. Radiother Oncol 2012;105:258–65.

[157] Matsui Y, Asano T, Kenmochi T, Iwakawa M, Imai T, Ochiai T. Effects of carbon-ion beams on human pancreatic cancer cell lines that differ in genetic status. Am J Clin Oncol 2004;27:24–8.

[158] Jinno-Oue A, Shimizu N, Hamada N, Wada S, Tanaka A, Shinagawa M, et al. Irradiation with carbon ion beams induces apoptosis, autophagy, and cellular senescence in a human glioma-derived cell line. Int J Radiat Oncol Biol Phys 2010;76:229–41.

[159] Tomiyama A, Tachibana K, Suzuki K, Seino S, Sunayama J, Matsuda KI, et al. MEK-ERK-dependent multiple caspase activation by mitochondrial proapoptotic Bcl-2 family proteins is essential for heavy ion irradiation-induced glioma cell death. Cell Death Dis 2010;1:e60.

[160] Fujita M, Otsuka Y, Imadome K, Endo S, Yamada S, Imai T. Carbon-ion radiation enhances migration ability and invasiveness of the pancreatic cancer cell, PANC-1, in vitro. Cancer Sci 2012;103:677–83.

[161] Takahashi Y, Teshima T, Kawaguchi N, Hamada Y, Mori S, Madachi A, et al. Heavy ion irradiation inhibits in vitro angiogenesis even at sublethal dose. Cancer Res 2003;63:4253–7.

[162] Kamlah F, Hanze J, Arenz A, Seay U, Hasan D, Juricko J, et al. Comparison of the effects of carbon ion and photon irradiation on the angiogenic response in human lung adenocarcinoma cells. Int J Radiat Oncol Biol Phys 2011;80:1541–9.

[163] Cui X, Oonishi K, Tsujii H, Yasuda T, Matsumoto Y, Furusawa Y, et al. Effects of carbon ion beam on putative colon cancer stem cells and its comparison with X-rays. Cancer Res 2011;71:3676–87.

[164] El Shafie RA, Habermehl D, Rieken S, Mairani A, Orschiedt L, Brons S, et al. In vitro evaluation of photon and raster-scanned carbon ion radiotherapy in combination with gemcitabine in pancreatic cancer cell lines. J Radiat Res 2013;54(Suppl. 1):i113–9.

[165] Shinoto M, Yamada S, Yasuda S, Imada H, Shioyama Y, Honda H, et al. Phase 1 trial of preoperative, short-course carbon-ion radiotherapy for patients with resectable pancreatic cancer. Cancer 2013;119:45–51.

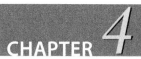

CHAPTER 4

The Role of Notch Signaling Pathway in the Progression of Pancreatic Cancer

Jiankun Gao[1], Fazlul H. Sarkar[2], Lucio Miele[3], Zhiwei Wang[4,5]

[1]Department of Basic Medical Sciences, Sichuan College of Traditional Chinese Medicine, Mianyang, Sichuan, China, [2]Department of Pathology and Oncology, Karmanos Cancer Institute, Wayne State University, Detroit, MI, USA, [3]University of Mississippi Cancer Institute, Jackson, MS, USA, [4]The Cyrus Tang Hematology Center, Jiangsu Institute of Hematology, the First, Affiliated Hospital, Soochow University, Suzhou, China, [5]Department of Pathology, Beth Israel Deaconess Medical Center, Harvard Medical School, Boston, MA, USA

Contents

Introduction	75
Notch Signaling Pathway	76
The Role of Notch in PC	77
Notch is Overexpressed in PC	78
Notch Promotes Cell Growth in PC	78
Notch Inhibits Cell Apoptosis in PC	79
Notch Regulates Cell Cycle in PC	79
Notch Regulates Tumor Cell Invasion in PC	79
Notch Regulates Tumor Angiogenesis in PC	80
Notch Predicts for Poor Prognosis in PC	80
Notch Regulates EMT in PC	80
Notch is Involved in Regulation of Cancer Stem Cells	81
Notch Crosstalks with miRNA in PC	82
Notch is Involved in Drug Resistance in PC	83
Notch Inhibition is a Novel Strategy for PC Treatment	83
Understanding Notch Signaling through Systems Biology	84
Conclusion	85
References	86

INTRODUCTION

Pancreatic cancer (PC) is a highly aggressive malignancy and ranks as the fourth leading cause of cancer-related death in the United States [1]. This high mortality is partly due to the absence of specific symptoms and signs, and the lack of early detection tests for PC, as well as the lack of effective

chemotherapies [2]. Although the molecular mechanisms of PC development remain largely unclear, many factors have been reported to be associated with increased incidence of PC [3]. For example, a history of diabetes
or chronic pancreatitis, chronic cirrhosis, a family history of PC, a high-fat
and high-cholesterol diet, tobacco smoking, alcohol and coffee intake, and
specific blood type have been found to contribute to PC development [4].
Accumulated evidence has demonstrated that many key genes and cell signaling pathways also play critical roles in pancreatic tumorigenesis [5–7].
Recently, some studies have demonstrated that the Notch signaling pathway
contributes to PC development and progression [8]. Therefore, in the following sections, we will discuss the roles of the Notch signaling pathway in
the regulation of cell proliferation, apoptosis, migration, invasion, metastasis,
angiogenesis, drug resistance, epithelial-to-mesenchymal transition (EMT),
and cancer stem cell (CSC) functions in PC.

NOTCH SIGNALING PATHWAY

It has been well documented that the Notch signaling pathway plays critical
mechanistic roles in the development of organs, tissue proliferation, differentiation, and apoptosis [8]. It is known that mammals express four transmembrane Notch receptors (Notch-1, Notch-2, Notch-3, and Notch-4)
and five canonical transmembrane ligands (Delta-like 1, Delta-like 3, Delta-
like 4, Jagged-1, and Jagged-2) [9]. All four Notch receptors are very similar,
although they have subtle differences in their extracellular and cytoplasmic
domains (Figure 4.1). The extracellular domains of the Notch proteins possess multiple repeats that are related to epidermal growth factor (EGF) and
are thought to participate in ligand binding. The amino-terminal EGF-like
repeats are followed by a cysteine-rich region termed the LNR (LIN-12/
Notch-related region), which prevents signaling when a ligand is absent
[10]. The cytoplasmic region of the Notch conveys the signal to the nucleus;
it contains a recombination signal-binding protein 1 for J-kappa (RBP-J)-
association molecule (RAM) domain, ankyrin (ANK) repeats, nuclear localization signals (NLS), a transactivation domain (TAD), and a region rich in
proline, glutamine, serine, and threonine residues (PEST) sequences [11].
Notch ligands have multiple EGF-like repeats in their extracellular domain
and a cysteine-rich region (CR) in serrate which are absent in delta [12].

The Notch signaling pathway is activated after Notch-ligand binding
followed by three consecutive proteolytic cleavages by multiple enzyme
complexes including γ-secretase complex [13]. This produces an active

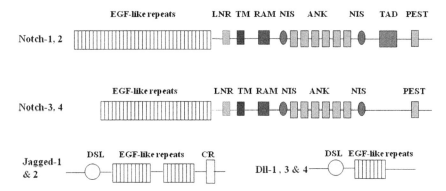

Figure 4.1 *Structure of Notch Receptors (1–4) and Ligands (Jagged-1, 2, Dll-1, 3, Four)*. Notch receptors and ligands contain multiple conserved domains. The extracellular domain contains EGF-like repeats and a cysteine-rich region. The intracellular domain contains the RAM domain, NLS, ANK, TAD and PEST domain. Notch ligands have multiple EGF-like repeats in their extracellular domain and a CR in Jagged which are absent in delta. (For color version of this figure, the reader is referred to the online version of this book.)

fragment, the Notch intracellular domain (NICD), which enters the nucleus and binds to CSL, displaces corepressors from CSL, and subsequently recruits a coactivator complex containing mastermind, p300, and other coactivators, leading to the activation of Notch target genes [8]. So far, many Notch target genes have been identified such as *hairy enhance of split (Hes) family, Hey family, Akt, cyclin D1, c-myc, cyclooxygenase-2 (COX-2), extracellular signal-regulated kinase (ERK), matrix metalloproteinase-9 (MMP-9), mammalian target of rapamycin (mTOR), nuclear factor-kappa B (NF-κB), p21, p27, p53, and vascular endothelial growth factor (VEGF)* [14]. Since these target genes are critically involved in tumorigenesis, the Notch signaling pathway plays a pivotal role in the development and progression of human cancers including PC via regulating its target genes [15].

THE ROLE OF NOTCH IN PC

It is worth mentioning that the function of Notch signaling in tumorigenesis can be either oncogenic or oncosuppressive, suggesting that its function is context dependent to some extent [16]. For example, one study has shown that Notch-1 has an oncosuppressive function in skin cancer [17]. In contrast, most studies have revealed that Notch activation is oncogenic in a variety of human cancers including PC [11]. In the following paragraphs, we will discuss how the Notch signaling pathway is involved in the development and progression of PC.

Notch is Overexpressed in PC

Aberrant Notch pathway activation has been implicated in the initiation and progression of PC [18]. For instance, Miyamoto et al. reported that Notch pathway components and Notch target genes are upregulated in invasive human PC [19]. Consistently, Terris et al. found that the Notch gene was highly expressed in human PC [20]. Similarly, Fukushima et al. also reported that Jagged-1 and Hes-1 were overexpressed in PC [21]. In line with this, Cavard et al. showed that members of the Notch pathway (Hey-1, Hey-2, Notch-2) were also upregulated in PC [22]. To further support the onco-genic role of Notch in PC, Büchler et al. found that Notch-3 and Notch-4 expressed at higher levels in human PC tissues compared with normal pan-creatic tissue [23]. They also found that Jagged-1, Jagged-2 and Dll-1 were significantly upregulated in PC tissue specimens [23]. In agreement with these findings, overexpression of Jagged-2 and Dll-4 has been reported in the vast majority of PC cell lines [24]. All of these reports clearly suggest the possible link between Notch gene overexpression and PC.

Notch Promotes Cell Growth in PC

Studies have demonstrated that Notch regulates cell proliferation in human cancers including PC. Our previously studies have documented the role of Notch-1 in controlling cell growth in PC [25]. Using MTT assay, we found that downregulation of Notch-1 expression by its siRNA caused cell growth inhibition in PC cell lines. Moreover, overexpression of Notch-1 by its cDNA transfection promoted cell growth in PC cells [25]. To further sup-port the role of Notch signaling pathway, one study has shown that blockade of delta-like ligand four inhibited tumor growth of pancreatic cancer [26]. Similarly, the suppression of Notch-3 expression inhibited cell growth in PC cells [27]. Moreover, genetic and pharmacologic inhibition of Notch signal-ing mitigated anchorage-independent growth in PC cells [24]. For example, MRK-003, a potent and selective γ-secretase inhibitor, treatment led to the downregulation of nuclear NICD and inhibition of anchorage-independent PC cell growth [28]. Treatment of PC cells with MRK-003 in cell culture significantly inhibited the subsequent engraftment in immunocompromised mice. Furthermore, MRK-003 treatment significantly blocked tumor growth in PC xenografts [28]. Mechanistically, it has been revealed that acti-vation of Notch-mediated cell growth may be mediated in part through the activation of NF-κB activity [29]. Taken together, the Notch signaling path-way that promotes tumor cell growth in PC is a scientific fact.

Notch Inhibits Cell Apoptosis in PC

It has been known that cell growth inhibitory effects are often partially associated with the induction of apoptosis. Indeed, it has been reported that the downregulation of Notch-1 induced apoptosis in PC cell lines, indicating that the growth inhibitory activity of Notch-1 depletion is partly attributed to an increase in cell death [25]. In line with this notion, over-expression of Notch-1 inhibited apoptosis in PC cell lines, suggesting that activation of the Notch signaling pathway could protect cells from apoptosis in PC [25]. Recently, it has been shown that the interaction of exosomal nanoparticles with PC cells led to decreased expression of Hes-1 and activation of the apoptotic pathway [30]. It is known that Bcl-2 plays a central role in cell apoptosis. One study has shown that the inhibition of Bcl-2 induced apoptosis is partly through downregulation of Notch-1 expression in PC [31]. Altogether, Notch could regulate the cell apoptosis in PC.

Notch Regulates Cell Cycle in PC

Accumulated evidence has revealed that Notch-1 controls the cell cycle in PC. For example, it has been shown that the downregulation of Notch-1 could induce cell cycle arrest in G_0-G_1 phase [29]. Specifically, Notch-1 knockdown by its siRNAs caused a typical G_0-G_1 phase arrest pattern in PC cells. In contrast, PC cells with overexpression of Notch-1 have a greater reduction in the fraction of cells at G_0-G_1 phase [29]. In line with the cell cycle arrest, expression of cyclin A1, cyclin D1, and cyclin-dependent kinase (Cdk)-2 was found to be decreased, while p21 and p27 expression was increased [29], suggesting that these cell cycle regulatory factors are involved in Notch-1-induced cell cycle progression and cell cycle arrest.

Notch Regulates Tumor Cell Invasion in PC

Emerging line of evidence has suggested that the Notch signaling pathway plays a critical role in the regulation of tumor invasion in PC. To support this concept, PC cells transfected with small interfering Notch-1 RNA showed a low level of penetration through the Matrigel-coated membrane, suggesting that downregulation of Notch-1 could decrease cell invasion [32]. In contrast, overexpression of Notch by its cDNA transfection led to increased tumor cell invasion by about 3.5 fold [32]. More importantly, it has been demonstrated that Notch-1-induced tumor cell invasion could in part be due to activation of NF-κB DNA-binding activity, which leads to the upregulation of NF-κB target genes, such as *MMP-9, VEGF, survivin,* and

COX-2 [32]. Moreover, inhibition of epidermal growth factor receptor signaling suppressed tumor cell invasion via downregulation of Notch-1 and its target genes in PC [33]. In support of the role of Notch in the regulation of cell invasion, it has been reported that PDGF-D downregulation was mechanistically associated with the downregulation of Notch-1, and its target genes such as *NF-κB, VEGF,* and *MMP-9,* resulting in the inhibition of tumor cell invasion in PC [34]. However, further in-depth studies are required to investigate the precise underlying mechanism of Notch-induced invasion in PC.

Notch Regulates Tumor Angiogenesis in PC

It is noteworthy that the Notch signaling pathway plays a critical role in tumor angiogenesis in PC. For example, blockade of delta-like ligand four (Dll-4) signaling inhibits angiogenesis of PC [26]. Dll-4 allele deletion or soluble Dll-4 treatment led to increased tumor vessel density, reduced vessel perfusion, resulting in reduced tumor size, suggesting that inhibition of Dll-4 is highly effective in disrupting tumor angiogenesis in PC [35] even though PC is not an angiogenic tumor in human. Recently, we found that downregulation of platelet-derived growth factor-D inhibits angiogenesis through inactivation of Notch-1 and NF-κB signaling and its target genes such as *MMP-9* and *VEGF* in PC cells [34]. Taken together, Notch signaling pathway is critically involved in governing tumor angiogenesis in PC.

Notch Predicts for Poor Prognosis in PC

Multiple studies have demonstrated that aberrant expression of the Notch signaling pathway could predict for poor prognosis in PC. Indeed, high Dll-4 expression is significantly associated with poor prognosis for surgically resected PC, advanced tumor stage, and lymph node metastasis [36]. Moreover, Notch-1, Notch-3, and Notch-4 were found to be significantly elevated in PC tumor tissues [37]. Higher nuclear expression of Notch-1, Notch-3, Notch-4, Hes-1, and Hey-1 was observed in advanced and metastatic PC tumors [37]. More importantly, nuclear Notch-3 and Hey-1 expression were correlated to reduced overall and disease-free survival following tumor resection with curative intent, suggesting that Notch-3 and Hey-1 could function as biomarkers for diagnosis, prognosis and treatment efficacy [37].

Notch Regulates EMT in PC

It has been documented that epithelial-to-mesenchymal transition (EMT) is a process where epithelial cells acquire a mesenchymal phenotype, leading to increased motility and invasion [38]. EMT is characterized by the loss of expression of epithelial markers such as E-cadherin and γ-catenin, and upregulation in the expression of mesenchymal molecular markers such as zinc-finger E-box binding homeobox (ZEB), snail, slug, vimentin, fibronectin, α-smooth muscle actin (SMA), and N-cadherin [39]. Recently, Notch has been reported to be involved in EMT processes [40]. Higher expression of Notch-2 and Jagged-1 has been observed in gemcitabine-resistant cells, which show the acquisition of EMT phenotype, as evidenced by elongated fibroblastoid morphology, downregulation of epithelial marker E-cadherin and upregulation of mesenchymal markers such as ZEB and vimentin [41]. Furthermore, depletion of Notch-2 and Jagged-1 by siRNA partially reversed the EMT phenotype, leading to the mesenchymal-to-epithelial transition; MET [41].

In order to directly address the role of Notch in EMT, Bao et al. demonstrated that forced overexpression of Notch-1 resulted in the acquisition of EMT phenotype by upregulation of mesenchymal cell markers, such as ZEB1, ZEB2, Snail2, and vimentin, and downregulation of epithelial cell marker E-cadherin in PC cells [42]. Consistent with this finding, Kang et al. found that overexpression of Dll-4 in PC cells upregulated the expression of Vimentin, ZEB and Snail, leading to EMT phenotype [43]. In line with these findings, it has been found that Midkine-Notch-2 interaction activated Notch signaling and subsequently induced EMT in PC cells [44]. Therefore, targeting Notch signaling would be able to inhibit the acquisition of EMT phenotype, which could result in the reversal of drug resistance which may be important in the treatment of metastatic disease.

Notch is Involved in Regulation of Cancer Stem Cells

Accumulating evidence has shown that there is a molecular link between Notch and cancer stem cells (CSCs) [45]. It is known that CSCs have been identified and isolated based on the expression of a specific molecule or combination of molecules such as CD24, CD34, CD44, CD133, epithelial-specific antigen (ESA), and aldehyde dehydrogenase (ALDH) [46]. Using these molecular markers, CSCs have been isolated from tumors of the hematopoietic system, breast, lung, prostate, colon, brain, head and neck, and pancreas [47]. Li et al. first described that $CD44^+/CD24^+/ESA^+$ pancreatic cancer cells show the stem cell properties consistent with self-renewal and increased tumorigenic potential [48]. Similarly, Hermann et al. reported that human pancreatic cancer tissue contains CSCs as defined by CD133 and

CXCR4 expression [49]. Moreover, ABCG2 and CD133 may also represent markers for pancreatic CSCs [50,51].

The Notch signaling pathway is believed to play a critical role in CSCs [52]. In support of such a claim, Wang et al. found that pancreatic CSCs show considerably higher levels of expression for Notch-1 [51]. Ji et al. also reported that pancreatic CSCs contain high levels of Notch-1 and Notch-2 [53]. These data suggest that the activation of Notch signaling may be involved in pancreatic CSCs self-renewal. Moreover, overexpression of Dll-4 in PC cells simultaneously stimulates the expression of Oct4 and Nanog, resulting in increased numbers of CSCs [10]. Our recent study showed that overexpression of Notch-1 in PC cells enhanced the formation of pancreatospheres consistent with a high level of CSC surface markers CD44 and EpCAM [42]. MRK-003, a potent and selective γ-secretase inhibitor, treatment resulted in the reduction of tumor-initiating cells that are capable of extensive self-renewal [28]. Taken together, activation of Notch signaling could contribute to CSC self-renewal capacity [54].

Notch Crosstalks with miRNA in PC

The Notch signaling pathway could be regulated by microRNAs (miRNAs) [55]. It is clear that miRNAs exert their inhibitory effects on gene expression through binding to the 3′ untranslated region of target mRNA [56]. Some miRNAs function as either an oncogene or a tumor suppressor gene [57]. In general, there are increased oncogenic miRNAs and decreased tumor suppressor miRNAs [58]. The extensive study of miRNAs over the past decades has demonstrated that miRNAs are frequently deregulated in PC and contribute to the pathogenesis and aggressiveness of the disease [59]. Since a single miRNA can affect a myriad of cellular processes, targeting miRNAs could become a promising strategy for aiding PC treatment [59].

Interestingly, miRNAs have been found to crosstalk with the Notch pathway in PC [53]. For example, miR-34a targeted the expression of Notch-1 and Notch-2 in PC cells [53]. Moreover, miR-34 has been found to be involved in pancreatic CSCs self-renewal through direct modulation of the Notch pathway [53]. To support the role of miRNA in regulating the Notch pathway, it has been revealed that miR-200 members target Notch pathway components, such as Jagged-1 and the mastermind-like coactivators Maml-2 and Maml-3 in PC cells [60]. Consistently, we found that overexpression of Notch-1 up-regulated miR-21 expression and downregulated the expression of miR-200b, miR-200c, and let-7 family in PC cells [42]. Altogether, these results demonstrated the crosstalks between Notch and miRNAs in PC.

Notch is Involved in Drug Resistance in PC

Although chemotherapy is an important therapeutic strategy for PC treatment, chemotherapy fails to eliminate all tumor cells because of intrinsic or acquired drug-resistance, which could lead to tumor recurrence and metastasis [61]. Increasing evidence has suggested that the Notch pathway plays a critical role in drug resistance in PC [62]. For instance, inhibition of Notch-3 enhances sensitivity to gemcitabine in PC through inactivation of PI3K/Akt-dependent pathway [27]. Kang et al. showed that over-activation of DLL-4/Notch pathway can simultaneously impair chemo-drug delivery and enhance chemoresistance in PC [43]. Moreover, it has been reported that gamma-secretase complexes regulate the responses of human PC cells to taxanes [63]. Our recent finding showed that Notch-2 and Jagged-1 are highly upregulated in gemcitabine-resistant PC cells [41]. Moreover, gemcitabine-resistant PC cells have shown acquired EMT phenotype with activation of Notch signaling pathway, suggesting that the activation of Notch signaling is mechanistically linked with the chemoresistance phenotype in PC [41]. CSCs have also been believed to play critical roles in drug-resistance partly because CSCs express drug transporters, leading to CSCs resisting resist the killing effects of the drug. Since the Notch signaling pathway regulates CSCs, targeting the Notch pathway could be a novel strategy to increase drug sensitivity through inhibiting CSCs function.

NOTCH INHIBITION IS A NOVEL STRATEGY FOR PC TREATMENT

The Notch signaling pathway is involved in cell growth, migration, invasion, EMT, CSCs and drug resistance. Thus, targeting the Notch pathway could be a novel strategy for the treatment of PC through inhibition of cell growth, reversal of EMT and eliminating CSCs as well as overcoming drug resistance [64]. Since Notch signaling is activated via the activity of γ-secretase, γ-secretase inhibitors (GSIs) could be useful for cancer therapy [9,65]. Indeed, emerging evidence has suggested that several forms of GSIs inhibited tumor cell growth, migration and invasion in various human cancers including PC [66]. For example, the inhibition of Notch activity by GSIs retarded tumor development in a murine model of PC [66]. Notably, GSI can block EMT, migration and invasion in PC cells, and suppress the tumor growth induced by pancreatic CSCs in a xenograft mouse model [67]. Although GSI has shown antitumor activity in human cancer, GSIs exhibit multiple side-effects. For instance,

GSIs could block the cleavage of all four Notch receptors and multiple other γ-secretase substrates, which could be important for normal cell survival [66]. Additionally, GSIs have unwanted cytotoxicity in the gastrointestinal tract [66].

To overcome the limitations of GSIs, several studies have used natural compounds, which are typically non-toxic to human cells, to inhibit the Notch signaling pathway in human malignancies. For example, natural agents such as genistein, curcumin, and sulforaphane have been reported to inhibit Notch expression [25,68]. Studies from our group have demonstrated that genistein and curcumin inhibited the expression of Notch-1 and its target genes including *Hes-1, Cyclin D1, Bcl-xL* and *NF-κB* in PC cells [25,68]. Recently, we further revealed that genistein inhibited cell growth, migration, invasion, EMT phenotype, and the formation of pancreatospheres via suppressing Notch-1 expression in PC cells [42]. We also observed that genistein could inhibit Notch-1 expression through upregulation of miR-34a in PC cells [69]. Sulforaphane, a natural compound derived from cruciferous vegetables, was shown to target the pancreatic CSCs [70–72]. Moreover, the synergistic activity of sulforaphane and sorafenib was found to be due to elimination of CSCs derived from PC cells [73]. Furthermore, sulforaphane increased the sensitivity of cells to chemotherapeutic agents such as cisplatin, gemcitabine, doxorubicin and 5-flurouracil through targeting CSCs mediated by the inactivation of Notch-1 in PC [70]. Studies from our group have also shown that curcumin inhibits cell growth and induced apoptosis in pancreatic cancer through inactivation of the Notch pathway [25]. Taken together, these findings suggest that natural compounds could function as non-toxic inhibitors of the Notch pathway in PC cells, and thus natural agents could be useful either alone or in combination with conventional therapeutics in the management of PC with better treatment outcome.

UNDERSTANDING NOTCH SIGNALING THROUGH SYSTEMS BIOLOGY

To understand the contributions of Notch signaling to normal development and cancer, a systematic identification of the different components in the pathway, the underlying control circuitries, and of the connections to other pathways is crucial. However, a major challenge for such comprehensive systems biology studies in human cells is the complexity and genetic redundancy in many of its pathways that make a systematic loss-of-function analysis difficult. This is especially true for Notch signaling, which is recognized to crosstalk with so many different parallel signaling. In this direction, Saj and colleagues using in vivo RNAi libraries for *Drosophila* dissected the complexity of Notch signaling on a genome-wide scale [74] Their binary expression system allowed for tissue-specific knockdown of genes. Using this systems they described a combined ex vivo and in vivo RNAi screening approach to identify regulators of Notch [74]. Their cell-based genome-wide RNAi screen selected a list of 900 potential modulators of Notch activity. These preselected candidates were then analyzed in vivo in a range of assays and allelic series, which enabled a large-scale confirmation of the data from the cell-based assay [74]. These studies lead to the establishment and analysis of a Notch interaction network. In summary, their results showed that such a systems approach can identify genes (401 in total) as regulators of Notch, and determined several cellular modules linking Notch and cancer [74]. This systems and network-deduced Notch interaction map opens up entirely new and interesting perspectives for the regulation of Notch signaling in development and diseases such as pancreatic cancer. Nevertheless, there is a need for more robust biological analyses, such as proteomic approaches, in order to place the interactors within the Notch pathway and to reveal the exact links to other pathways and the cellular metabolic network.

CONCLUSION

In summary, evidence has convincingly shown that the Notch signaling pathway plays a central role in the development and progression of PC through regulation of cell growth, apoptosis, migration, invasion, angiogenesis, and metastasis (Figure 4.2). Moreover, the Notch pathway is critically involved in controlling the acquisition of EMT phenotype and the formation of CSCs in PC. More importantly, Notch signaling is associated with drug resistance in PC (Figure 4.2). Therefore, due to its multiple functions, targeting the Notch pathway could become a promising strategy for the treatment of PC. To that end, natural compounds could become a major player because they are less toxic or non-toxic to humans. Therefore, these natural agents could be useful for the prevention of tumor progression and/or for successful treatment of PC mediated through inactivation of the Notch signaling pathway. However, further pre-clinical and clinical studies are warranted.

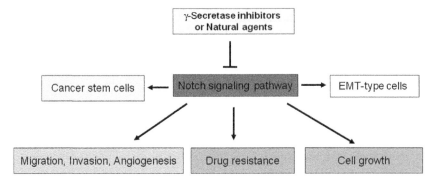

Figure 4.2 *The Role of Notch Signaling Pathway in the Development and Progression of Cancer.* Natural agents and γ-secretase inhibitors could be useful for targeting the Notch signaling pathway. (For color version of this figure, the reader is referred to the online version of this book.)

REFERENCES

[1] Siegel R, Naishadham D, Jemal A. Cancer statistics, 2013. CA Cancer J Clin 2013;63: 11–30.

[2] Werner J, Combs SE, Springfeld C, Hartwig W, Hackert T, Buchler MW. Advanced-stage pancreatic cancer: therapy options. Nat Rev Clin Oncol 2013;10:323–33.

[3] Hackert T, Buchler MW. Pancreatic cancer: advances in treatment, results and limitations. Dig Dis 2013;31:51–6.

[4] Hidalgo M. Pancreatic cancer. N Engl J Med 2010;362:1605–17.

[5] Zavoral M, Minarikova P, Zavada F, Salek C, Minarik M. Molecular biology of pancreatic cancer. World J Gastroenterol 2011;17:2897–908.

[6] Hong SM, Park JY, Hruban RH, Goggins M. Molecular signatures of pancreatic cancer. Arch Pathol Lab Med 2011;135:716–27.

[7] Krautz C, Ruckert F, Saeger HD, Pilarsky C, Grutzmann R. An update on molecular research of pancreatic adenocarcinoma. Anticancer Agents Med Chem 2011;11: 411–7.

[8] Wang J, Han F, Wu J, Lee SW, Chan CH, Wu CY, et al. The role of Skp2 in hematopoietic stem cell quiescence, pool size, and self-renewal. Blood 2011;118:5429–38.

[9] Miele L. Notch signaling. Clin Cancer Res 2006;12:1074–9.

[10] Radtke F, Raj K. The role of Notch in tumorigenesis: oncogene or tumour suppressor? Nat Rev Cancer 2003;3:756–67.

[11] Bray SJ. Notch signalling: a simple pathway becomes complex. Nat Rev Mol Cell Biol 2006;7:678–89.

[12] Wang Z, Li Y, Sarkar FH. Notch signaling proteins: legitimate targets for cancer therapy. Curr Protein Pept Sci 2010;11:398–408.

[13] Espinoza I, Miele L. Deadly crosstalk: Notch signaling at the intersection of EMT and cancer stem cells. Cancer Lett 2013;341:41–5.

[14] Ranganathan P, Weaver KL, Capobianco AJ. Notch signalling in solid tumours: a little bit of everything but not all the time. Nat Rev Cancer 2011;11:338–51.

[15] Espinoza I, Pochampally R, Xing F, Watabe K, Miele L. Notch signaling: targeting cancer stem cells and epithelial-to-mesenchymal transition. Onco Targets Ther 2013;6:1249–59.

[16] Dotto GP. Notch tumor suppressor function. Oncogene 2008;27:5115–23.

[17] Nicolas M, Wolfer A, Raj K, Kummer JA, Mill P, van Noort M, et al. Notch1 functions as a tumor suppressor in mouse skin. Nat Genet 2003;33:416–21.

[18] Ristorcelli E, Lombardo D. Targeting Notch signaling in pancreatic cancer. Expert Opin Ther Targets 2010;14:541–52.

[19] Miyamoto Y, Maitra A, Ghosh B, Zechner U, Argani P, Iacobuzio-Donahue CA, et al. Notch mediates TGF alpha-induced changes in epithelial differentiation during pancreatic tumorigenesis. Cancer Cell 2003;3:565–76.

[20] Terris B, Blaveri E, Crnogorac-Jurcevic T, Jones M, Missiaglia E, Ruszniewski P, et al. Characterization of gene expression profiles in intraductal papillary-mucinous tumors of the pancreas. Am J Pathol 2002;160:1745–54.

[21] Fukushima N, Sato N, Prasad N, Leach SD, Hruban RH, Goggins M. Characterization of gene expression in mucinous cystic neoplasms of the pancreas using oligonucleotide microarrays. Oncogene 2004;23:9042–51.

[22] Cavard C, Audebourg A, Letourneur F, Audard V, Beuvon F, Cagnard N, et al. Gene expression profiling provides insights into the pathways involved in solid pseudopapillary neoplasm of the pancreas. J Pathol 2009;218:201–9.

[23] Buchler P, Gazdhar A, Schubert M, Giese N, Reber HA, Hines OJ, et al. The Notch signaling pathway is related to neurovascular progression of pancreatic cancer. Ann Surg 2005;242:791–800, discussion 800–1.

[24] Mullendore ME, Koorstra JB, Li YM, Offerhaus GJ, Fan X, Henderson CM, et al. Ligand-dependent Notch signaling is involved in tumor initiation and tumor maintenance in pancreatic cancer. Clin Cancer Res 2009;15:2291–301.

[25] Wang Z, Zhang Y, Banerjee S, Li Y, Sarkar FH. Notch-1 down-regulation by curcumin is associated with the inhibition of cell growth and the induction of apoptosis in pancreatic cancer cells. Cancer 2006;106:2503–13.

[26] Oishi H, Sunamura M, Egawa S, Motoi F, Unno M, Furukawa T, et al. Blockade of delta-like ligand 4 signaling inhibits both growth and angiogenesis of pancreatic cancer. Pancreas 2010;39:897–903.

[27] Yao J, Qian C. Inhibition of Notch3 enhances sensitivity to gemcitabine in pancreatic cancer through an inactivation of PI3K/Akt-dependent pathway. Med Oncol 2010;27:1017–22.

[28] Mizuma M, Rasheed ZA, Yabuuchi S, Omura N, Campbell NR, de Wilde RF, et al. The gamma secretase inhibitor MRK-003 attenuates pancreatic cancer growth in preclinical models. Mol Cancer Ther 2012;11:1999–2009.

[29] Wang Z, Zhang Y, Li Y, Banerjee S, Liao J, Sarkar FH. Down-regulation of Notch-1 contributes to cell growth inhibition and apoptosis in pancreatic cancer cells. Mol Cancer Ther 2006;5:483–93.

[30] Ristorcelli E, Beraud E, Mathieu S, Lombardo D, Verine A. Essential role of Notch signaling in apoptosis of human pancreatic tumoral cells mediated by exosomal nanoparticles. Int J Cancer 2009;125:1016–26.

[31] Wang Z, Azmi AS, Ahmad A, Banerjee S, Wang S, Sarkar FH, et al. TW-37, a small-molecule inhibitor of Bcl-2, inhibits cell growth and induces apoptosis in pancreatic cancer: involvement of Notch-1 signaling pathway. Cancer Res 2009;69:2757–65.

[32] Wang Z, Banerjee S, Li Y, Rahman KM, Zhang Y, Sarkar FH. Down-regulation of notch-1 inhibits invasion by inactivation of nuclear factor-kappaB, vascular endothelial growth factor, and matrix metalloproteinase-9 in pancreatic cancer cells. Cancer Res 2006;66:2778–84.

[33] Wang Z, Sengupta R, Banerjee S, Li Y, Zhang Y, Rahman KM, et al. Epidermal growth factor receptor-related protein inhibits cell growth and invasion in pancreatic cancer. Cancer Res 2006;66:7653–60.

[34] Wang Z, Kong D, Banerjee S, Li Y, Adsay NV, Abbruzzese J, et al. Down-regulation of platelet-derived growth factor-D inhibits cell growth and angiogenesis through inactivation of Notch-1 and nuclear factor-kappaB signaling. Cancer Res 2007;67:11377–85.

[35] Djokovic D, Trindade A, Gigante J, Badenes M, Silva L, Liu R, et al. Combination of Dll4/Notch and Ephrin-B2/EphB4 targeted therapy is highly effective in disrupting tumor angiogenesis. BMC Cancer 2010;10:641.

[36] Chen HT, Cai QC, Zheng JM, Man XH, Jiang H, Song B, et al. High expression of delta-like ligand 4 predicts poor prognosis after curative resection for pancreatic cancer. Ann Surg Oncol 2012;19(Suppl. 3):S464–74.

[37] Mann CD, Bastianpillai C, Neal CP, Masood MM, Jones DJ, Teichert F, et al. Notch3 and HEY-1 as prognostic biomarkers in pancreatic adenocarcinoma. PloS One 2012;7:e51119.

[38] De Craene B, Berx G. Regulatory networks defining EMT during cancer initiation and progression. Nat Rev Cancer 2013;13:97–110.

[39] Nauseef JT, Henry MD. Epithelial-to-mesenchymal transition in prostate cancer: paradigm or puzzle? Nat Rev Urol 2011;8:428–39.

[40] Wang Z, Li Y, Kong D, Sarkar FH. The role of Notch signaling pathway in epithelial-mesenchymal transition (EMT) during development and tumor aggressiveness. Curr Drug Targets 2010;11:745–51.

[41] Wang Z, Li Y, Kong D, Banerjee S, Ahmad A, Azmi AS, et al. Acquisition of epithelial-mesenchymal transition phenotype of gemcitabine-resistant pancreatic cancer cells is linked with activation of the notch signaling pathway. Cancer Res 2009;69:2400–7.

[42] Bao B, Wang Z, Ali S, Kong D, Li Y, Ahmad A, et al. Notch-1 induces epithelial-mesenchymal transition consistent with cancer stem cell phenotype in pancreatic cancer cells. Cancer Lett 2011;307:26–36.

[43] Kang M, Jiang B, Xu B, Lu W, Guo Q, Xie Q, et al. Delta like ligand 4 induces impaired chemo-drug delivery and enhanced chemoresistance in pancreatic cancer. Cancer Lett 2013;330:11–21.

[44] Gungor C, Zander H, Effenberger KE, Vashist YK, Kalinina T, Izbicki JR, et al. Notch signaling activated by replication stress-induced expression of midkine drives epithelial-mesenchymal transition and chemoresistance in pancreatic cancer. Cancer Res 2011;71:5009–19.

[45] Wang J, Sullenger BA, Rich JN. Notch signaling in cancer stem cells. Adv Exp Med Biol 2012;727:174–85.

[46] Xia J, Chen C, Chen Z, Miele L, Sarkar FH, Wang Z. Targeting pancreatic cancer stem cells for cancer therapy. Biochim Biophys Acta 2012;1826:385–99.

[47] Martin-Belmonte F, Perez-Moreno M. Epithelial cell polarity, stem cells and cancer. Nat Rev Cancer 2012;12:23–38.

[48] Li C, Heidt DG, Dalerba P, Burant CF, Zhang L, Adsay V, et al. Identification of pancreatic cancer stem cells. Cancer Res 2007;67:1030–7.

[49] Hermann PC, Huber SL, Herrler T, Aicher A, Ellwart JW, Guba M, et al. Distinct populations of cancer stem cells determine tumor growth and metastatic activity in human pancreatic cancer. Cell Stem Cell 2007;1:313–23.

[50] Matsuda Y, Kure S, Ishiwata T. Nestin and other putative cancer stem cell markers in pancreatic cancer. Med Mol Morphol 2012;45:59–65.

[51] Wang YH, Li F, Luo B, Wang XH, Sun HC, Liu S, et al. A side population of cells from a human pancreatic carcinoma cell line harbors cancer stem cell characteristics. Neoplasma 2009;56:371–8.

[52] Takebe N, Harris PJ, Warren RQ, Ivy SP. Targeting cancer stem cells by inhibiting Wnt, Notch, and Hedgehog pathways. Nat Rev Clin Oncol 2011;8:97–106.

[53] Ji Q, Hao X, Zhang M, Tang W, Yang M, Li L, et al. MicroRNA miR-34 inhibits human pancreatic cancer tumor-initiating cells. PloS One 2009;4:e6816.

[54] Wang Z, Ahmad A, Li Y, Azmi AS, Miele L, Sarkar FH. Targeting notch to eradicate pancreatic cancer stem cells for cancer therapy. Anticancer Res 2011;31:1105–13.

[55] Mo YY, Tang H, Miele L. Notch-associated microRNAs in cancer. Curr Drug Targets 2013;14:1157–66.

[56] Kasinski AL, Slack FJ. Epigenetics and genetics. MicroRNAs en route to the clinic: progress in validating and targeting microRNAs for cancer therapy. Nat Rev Cancer 2011;11:849–64.

[57] Ryan BM, Robles AI, Harris CC. Genetic variation in microRNA networks: the implications for cancer research. Nat Rev Cancer 2010;10:389–402.

[58] Calin GA, Croce CM. MicroRNA signatures in human cancers. Nat Rev Cancer 2006;6:857–66.

[59] Pai P, Rachagani S, Are C, Batra SK. Prospects of miRNA-based therapy for pancreatic cancer. Curr Drug Targets 2013;14:1101–9.

[60] Brabletz S, Bajdak K, Meidhof S, Burk U, Niedermann G, Firat E, et al. The ZEB1/miR-200 feedback loop controls Notch signalling in cancer cells. EMBO J 2011;30:770–82.

[61] Wang Z, Li Y, Ahmad A, Azmi AS, Kong D, Banerjee S, et al. Targeting miRNAs involved in cancer stem cell and EMT regulation: an emerging concept in overcoming drug resistance. Drug Resist Updat 2010;13:109–18.

[62] Wang Z, Li Y, Ahmad A, Banerjee S, Azmi AS, Kong D, et al. Pancreatic cancer: understanding and overcoming chemoresistance. Nat Rev Gastroenterol Hepatol 2011;8 :27–33.

[63] Tasaka T, Akiyoshi T, Yamaguchi K, Tanaka M, Onishi H, Katano M. Gamma-secretase complexes regulate the responses of human pancreatic ductal adenocarcinoma cells to taxanes. Anticancer Res 2010;30:4999–5010.

[64] Wang Z, Li Y, Ahmad A, Azmi AS, Banerjee S, Kong D, et al. Targeting Notch signaling pathway to overcome drug resistance for cancer therapy. Biochim Biophys Acta 2010;1806:258–67.

[65] Miele L, Miao H, Nickoloff BJ. NOTCH signaling as a novel cancer therapeutic target. Curr Cancer Drug Targets 2006;6:313–23.

[66] Espinoza I, Miele L. Notch inhibitors for cancer treatment. Pharmacol Ther 2013; 139:95–110.

[67] Palagani V, El Khatib M, Kossatz U, Bozko P, Muller MR, Manns MP, et al. Epithelial mesenchymal transition and pancreatic tumor initiating CD44+/EpCAM+ cells are inhibited by gamma-secretase inhibitor IX. PloS One 2012;7:e46514.

[68] Wang Z, Zhang Y, Banerjee S, Li Y, Sarkar FH. Inhibition of nuclear factor kappab activity by genistein is mediated via Notch-1 signaling pathway in pancreatic cancer cells. Int J Cancer 2006;118:1930–6.

[69] Xia J, Duan Q, Ahmad A, Bao B, Banerjee S, Shi Y, et al. Genistein inhibits cell growth and induces apoptosis through up-regulation of miR-34a in pancreatic cancer cells. Curr Drug Targets 2012;13:1750–6.

[70] Kallifatidis G, Labsch S, Rausch V, Mattern J, Gladkich J, Moldenhauer G, et al. Sulforaphane increases drug-mediated cytotoxicity toward cancer stem-like cells of pancreas and prostate. Mol Ther 2011;19:188–95.

[71] Li SH, Fu J, Watkins DN, Srivastava RK, Shankar S. Sulforaphane regulates self-renewal of pancreatic cancer stem cells through the modulation of Sonic hedgehog-GLI pathway. Mol Cell Biochem 2013;373:217–27.

[72] Srivastava RK, Tang SN, Zhu W, Meeker D, Shankar S. Sulforaphane synergizes with quercetin to inhibit self-renewal capacity of pancreatic cancer stem cells. Front Biosci (Elite Ed) 2011;3:515–28.

[73] Rausch V, Liu L, Kallifatidis G, Baumann B, Mattern J, Gladkich J, et al. Synergistic activity of sorafenib and sulforaphane abolishes pancreatic cancer stem cell characteristics. Cancer Res 2010;70:5004–13.

[74] Saj A, Arziman Z, Stempfle D, van Belle W, Sauder U, Horn T, et al. A combined ex vivo and in vivo RNAi screen for notch regulators in *Drosophila* reveals an extensive notch interaction network. Dev Cell 2010;18:862–76.

Gene Expression Profiling and Bioinformatics Analysis in Pancreatic Cancer

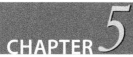

CHAPTER 5

Bioinformatics Analysis of Pancreas Cancer Genome in High-Throughput Genomic Technologies

Enrique Carrillo-de Santa Pau, Francisco X. Real, Alfonso Valencia
Spanish National Cancer Research Center (CNIO), Madrid, Spain

Contents

Introduction	94
Heterogeneity and Quality of Samples for High-Throughput Genomic Technologies	95
Microarrays	96
Technique	96
Bioinformatic Analysis	96
Microarrays in the Pancreas	99
Expression Microarrays	99
Genotyping Microarrays	100
Next-Generation Sequencing	101
ChIP-seq	101
Technique	101
ChIP-seq Encyclopedia of DNA Elements Guidelines	102
Bioinformatics Analysis	102
Further ChIP-seq Applications	105
ChIP-seq Analysis of Pancreatic Cancer	107
RNA-seq	107
Technique	107
RNA-seq ENCODE Guidelines	108
Bioinformatic Analysis	108
RNA-seq in the Pancreas	110
Cancer Genome Sequencing	111
Genome–Exome Sequencing Studies in the Pancreas	114
Databases and Resources	115
Sequence Read Archive	116
GenBank and the European Nucleotide Archive	116
The ENCODE Project	116
Gene Expression Omnibus	117
Array-Express	117

Oncomine   118
IntOGen   122
The Gene Expression Barcode   122
The Single-Nucleotide Polymorphism Database   122
The Catalogue of Somatic Mutations in Cancer   122
The cBioPortal for Cancer Genomics   123
The Cancer Genome Atlas   124
The International Cancer Genome Consortium   124
The 1000 Genomes Project   124
The Cancer Cell Line Encyclopedia   125
The Pancreatic Expression Database   125
Conclusion and Future Perspectives   125
References   126

INTRODUCTION

The technology revolution by the Human Genome Project from 1986 to 2003 [1] has propelled the field of bioinformatics into a new era, with the formidable challenge of organizing, classifying, making available, and interpreting complex genomic data within the context of large biological databases and repositories containing the accumulated information.

The major advances in experimental methods for genome characterization based on deoxyribonucleic acid (DNA)/ribonucleic acid (RNA) microarrays and DNA sequencing—for example, capillary-based DNA Sanger sequencing and, more recently, next-generation sequencing (NGS)—make analysis mutations, gene expression, and copy number alterations possible in a large number of cancer genomes [2]. Indeed, 21st-century sequencing-based experiments generate substantially more data and are more broadly applicable than microarray technology, allowing for various novel functional assays, including quantification of protein–DNA binding or histone modifications (chromatin immunoprecipitation followed by sequencing, ChIP-seq), transcript levels using RNA sequencing (RNA-seq), and genome (WGS) and exome sequencing (WES) variant discovery.

New genomic technology has come at a cost, however, resulting in a greater challenge for associated bioinformatics analyses. The fast development of bioinformatics and the complex combination of related biology, computer science, and information technology often make it difficult for biomedical researchers to use the available technology to its fullest and, in many cases, even to select the appropriate tools and computational resources.

This chapter provides an overview of the high-throughput genomics technologies (with an emphasis in NGS), the data currently available (cancer-related databases) and the types of bioinformatic analyses that need to be applied. It emphasizes the specific challenges posed by the analysis of pancreatic samples and provides specific examples.

HETEROGENEITY AND QUALITY OF SAMPLES FOR HIGH-THROUGHPUT GENOMIC TECHNOLOGIES

Standardized protocols for sample quality are essential to ensure reproducible results and comparability. In general, clinical sample experiments are complicated due to the differences in sample quantity, quality and purity. Tumor samples often include substantial fractions of necrotic or apoptotic cells as well as a mixture of malignant and nonmalignant cells. Also, nucleic acids isolated from cancer are often of lower quality than those purified from peripheral blood. Along this line, tumors may be highly heterogeneous and composed of different clones with different genomes [3,4]. Furthermore, the control samples are also problematic because peripheral blood provides only an imperfect reference and surgical resections are difficult to obtain. Bioinformatics methods are being designed to alleviate most of these issues, but they still impose constraints that have to be taken into account during the organization and interpretation of cancer genome projects.

Aside from the pancreatic tissue samples, cellular components and their function pose additional challenges to the analysis. The pancreas is composed of three major cell types (acinar, ductal, and endocrine). The acinar component is the largest in normal tissue, accounting for about 80% of all cells. Therefore, a comparison of different origin tumors with the normal pancreas is not fully suited per se. Moreover, pancreatic tumors are characterized by a massive desmoplastic reaction and "contamination" from inflammatory/stromal components, which often result in a tumor mass that contains around 38% (ranging from 5% to 85%) of cancer cells [5]. Unlike other neoplasms, histological evaluation of the cellular composition of the specimens used for analyte isolation is essential. In addition, the exocrine pancreas produces large amounts of hydrolytic enzymes, which prevent quality samples from being obtained for analysis. Appropriate controls should be used to examine analyte degradation. It is a fact that an RNA integrity number (RIN) score higher than 7, as recommended for RNA-seq experiments, is hard to obtain in human pancreas samples.

The purity and quality of the material (DNA/RNA) required will have a decisive influence on the quality of the raw data obtained and should be taken into account during the design of the analysis, selection of algorithms, and the follow-up interpretation of the results. The basic bioinformatics approaches applied to the initial raw data are described in detail in the following section.

MICROARRAYS

The development of the microarray technology at the end of the past century was a revolution in the molecular biology field. Microarrays allowed multiple hypotheses to be interrogated simultaneously with robust methods, thereby leading to an application in gene discovery, gene regulation, biomarker determination, and disease classification. Microarrays have been used widely in research, and they commonly are found in the facilities of many academic institutions and biotechnology companies.

Technique

Microarrays are hybridization based and commonly are used to measure the binding of a nucleic acid analyte on the basis of sequence complementarity. This allows both analysis of expression and genotyping. cDNA (two colors) and oligonucleotide (single color) microarrays are the two main microarrays platforms and both have been used widely. cDNA microarrays are useful to measure transcript abundance and are based in printed cDNA with size ranging from a few 100 bases to several kilobases. In two-color arrays, the test and reference samples are labeled with fluorescent Cy5 or Cy3 dyes, using reverse transcriptase, and subsequently are hybridized. The slides are scanned to measure fluorescence, and the signal is relative to the abundance hybridized transcripts. In oligonucleotide microarrays, the probes are directed synthesized on glass slides using photolithography technology. The probes are usually 9–50 nucleotide oligonucleotides that hybridize with samples labeled with biotin or Cy3 dye (single-color arrays).

Bioinformatic Analysis

The first step in the analysis of microarray data is normalization, which is aimed at compensating differences in labeling, hybridization, and detection methods. Data normalization is essential for comparison of different experiments. The selection of the appropriate method depends on the type of array and expected biases. Total intensity normalization assumes that the total hybridization intensities summed over all elements in the arrays should be the same for each sample. In addition, there are a number of alternative approaches to the total intensity normalization method, including linear regression analysis, log centering, rank invariant methods, and others. Because these methods can have a systematic dependence on intensity, the effect of which is often nonlinear and can vary from different slides, locally weighted linear regression normalization has been proposed as a method to remove intensity-dependent effects, taking into account individual slides to remove slide-dependent dye effect [6].

Most normalization algorithms can be applied to the entire data set (global normalization) or to some subset of the data (local normalization). Local normalization helps to correct spatial variations in the array, such as variability in slide surface or slight differences in hybridization conditions across the arrays. Then the variability between regions of an array or between arrays should be corrected so that their variance is the same, normally achieved by adjusting the log2 (ratio) measurements [6].

Housekeeping genes frequently have been used to normalize microarray expression data under the assumption that they display stable levels across samples. This is not always the case, however, leading to erroneous conclusions as shown by Welsh et al. [7] and Yu et al. [8]. Other strategies have been proposed to overcome the housekeeping limitations based on identifying genes that are not expressed differentially across different biological samples in the same data set, to normalize the data. A major normalization effort should be made using standardized spike-in controls of known concentration, defined length, and guanine–cytosine (GC) content [9]. Finally, visual inspection is recommended using box plots, scatter plots, or MA plots—plots of the distribution of the Cy5/Cy3 intensity ratio ('M') versus the average intensity ('A')—to identify possible errors introduced during the normalization procedure. Even though many normalization algorithms have been developed, the Limma package [10] has gained wide acceptance and includes all of the necessary tools for the analysis of the different types of array-based experiments. Limma is part of Bioconductor (http://www.bioconductor.org/), an open-source package based on the R programming language for the analysis of high-throughput genomic data, including microarrays.

After data normalization, the analysis of expression microarrays can be carried out with supervised or unsupervised methods. Supervised methods identify differential gene expression (DGE) patterns between samples of known phenotypes—for example, cells that are exposed or not exposed to experimental manipulation. A number of statistical tests are applied—such as the t-test, Wilcoxon rank-sum test, or significant analysis of microarray—to identify the DGE between two groups or tests based on analysis of variance to identify differential expression between multiple groups. Microarrays test multiple hypotheses in a single experiment and can produce hundreds of false-positive results. These false positives that result from multiple comparisons are controlled by family-wise error rate or the false discovery rate (FDR) estimations. The first represents the probability of having at least one false-positive result for all the tests and the second is less stringent and provides the expected proportion of false positives among the significant results.

Unsupervised methods group samples or genes based on their expression distance, without using information about the associated phenotypes. The most common method used is hierarchical clustering, which groups the samples that have similar expression patterns, genes that are highly correlated, or both, producing dendrograms in which the length of the branches is inversely proportional to the similarity between samples or genes. Other unsupervised methods are K-means, principal component analysis, or self-organizing maps.

Moreover, the unit of analysis can be "gene modules" instead of individual genes, as the latter can be grouped based on previous biological knowledge. The genes can be grouped according to biological pathway, motif sharing, or tissue expression. This kind of analysis has been termed "functional analysis". Three types of methods follow this strategy. One is the singular enrichment analysis (SEA), which is the best strategy established for enrichment analysis and is based on a preselected list of genes defined by the user. This is measured by different statistics, such as chi-squared, Fisher's, binomial, or hypergeometric tests. Another is the Gene-Set Enrichment Analysis (GSEA), which is based on a ranked list of genes and Kolmogorov–Smirnov statistics. This method has the advantage of not requiring arbitrary cutoffs. The third method is the modular enrichment analysis, which incorporates extra network discovery algorithms into the SEA methodology.

In the case of microarrays used for genotyping, the software provided by the manufacturers normally is used for the normalization and genotype analysis step. Currently, microarrays are able to genotype more than a million single-nucleotide polymorphisms (SNPs) simultaneously. The first step is to summarize the probe intensities for each SNP, followed by a call based on the summarized intensities. There are three possible genotypes (assuming diploidy): AA, BB (homozygous), and AB (heterozygous), where A and B denote the two possible alleles. Further steps include linkage disequilibrium and phasing, where alleles at two or more loci appear together in the same individual more often than would be expected by chance.

Genome-wide association studies (GWAS) use germline DNA to identify genetic variants that are more common in individuals with a given phenotype than in the control population. They provide a powerful tool to analyze genetic variation but are limited by the false-positive rate derived from the large number of comparisons performed. To acquire statistical significance—in the case of common, low-penetrance, alleles—large numbers of affected (cases) and unaffected (controls) individuals are needed. In microarray genotyping, the signal intensity is related with the DNA amount harboring the region interrogated by the probe. Therefore, the probe intensity can be used for further analyses, including DNA copy changes, the detection of loss of heterozygosity (LOH) and uniparental disomies, and other structural alterations. Algorithms for copy number—such as WaviCGH [11]—follow similar steps, including the summarization of the intensity of consecutive probes (2–40) into a single measure, followed by segmentation to infer chromosomal segments of constant copy number, the calling of gains and losses regions, and the identification of minimal common regions over a set of samples.

Microarrays in the Pancreas
Expression Microarrays
Microarrays have been used widely in the cancer field for more than a decade for detection of biomarkers, sample classification, response to treatment, and drug screening. Unlike with other tumor types, the number of data sets and samples available in pancreatic cancer is limited. For example, across the 715 microarray data sets and 87,633 samples included in Oncomine (see description in databases and resources section) only 29 data sets with 606 samples referred to pancreatic cancer. In contrast, other frequent tumors (such as colorectal, breast, lung, or brain) are represented by more than twice the number of the data sets, with up to 132 data sets, which include 14,277 samples, in the breast. This reflects the difficulty of accessing pancreatic samples and obtaining sufficient quantity and quality compared with other tumor types as noted in the previous sections.

The earliest studies using expression microarrays focused on the use of gene expression profiles to characterize pancreatic ductal adenocarcinoma (PDAC) [12–15]. These studies identified sets of genes differentially expressed between PDAC and normal samples ranging from 75 to 587 genes. Grutzmann et al. [16] carried out the first meta-analysis, which showed 568 deregulated genes in pancreatic cancer, of which only 22% had been described previously. Following these studies, Badea et al. [17] defined their own DGE set in 36 pancreatic tumor tissues, and compared the list with previous results on pancreatic cancer and microarrays from 25 different publications, to define a list of target genes involved in pancreatic cancer. This strategy allowed the identification of 135 genes of the 239 from its data set in any of the other studies, some of them with prognosis and survival implications. Collisson et al. (128) were the first to use transcriptomic data to identify subtypes of pancreatic adenocarcinoma, characterized on the basis of their gene expression profiles, with potential implications for therapeutic response [18,19]. These studies need to be validated in independent series. Expression microarrays also have been applied to assess the drug response of pancreatic cancer cell lines, primary cultures, or xenografts. These approaches have identified genes such as *Rrm1, Top2a, Casp3,* and others that have shown resistance to gemcitabine, the standard treatment for advanced pancreatic cancer. A review on gene expression profiling and pancreatic cancer can be consulted in reference [20]. Recently, Gadaleta et al. [21] performed the most significant integrated analysis in pancreas cancer to date using microarrays expression data, for a total of 309 samples from different studies and sources (cancer pancreas samples, cell lines, xenografts) using the same microarray platform. The main findings of this study pointed out that normal samples adjacent to tumors often display transcriptomic changes, and the xenografts and cell line models do not fully recapitulate the transcriptome of primary tumors (detailed results can be consulted in the Pancreatic Expression Database (PED)). This may explain the differences between studies and the difficulty in moving gene expression profiles to the clinic. Another interesting resource for pancreatic cancer studies is the microarray transcriptome characterization in islets of healthy human donors carried out by Dorrel et al. [22]. These authors used cell type-specific surface-reactive antibodies to capture dispersed single cells and to characterize the transcriptome of alpha, beta, large-duct, small-duct, and acinar cells.

Genotyping Microarrays

The largest GWAS conducted in pancreatic cancer was reported by Petersen et al. [23]. This report included 3851 cases and 3934 controls from 20 studies and identified eight SNPs overlapping with three regions associated with pancreatic cancer risk (1q32.1, 5p15.33, and 13q22.1). The region 1q32.1 includes five specific SNPs associated with pancreatic cancer susceptibility for gene *LRH1/NR5A2*, an "orphan" nuclear receptor critical in development. Another SNP identified in 5p15.33 was placed in *CPTM1L-TERT* locus, genes that have been implied in carcinogenesis. The region 13q22.1 is a large nongenic region with two associated SNPs that appear to be specific to pancreatic cancer. As commented previously, genotyping microarrays have been used widely in pancreatic cancer to assess copy number aberrations. Several amplifications have been described in different studies, but those related to oncogenes, such as *KRAS, MYC, or AKT2*, have been described in multiple cases, as well as deletions affecting tumor suppressors, such as *TP53, CDKN2A*, and *SMAD4*. Unfortunately, until now neither RNA- nor DNA-based studies have provided the basis for improved diagnostic or predictive tools. Lack of replication studies together with the challenges related to the disease and the need to obtain samples using invasive procedures contribute to this slow progress. In fact, access to clinical samples is difficult because only 20% of cases with pancreatic cancer undergo surgery and most patients are very sick at the time of diagnosis and have an extremely short life expectancy.

NEXT-GENERATION SEQUENCING

Next-generation sequencing (NGS) is used for the identification of protein binding to chromatin, quantification of RNA levels, and identification of mutations, as well as for other applications. Some bioinformatic processing of the data is common to all of these, as seen in the schematic workflow provided in Figure 5.1.

ChIP-seq

One of the earliest applications of NGS is ChIP-seq. This technique generates genome-wide profiling of DNA-bound proteins by sequencing the DNA fragments hybridized to the proteins recognized by the antibodies. Proteins are therefore in contact with the DNA directly or as part of larger protein complexes [24,25]. ChIP-seq outperforms previous techniques (e.g., ChIP–ChIP microarrays) in terms of resolution, coverage, and dynamic range. It also presents fewer artifacts, for small- and large-scale approaches, including the first genome-scale view of DNA–protein interactions [26], and for these reasons, it has become widely used.

Technique
Briefly, the DNA-binding protein is cross-linked to DNA sheared into small fragments (200–600 bp) and immunoprecipitated with an antibody specific to the protein of interest. The immunoprecipitated DNA fragments then are used as the input for the sequencing library preparation protocol and finally are sequenced. Although the Illumina/Solexa Genome analyzers dominate the NGS market, multiple platforms have been developed.

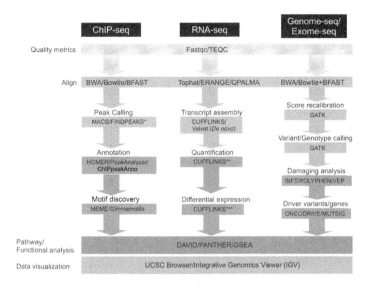

Figure 5.1 *Bioinformatic Analysis Workflow in Next-Generation Sequencing Approaches.* *Additional software in references [17,22,23]. **Additional softwares in references [57,58]. ***Additional software in reference [59]. (For color version of this figure, the reader is referred to the online version of this book.)

ChIP-seq Encyclopedia of DNA Elements Guidelines

Guidelines for good practices and quality metrics for ChIP-seq experiments have been developed by the Encyclopedia of DNA Elements (ENCODE) consortium [27]. In brief, ideally the objective is (1) to obtain ≥10 million uniquely mapping reads per replicate experiment, (2) to generate and sequence a control ChIP library for each experiment (cell type, tissue, or embryo collection), and (3) to perform experiments at least twice to ensure reproducibility.

Bioinformatics Analysis

The first step of the bioinformatics analysis workflow is a quality check, beginning with the use of a browser for the direct inspection of the quality of the raw sequence data. Fastqc [28] or TEQC [29] algorithms are used to assess sequencing error rates, per-base/read Phred scores (a quality score related to the probability of an erroneous call per nucleotide), total number and distribution of the reads along the genome, and read duplication (a potential polymerase chain reaction (PCR) artifact introduced during library construction). These initial quality analyses constitute essential steps for any genome analysis exercise.

Following quality analysis, the raw sequenced reads are aligned to the reference genome. The regions of the genome with repeats, poor quality reads, possible sequencing artifacts, and reads that do not match the reference genome are common problems and can be present at different levels. The obvious recommendation is to use the latest stable release of the reference genome, although in many cases the need to take previous publications into account makes the use of previous versions necessary. Genome references can be downloaded from databases, such as Ensembl [30] or University of California, Santa Cruz (UCSC) [31,32], and visualized using the corresponding browsers.

The vast amount of NGS data has required the development of specific alignment strategies. The most commonly used ones among these are Burrows–Wheeler Aligner (BWA) [33], Bowtie [34], and BLAT-Like Fast Accurate Search Tool (BFAST) [35]. The first two methods are faster than BFAST, although BFAST is more accurate and consumes more memory.

After aligning the reads, a preprocessing step is required to analyze the data. Reads with aligned gaps, more than two mismatches, or multiple alignments in the genome as well as duplicate reads (a potential PCR artifact) are removed for further analysis. Once again, direct visualization of the data in a genome browser is important to assess the quality of the resulting alignments. Moreover, data visualization helps to choose the most appropriate peak caller for the type of signal obtained, to identify the binding regions of the transcription factor (TF) of interest. DNA-bound proteins can provide different binding patterns, while most TFs have narrow signals, others such as chromatin modifications tend to be broader. These differences in the signal patterns require the use of specific algorithms for a correct identification of the true binding sites.

Dozens of peak callers have been developed for the identification of true protein-binding sites from the background of spurious sequence reads. Briefly, DNA fragments pulled down from sense and antisense strands in the immunoprecipitation typically are sequenced as single-ended reads and, therefore, local enrichment is expected in both strands in similar reads. This pattern results in a strand-dependent bimodality of read-density that shifts from the source point (i.e., actual binding site, "summit") by half the average sequenced fragment length and that typically is referred to as the "shift". The reads from both strands will form a single peak where the summit corresponds closely to the binding site [36].

In the typical ChIP-seq experiment, a relatively small number of reads will align directly in true binding sites (peaks), while most of them will represent unspecific binding and can be considered as background. To minimize the prediction of false-positive binding sites, peak callers incorporate different modalities of background correction. In some cases, ChIP-seq experiments use control samples to model the background distribution of reads, in others, the computational methods estimate the background distribution using the experimental data directly. Although both nonspecific immunoglobulin G (IgG) antibodies and random sheared chromatin fragments without previous antibody immunoprecipitation ("input chromatin") have been used as controls, IgG is less recommended because "input chromatin" provides greater, more evenly distributed coverage of the genome [37]. If IgG antibodies are used, they should be of the same species as the relevant antibody; moreover IgG immunoprecipitates much less DNA than specific antibodies. The use of control samples allows for the estimation of the statistical significance of the peaks on the basis of an empirical background. Although different biases have been described in control libraries [38], control samples are important, as open chromatin regions are easier to shear than closed regions and they tend to generate more reads and a higher background signal [39]. Moreover, the heterogeneous efficiency of sequencing in different genome regions and the variable specificity and cross-reactivity of the antibodies [37] complicates the results.

Once the candidate peaks are selected, the main criterion to select the binding sites is the statistical significance of the enrichment relative to the background.

Because the number, size, and position of the detected binding sites, as well as the associated statistical significance, can vary greatly, the choice of a peak detection algorithm is a key question. Even if the default parameters of the peak callers work well in most cases, they might not be optimal for particular cases. The large number of adjustable parameters is, without a doubt, a major complication for the users of peak detection methods. References [36,40,41] describe efforts to compare peak callers.

The predicted binding regions are the entry point for downstream functional analysis, such as motif discovery and annotation. Sequence motifs for DNA-binding proteins are recurrent nucleotide patterns that indicate sequence-specific binding sites, with a presumed biological function. The analysis on DNA sequence motifs has become important because of its role in DNA three-dimensional (3D) structure and gene regulation. In the case of TF with well-defined canonical binding motifs, this information can be used to facilitate the analysis of the quality and confidence of the ChIP-seq peaks. In this sense, motif databases, such as TRANSFAC [42] and JASPAR

[43], can be used to assess the results of the different algorithms. The Multiple Em for Motif Elicitation (MEME) Suite is a good example of a software tool kit that allows for different types of motif analysis, such as motif discovery, motif–motif database searching, motif-sequence database searching, and function assignment [44].

For the exploration of the biological significance of the predicted binding sites, the annotation of the associated genomic features are combined and explored. This process of annotation can be carried out with multiple algorithms [45,46]. Annotations, usually in gene transfer format (GTF), are obtained from Ensembl [30] or UCSC [31] genome references. The methods then carry out the assignment of the peaks to the annotated features—transcription start site (TSS), transcription termination site (TTS), Exon (Coding), 5′ untranslated region (UTR) Exon, 3′ UTR Exon, Intronic, or Intergenic—using a variety of distance statistics. The resulting associations between TF (or other DNA-binding proteins) and genes (or gene features) are then subject to enrichment analysis strategies, as mentioned in the microarrays section, which are applied to such classes as gene ontologies, pathways, disease annotations, or drug target identification. Methods to perform enrichment analysis include the Database for Annotation, Visualization, and Integrated Discovery (DAVID) [47] or the Molecular Signatures Database from GSEA [48]. Finally, in many cases, it is useful to complement the downstream analysis with the direct visualization of the distribution of aligned reads using density heat-map plot methods, such as EpiChIP [49] or SeqMiner [50].

Further ChIP-seq Applications

Further applications of ChIP-seq technology are based on the recognition of other DNA-binding proteins in addition to TFs, including histone modifications, polymerases, and cytosine modifications, which are all of particular interest in epigenomics. Even if all of these applications are technically similar, important differences should be taken into account during the interpretation of the results of the peak callers. TF peaks tend to be narrow, covering a few hundred base pairs, whereas peaks of histone modifications such as H3K27me3 (mark of repression) or H3K36me3 (mark of transcription elongation) tend to be broad and can occupy several kilobases, and Pol II peaks show both patterns, narrow and broad peaks. As noted, the selection of the appropriate peak caller for each type of signal is a key step in the analysis and interpretation of the results, and data visualization can help to choose the best strategy.

Nucleosome positioning plays a key role in organizing higher order chromatin structures in eukaryotic cells. The organization of nucleosomes is important to expose selectively functional important sequence domains and to allow the interaction between DNA and binding proteins that regulate or prevent gene expression. Modifications to ChIP-seq protocols have been developed to identify specific DNA regions potentially associated with nucleosome positioning and regulation of gene expression.

DNase I hypersensitive sites sequencing (DNase-seq) is based on the genome-wide sequencing of free-histone regions sensitive to cleavage by DNase I [51] and requires the permeabilization of cells or isolation of cell nuclei. Alternatively, Formaldehyde-Assisted Isolation of Regulatory Elements sequencing (FAIRE-seq) [52] cross-links the chromatin with formaldehyde, sequestering the DNA linked to histones and leaving histone-free DNA fragments for sequencing. These techniques help to identify DNA regions with nucleosome depletion associated with regulatory chromatin domains. In principle, FAIRE-seq is more adequate to detect distal regulatory elements, whereas DNase-seq is better for detecting promoter regions. Actually, algorithms to handle this type of data are not well established and ChIP-seq peak finders are used in the absence of specific algorithms. Therefore, these algorithms do not completely fit the patterns formed in a DNase-seq or FAIRE-seq experiment. To date, F-seq [53] is considered the most appropriate algorithm to handle this kind of data, but it is limited as it does not have any available statistical assessment and it does not allow for the inclusion of control samples in the analysis.

One more method to determine nucleosome positioning is Micrococcal Nuclease sequencing (MNase-seq), based on the capacity of the micrococcal nuclease restriction enzyme to degrade genomic DNA that is not protected by histones [54]. The sequencing of the remaining DNA reveals the sections of the genome occupied by nucleosomes. MNase-seq can be combined with ChIP-seq to map nucleosomes that contain specific histone modifications. A complete list of software to infer nucleosome positioning from MNase-seq and ChIP-seq histone modifications experiments can be consulted at http://generegulation.info/index.php/nucleosome-positioning.

Once the position of TFs, histone marks, or nucleosomes have been determined, the information can be combined to determine the segmentation of the genome in regions with different levels of regulatory or transcriptional activity. ChromHmm [55] or Segway [56], based on hidden Markov models, are the first generation of methods able to generate genome segmentation corresponding to potential cell type–specific activity patterns.

ChIP-seq Analysis of Pancreatic Cancer

Very little genomic information is available using genome-wide ChIP-seq profiling of pancreatic cancer. Several studies have assessed the occupancy of TFs in normal exocrine pancreas: PTF1A, a TF that regulates exocrine pancreas-specific gene expression, and LRH1/NR5A2 a member of the nuclear receptor family that is required for exocrine differentiation. Holmstrom et al. [24] identified 17,108 binding sites for LRH1, 62% of which were mapped in gene bodies predominantly around the TSS. These genes revealed enrichment for exocrine pancreas-related processes, including digestion, secretion, and mitochondrial metabolism. Out of 17,108 binding sites for LRH1, 1533 colocalized with PRF1 and RBPJL (components of the PTF1-L complex). Further analysis confirmed that LRH1 and the PTF1-L complex cooperate in activating acinar-specific gene transcription [24].

Recently, Tzatsos et al. [25] showed that KDM2B, an H3K36me2 demethylase, promotes tumor development through Polycomb Repressive Complex 2 (PRC2)–mediated gene repression through integral roles in both Polycomb group- and v-myc avian myelocytomatosis viral oncogene homolog (MYC)-mediated transcriptional regulation.

RNA-seq

Expression microarrays have been the standard tool for gene expression quantification for more than a decade, but they now are being replaced by RNA-seq (whole-transcriptome shotgun sequencing), an NGS technology that is able to discover, map, and quantify transcripts. Although both technologies have similar results in terms of relative gene expression quantification, RNA-seq has clear advantages because it covers a wider range of expression values [57,58], it does not have the problems of cross-hybridization typical of microarrays, it provides information about RNA splice events that cannot be obtained by standard expression microarrays, and in general it has the capacity to explore new genome features instead of analyzing only a predetermine version of the genome as occurs with expression arrays [59].

Technique

In general, a population of RNAs, whether total or fractionated, such as poly(A)+, microRNAs (miRNAs), Piwi-interacting RNAs (piRNAs) or short interfering RNAs (siRNAs), is converted to a library of cDNA fragments. During library preparation, cDNA is fragmented into smaller pieces to obtain short sequences that serve as the template for sequencing with or without amplification (to increase the number of DNA copies), from one end (single-end sequencing), which frequently is used for quantification, or from both ends (pair-end sequencing), which is more appropriate for transcript assembly. The usual steps of RNA fragmentation and size selection for 200-base-pair fragments should be taken with care because they may underrepresent the shortest transcripts [60,61].

The typical reads are 30–400 bp, depending on the RNA-seq purpose. For example, short reads (30–60 bp) are more adequate for gene expression quantification, whereas longer (70–400 bp) and pair-end reads are better for detecting connectivity between multiple exons, to interrogate transcriptome isoforms, or to map splicing sites.

RNA-seq ENCODE Guidelines

As with ChIP-seq, the ENCODE consortium developed guidelines, practices, and quality metrics for RNA-seq experiments [62]. To ensure that the data are reproducible, the experiments should be performed with at least two biological replicates having a typical R-squared correlation of gene expression between 0.92 and 0.98 for cell lines, as some variation between biological replicates under the same conditions is expected because of slight technical variations in library preparation, sequencing efficiency, mapping, and others. The correlation can be lower for individuals or samples from transgenic animals or embryos because of differences between individuals.

For experiments that are to evaluate the similarity between the transcriptional profiles of two samples, only modest sequencing depths may be required, for example, one lane yielding 30 million of which 20–25 million reads are mappable. Experiments with the objective of discovering novel transcribed elements will require more extensive sequencing. The ability to detect reliably low-copy-number transcripts depends on the depth of sequencing. Toung et al. [63] stated that in B cells, the expression values of the highly expressed isoforms increased with higher sequencing depths, whereas the isoform with the lowest level of expression was fairly constant. The authors claimed that although 100 million reads are enough to detect most expressed genes and transcripts, about 500 million reads are needed to measure their expression levels accurately.

Bioinformatic Analysis

The steps of quality assessment of the raw sequence are the same for bioinformatic analysis as described for the ChIP-seq experiments. Further steps can include the alignment of the reads to the reference genome or to the proposed reference set of transcripts to produce a genome-scale transcription map or to quantify the level of expression of specific genes.

The alignment methods for available reference genomes are similar to ChIP-seq with the main difference being the alignment of reads across splice junctions. The primary approach is to map the ungapped sequence reads across sequences, representing known splice junctions. This also can be supplemented with any set of predicted splice junctions from spliced expressed sequence tags (ESTs) or gene-finder predictions, such as those implemented by Enhanced Read Analysis of Gene Expression (ERANGE) [59]. All of these approaches, however, ultimately are limited to recovering previously documented splice variants. Alternatively, packages such as TopHat [64] first identify enriched regions representing transcribed fragments (transfrags) and build candidate exon–exon splice junctions to map additional reads across samples. These strategies work much better with data from RNA-seq libraries that preserve information about which strand originally was transcribed. This strategy provides information about adjacent genes transcribed in different strands or antisense transcripts (noncoding) with potential regulatory roles overlapping coding genes. De novo transcriptome assemblies, applying programs such as Velvet [65], are useful to detect chimeric transcripts from chromosomal rearrangements typical of tumors, a complex process that can consume substantial computational resources.

After mapping reads, a final goal is to measure relative gene expression abundance or to capture DGE across multiple samples, even if, in principle, it could be assumed that transcript abundance would be directly proportional to the number of reads aligned on the corresponding transcript or gene. A number of factors, however, have to be taken into account, namely, the length of the transcripts or genes, and the differences in sequencing depth and quality of the compared samples. Reads/fragments per kilobase per million (RPKM/FPKM) is the simplest way to normalize the read count using the length of the transcript or gene and the number of million reads that can be mapped. Therefore, transcript or gene RPKMs/FPKMs allow samples to be directly comparable by providing a relative ranking of expression. To ensure comparability across transcripts, samples, protocols, and platforms, a major normalization effort should be made using standardized spike-in RNA controls of known concentration, defined length, and GC content [9]. A big issue in pancreas RNA-seq experiments is the high levels of expression in acinar genes, which affect the analyses for gene expression, detection, and quantification.

Finally, it is important to find a statistical distribution approximating the nature of the data to compare gene expression across samples. RNA-seq data can be described by a Poisson distribution, but library preparation and mapping errors can increase the variance of the expected distribution (over dispersion). The development of methods to estimate over dispersion is an active field of research and new methods are being developed. So far, RPKMs values can differ between different algorithms and the first comparisons between available methods are now available [66,67]. At the same time, there are different statistical methods to estimate DGE and to provide a statistical measure of the differences between treatments or populations (*p*-values, *q*-values, FDRs, etc.) [68].

In general, the list of genes with differential expression that can be obtained from these experiments have limited interest, and external information is required to infer biological functions. Functional enrichments analysis or network interactions [69,70] based on the list of DGE is the usual procedure, in a similar way to that described previously for microarrays or ChIP-seq experiments. In addition, the GSEA discussed in the microarrays section can be applied in DGE analysis derived from RNA-seq.

RNA-seq in the Pancreas

RNA-seq has been applied to characterize different pancreatic cell populations. Ku et al. [71] characterized the pancreatic β-cell transcriptome in mice providing a useful resource for further analysis. The de novo assembly approach used by these authors not only provided information about gene expression but also allowed the description of promoters and cell-specific patterns of alternative splicing. In addition, these authors described more than 1000 lincRNA expressed in β-cells, most of them β-cell specific. Other interesting resources include the characterization of the pancreatic islet transcriptome carried out by Eizirik et al. [72] or Bramswig et al. [73] and the lncRNAs analyses carried out by Moran et al. [74] in human islet cells. These pancreatic RNA-seq resources might be useful as references for direct comparison with cancer. Studies by Rodriguez-Seguel [75] comparing transcriptomes in hepatic and pancreatic progenitors, isolated from mouse embryo, described gene expression programs in liver and pancreatic progenitors. Moreover, the wingless-type MMTV integration site family (WNT) pathway was described as a potential regulator to reprogram adult hepatic cells into pancreatic cells, whereas at the same time, the WNT pathway has had implications in pancreatic metastases by applying the RNA-seq technique to pancreatic circulating tumor cells [76].

Cancer Genome Sequencing

A large number of articles have been published in the past few years identifying somatic mutational signatures in various cancers based on full cancer genome-sequencing biology.

The technique is based on complete DNA fragmentation of an individual sample, sequencing, and accurate alignments. An alternative to whole-genome sequencing is to target only specific regions of the genome, by selecting them using a specific capture technology. Today's technology can capture up to 70 Mb of exons, noncoding RNAs, noncoding regions with high regulatory potential, or other regions of specific interest. Exome sequencing reduces the cost of sequencing and increases the sensitivity of detection, but it misses variants in regions nontargeted by the capture methods.

Variant calling is highly dependent on alignment quality, which can be improved by the combination of fast aligners, such as BWA with sensitive aligners like BFAST [77]. In addition, a common strategy is to use long and paired-end reads (reads from the 5′ and 3′ ends of the same DNA fragment) to improve the quality of the alignments, particularly in the regions that present a higher variability with respect to the reference genome. Incorrectly aligned reads will imply wrongly predicted variants or wrongly assigned genotypes.

Systems such as the Integrative Genomics Viewer (IGV) [78] commonly are used for the downstream steps of alignment visualization and inspection of specific positions. IGV is a light-weight, high-performance visualization tool that enables intuitive real-time exploration of diverse, large-scale genomic data sets. IGV manage large alignment files in an efficient and fast way. Moreover, IGV provides a summary including the reads supporting the reference and the variant nucleotide in the selected positions.

On the basis of the short-read sequence alignments, variant calling algorithms will determine the positions presenting nucleotide changes, insertions, or deletions with respect to the reference genome. Genotype calling will use these positions to assign genotypes. Variants or genotypes of higher confidence are obtained by combining quality scores and number of reads covering the base or supporting each allele. Other filtering criteria include the differences in quality scores for major and minor alleles; extreme read depths, due to PCR artifacts; and strand bias, different proportion of reads covering the base between strands.

Somatic variants are obtained after comparing the list of variants obtained from tumor and "normal" samples. Variants in both samples are considered as germline variants, whereas variants exclusive of the tumor sample are considered somatic. In solid tumors, "normal" samples frequently are obtained from peripheral blood mononuclear cells, but surgical margins or proximal lymph nodes also commonly are used. In both cases, contaminations cannot be completely disregarded, peripheral blood may contain circulating tumor DNA or tumor cells and marginal tissues might include residual disease or early tumor cells.

Somatic variants include not only single-nucleotide changes but also copy number variations (CNVs), copy-neutral regions of loss of heterogeneity (cnLOH), and inversions and translocations among others. The list of somatic variants from the primary analysis then will be analyzed in a further step to identify potential functional alterations of the corresponding gene and protein products. Single-nucleotide variants in an exon that would change the coding frame or replace a key residue (nonsynonymous mutations) can strongly affect the catalytic function of a given protein and its associated biological function. Even if the prediction of the consequences of point mutations in coding regions is still an area of intense research activity, a number of methods commonly are used to predict the potential pathogenicity of point mutations [79–81].

A second indicator of the importance of the mutations is their accumulation in key genes and mutational hot spots. Indeed, the combination of the damaging potential of the mutations and statistical accumulation (mutation recurrence in a cohort) are the main indicators for the selection potential of driver mutations and drivers genes.

Additionally, some algorithms can include information on copy number alterations and gene expression (RNA-seq to improve the predictions of genes and mutations that could be cancer drivers) [82,83]. A note of caution is necessary in many cases, because genome discovery cohorts often are limited in size and the statistical value of their conclusions should not be overestimated.

Once a list of variants or genes is selected for interpretation, the first approach is to look for known recurrent mutated genes in cancer as *TP53* or *KRAS*. Usually, these lists include a higher number of nonrecurrent mutations that make further interpretations difficult. The upper interpretation step to overcome this issue is to link variations or genes with signaling pathways, protein networks, or a gene ontology database to assess enrichment for functional interpretation. The enrichment is measured by different statistical methods and implemented in algorithms, such as those cited in the microarrays and ChIP-seq sections.

The GSEA method can be applied in gene-ranked lists obtained from Oncodrive [82] or MutSigCV [83]. These methods rank the genes using a score based in sample recurrence or predicted damaging of the variants for each gene, but large cohorts are required for effective results. In addition, variants can be associated with coding regions so that with protein domains, an enrichment analysis can be conducted in protein families with similar domains. The information contained in the Pfam database [84], a database of protein domains, is used. More complex analysis on how the variants affect protein–protein interactions or protein 3D structure can be performed. A revision on cancer genome analysis can be visited in reference [85].

Recently, other tasks such as clonal evolution characterization have led to characterizing cancer types or subtypes [3,4], but the methodology and the bioinformatics approaches that are available are naïve and future improvements are required to address these kind of questions. Moreover, thanks to NGS technology and bioinformatics development, the sequencing genome studies have allowed previously unknown mutational phenomena to be identified, together with descriptions of new variants, driver genes for diseases, and their functional impact.

The novel mutational phenomenon called "kataegis" was first described by Nik-Zainal et al. [3]. This process is characterized by a pattern of hypermutation clusters with the same nucleotide substitution in small genomic regions. Kataegis has been related to defects within the APOBEC protein family, and further studies to determine its role and functional impact in disease are required in the near future. Another new phenomenon described by Stephens et al. [86] is called "chromothripsis". Chromothripsis describes a massive genomic rearrangement in one or more chromosomes in a single catastrophic event during the cells' history, but the mechanism and the functional impact remain unclear. Bioinformatic tools or algorithms to explore these types of processes have not yet been standardized and well-trained bioinformaticians are required to conduct this type of analysis.

The expectations regarding personalized medicine that have been generated over the past few years have increased because of the power of sequencing together with bioinformatic development identifying variants linked to diseases in whole–exome genomes. The main challenge of bioinformatics in this field is to improve the effectiveness of the analysis and interpretation steps, together with a decrease in the variant–gene target identification times and treatment options before deciding on a patient treatment. The combination of information of a different nature, such as the potential disease variants and their altered function, the knowledge about drug targets, and pathological and clinical information could help clinical decisions in the future, as demonstrated by Villarroel et al. [87] and discussed in the next section.

Genome–Exome Sequencing Studies in the Pancreas

A group at Johns Hopkins led the pathway to cancer exome sequencing using the first-generation techniques of PCR amplification of exons and Sanger sequencing analysis. Jones et al. [88] were the first to describe mutational patterns in 24 advanced cases of PDAC. These authors found 39 genes recurrently mutated across the samples; only 4 of these samples, previously known to be involved in pancreatic cancer, showed a probability of harboring passenger mutations <0.001: *KRAS*, *INK4A*, *SMAD4*, and *TP53*. The 39 recurrently mutated genes were further assessed in a prevalence screen, including xenografts, leading to the identification of 12 pathways that were altered consistently in 67% of the cases analyzed as *KRAS*, TGF-β, and Wnt/Notch signaling. A reanalysis of the data that considered familial history of pancreatic cancer led to the identification of a new breast cancer 2, early onset (*BRCA2*)-related pancreatic cancer susceptibility gene: the partner and localizer of *BRCA2* (*PALB2*) [89]. Moreover, Villarroel et al. [87] reported a patient with pancreatic cancer and a germline *PALB2* mutation, identified by sequencing, who was an exceptional responder to the DNA cross-linking agent mitomycin C. These pioneering studies showed the potential of the genome-wide mutational analyses to identify new cancer driver genes that could lead therapeutic intervention in personalized medicine. Subsequent analyses carried out by Roberts et al. [90], sequencing 38 cases of pancreatic cancer from 16 families, identified ataxia telangiectasia mutated (*ATM*) as another familial pancreatic cancer predisposition gene.

The largest sequencing study, carried out using second-generation technology, on 99 pancreatic cancer cases was published by the International Cancer Genome Consortium (ICGC) [5]. Again, this study revealed the predominant involvement of the four major pancreatic cancer genes across tumors with the additional contribution of other genes with a low overall frequency. This study further highlighted the importance of damage repair mechanisms in sporadic PDAC—including both the BRCA and ATM-related pathways—as well as familial disease. Biankin et al. [5] also described a pathway analysis revealing axon guidance as a novel biological function altered in this tumor, related with the activity of the met proto-oncogene (MET) and WNT pathways, possibly providing new therapeutic opportunities. The ICGC also has underscored the difficulties in the genomic study of PDAC, resulting from the associated desmoplasia and the biases derived from the use of samples from patients with resectable tumors.

The analysis of the genome of rare types of pancreatic tumors also has unveiled new drivers involved therein. Studies using fluid from neoplastic pancreatic cysts showed that mutations in five genes (*VHL, RNF43, CTNNB1, GNAS,* and *KRAS*) are able to distinguish among cystic tumor subtypes [91]. Although *VHL* mutations are exclusive in serous cystadenomas and *CTNNB1* are exclusive for solid pseudopapillary neoplasms, intraductal papillary mucinous neoplasms (IPMNs) never have mutations in these genes, and mucinous cystic neoplasms carry exclusively *KRAS* or *RNF43* mutations. Functional annotation has revealed the involvement of genes involved in protein degradation is as important in cystic tumors. The limited number of samples (eight per cyst type) included in these studies calls for independent replication before their application in clinical studies. In fact, the prevalence of *GNAS* and *KRAS* mutations in the IPMN samples study was higher than those performed by Furukawa et al. [92]. The ICGC now has a project dealing with rare and neuroendocrine pancreatic tumors, and it is expected that in the next few years, their genomic landscape will be revealed.

Regarding neoplastic progression, Yachida et al. [93] studied seven metastatic pancreatic cancers with matched primary tumors. These authors were able to define the genomic changes that drive the progression from invasive cancer to widespread metastases. They observed that genetic heterogeneity in metastases is represented and evolved from the original primary tumor. Moreover, timing analysis of the genetic changes from the initial mutation in a cell to the acquisition of metastatic properties takes a long period, more than 10 years. These findings suggest a broad window of opportunity for early pancreatic tumor detection. Similar results were described by Campbell et al. [94] that focused on rearrangements. Many of them in the metastases were present in the primary tumor. Moreover, rearrangements occurred at early stages of the metastases driving clonal expansion. Afterward, a model of PDAC kinetics of metastasis was proposed by Haeno et al. [95].

DATABASES AND RESOURCES

The vast amount of cancer genomic data generated has to be collected, processed, and integrated to be accessible and manageable by the scientific community. This part of the chapter introduces some of the basic resources, placing special emphasis on pancreas data.

Sequence Read Archive

The Sequence Read Archive (SRA) store raw sequence data from NGS tech-nologies. The data stored in this database have increased from ~2Tb of infor-mation in 2009 to more than 1000Tb. The SRA now includes more than 100 different pancreas entries, including ChIP-seq, FAIRE-seq, and RNA-seq experiments among others. The dbGaP study "Expressed Pseudogenes in the Transcriptional Landscape of Human Cancers" includes 28 neoplasms and 25 non-neoplasm samples from the pancreas of human participants. In this study, the authors described a systematic analysis of pseudo-gene transcription from an RNA-seq resource of 293 samples from 13 cancer and normal tissue types, including the pancreas [96]. Another dbGaP study that includes pancreas sam-ples in te SRA, is the Genotype-Tissue Expression (GTEx). Its main goal is to create a data resource to allow for the systematic study of genetic variation and the regulation of gene expression in multiple reference human tissues [97]. Other pancreas-related resources include ChIP-seq data for different TFs related to pancreas development, such as Ptf1a [24,98] or Lrh1 [24], and FAIRE-seq for open chromatin from the ENCODE consortium.

Website: http://www.ncbi.nlm.nih.gov/sra

GenBank and the European Nucleotide Archive

In the GenBank and the European Nucleotide Archive (ENA) repositories are annotated collections of publicly available DNA sequences, such as the SRA GenBank, which have increased the number of DNA sequences from the NGS experiments to more than 167 million sequences, 13,206 of which include the annotation of pancreas. GenBank is divided into three divisions: the main collection called CoreNucleotide; dbEST, which is a collection of short single-read transcript sequences from GenBank, which provides a resource to evaluate gene expression, find potential variation, and annotate genes, with 432,972 annotated for pancreas; and dbGSS (Genome Survey Sequences), which is a collection of unannotated short single-read primar-ily genomic sequences from GenBank, including random survey sequences, clone-end sequences, and exon-trapped sequences.

Website GenBank: http://www.ncbi.nlm.nih.gov/genbank/

Website ENA: http://www.ebi.ac.uk/ena/

The ENCODE Project

The ENCODE project is an international collaboration with the aim of iden-tifying all functional elements in the human genome sequence. The ENCODE project has systematically mapped regions of transcription, TF association, chromatin structure, and histone modification in 147 different cell types. The elements mapped (and approaches used) include RNA transcribed regions (RNA-seq, Cap analysis gene expression, RNA paired-end tags, and manual annotation), protein-coding regions (mass spectrometry), transcription-factor-binding sites (ChIP-seq and DNase-seq), chromatin structure (DNase-seq, FAIRE-seq, histone ChIP-seq, and MNase-seq), and DNA methylation sites (Reduced representation bisulfite sequencing assay). The 9 years of research are summarized in more than two dozen articles published in *Nature*, *Science*, and other journals showing that 80% of DNA has a function (see the *Nature* ENCODE explorer website). All data generated is accessible to download or can be viewed directly in the UCSC browser, enabling researches to integrate the ENCODE with their own data. Table 5.1 shows and describes the seven pancreas cell lines included in the project and Table 5.2 shows the data available for each one with the accession codes, if available.

Website: http://www.genome.gov/10005107

Nature ENCODE explorer website: http://www.nature.com/encode/#/threads

ENCODE at UCSC website: http://genome.ucsc.edu/ENCODE/

Gene Expression Omnibus

The Gene Expression Omnibus (GEO) is a public repository of high-through-put data from microarrays and NGS technologies. This database contains primary data as expression values from RNA-seq experiments or binding sites (peaks) from ChIP-seq. In addition to download data, GEO allows researchers to perform basic analysis. The GEO Profiles database stores gene expression profiles derived from curated GEO DataSets. Each profile is presented as a chart that displays the expression level of one gene across all samples within a data set. Moreover, GEO2R allows for a comparison of two or more groups of samples to identify genes that are differentially expressed across experimental conditions. Currently, 260 entries from among the more than 1400 entries with a pancreas term are studies related to pancreatic cancer.

Website: http://www.ncbi.nlm.nih.gov/geo/

Array-Express

ArrayExpress is the European version of GEO, a database of functional genomics experiments that includes gene expression data from microarrays and high-throughput sequencing studies with public access for the scientific community to download data for downstream analysis.

Website: http://www.ebi.ac.uk/arrayexpress/

Table 5.1 Pancreas Cell Lines Included in the ENCODE Project (17/09/2013)

Cell Type	Description
8988T	Pancreas adenocarcinoma (PA-TU-8988T), "established in 1985 from the liver metastasis of a primary pancreatic adenocarcinoma from a 64-year-old woman"—DSMZ.
BC_Pancreas_H12817N	Pancreas, donor H12817N, age 71 years, Caucasian.
HPDE6-E6E7	Pancreatic duct cells immortalized with E6E7 gene of HPV.
PANC-1	Pancreatic carcinoma, (PMID: 1140870) PANC-1 was established from a pancreatic carcinoma, which was extracted via pancreatico-duodenectomy specimen from a 56-year-old Caucasian individual. Malignancy of this cell line was verified via in vitro and in vivo assays.
Pancreas_OC	Primary frozen pancreas tissue from NCTC donor IDs 09-0144A (Rep B1) and 10-0021A (Rep B2).
PanIsletD	Dedifferentiated human pancreatic islets from the National Disease Research Interchange (NDRI), same source as PanIslets.
PanIslets	Pancreatic islets from two donors, the sources of these primary cells are cadavers from the NDRI and another sample isolated as in Bucher et al., assessment of a novel two-component enzyme preparation for human islet isolation and trans-plantation. *Transplantation* 79, 917 (2005).

Oncomine

Oncomine is a cancer-profiling database containing published data, which has been collected, standardized, annotated, analyzed, and presented to the end user. This database contains data sets available from the GEO and the Stanford Microarray Databases, but of greatest interest is the fact that it includes more downstream analysis than other databases. Differential expression analysis, either in one study or across multiple independent studies, can be performed between cancer and "normal" tissues, high versus low grade, and different outcomes. Further analysis that easily may be performed by researchers includes coexpression or cancer outlier profile analysis (COPA), which searches for the gene expression profiles that display the most profound over-expression in a subset of tumors. Twenty-nine pancreatic cancer microarray data sets are present in this database out of 715 included. Half are from cell lines and the others are from human samples, ranging from 6 to 78 cases.

Website: https://www.oncomine.org/resource/login.html

Table 5.2 Data Type Available in the ENCODE Project for Pancreas Cell Lines (17/09/2013)

Data_Type	Cell_Type	Experimental_Factors	Lab	GEO_Accession	DCC_Accession	Date_Unrestricted
DNase-seq	89988T	none	Duke	GSM816667	wgEncodeEH001103	8/1/2011
Exon Array	89988T	Version=V2	Duke		wgEncodeEH001057	9/16/2010
Exon Array	89988T	none	Duke		wgEncodeEH001057	9/14/2011
Methyl Array	BC_Pancreas_H12817N	LabVersion=Methyl27	HudsonAlpha	GSM999429	wgEncodeEH000870	10/19/2011
Methyl RRBS	BC_Pancreas_H12817N	none	HudsonAlpha	GSM816639	wgEncodeEH001392	12/21/2011
DNase-seq	BC_Pancreas_H12817N	none	Duke		wgEncodeEH001106	9/6/2011
Exon Array	HPDE6-E6E7	Version=V2	Duke		wgEncodeEH001065	9/16/2010
Exon Array	HPDE6-E6E7	none	Duke		wgEncodeEH001065	9/14/2011
ChIP-seq	PANC-1	Antibody=H3K27ac Control=UCDavis Input Control	USC	GSM818826	wgEncodeEH002080	6/19/2012
ChIP-seq	PANC-1	Antibody=H3K4me1_ (pAb-037-050) Control=UCDavis Input Control	USC		wgEncodeEH002081	6/19/2012
ChIP-seq	PANC-1	Antibody=H3K4me3 Control=UCDavis Input Control	UW	GSM945261	wgEncodeEH001911	3/24/2012
ChIP-seq	PANC-1	Antibody=H3K4me3B Control=UCDavis Input Control	USC	GSM945856	wgEncodeEH002876	12/29/2012
ChIP-seq	PANC-1	Antibody=Input	UW		wgEncodeEH001900	3/24/2012
ChIP-seq	PANC-1	Antibody=Input Control=UCDavis Input Control	USC		wgEncodeEH002070	6/19/2012

Continued

Table 5.2 Data Type Available in the ENCODE Project for Pancreas Cell Lines (17/09/2013)—cont'd

Data_Type	Cell_Type	Experimental_Factors	Lab	GEO_Accession	DCC_Accession	Date_Unrestricted
ChIP-seq	PANC-1	Antibody=NRSF Protocol=ChIP AMpure XP	HudsonAlpha	GSM1010859	wgEncodeEH003285	4/28/2013
ChIP-seq	PANC-1	Antibody=NRSF Protocol=PCR 2-round	HudsonAlpha			4/19/2010
ChIP-seq	PANC-1	Antibody=NRSF Protocol=PCR 2-round	HudsonAlpha	GSM803370	wgEncodeEH001552	5/6/2011
ChIP-seq	PANC-1	Antibody=NRSF Protocol=biorupter, PCR 1-round	HudsonAlpha	GSM1010792	wgEncodeEH002280	3/29/2012
ChIP-seq	PANC-1	Antibody=Pol2-4H8 Protocol=biorupter, PCR 1-round	HudsonAlpha	GSM1010788	wgEncodeEH002265	3/27/2012
ChIP-seq	PANC-1	Antibody=RevXlinkChromatin Protocol=ChIP AMpure XP	HudsonAlpha	GSM1010853	wgEncodeEH003429	5/1/2013
ChIP-seq	PANC-1	Antibody=RevXlinkChromatin Protocol=PCR 2-round	HudsonAlpha			4/19/2010
ChIP-seq	PANC-1	Antibody=RevXlinkChromatin Protocol=PCR 2-round	HudsonAlpha	GSM803394	wgEncodeEH001525	10/20/2011
ChIP-seq	PANC-1	Antibody=RevXlinkChromatin Protocol=biorupter, PCR 1-round	HudsonAlpha	GSM1010796	wgEncodeEH002285	4/18/2012

ChIP-seq	PANC-1	Antibcdy=Sin3Ak-20 Protocol=biorupter, PCR 1-round	HudsonAlpha	GSM1010785	wgEncodeEH002266	3/27/2012
ChIP-seq	PANC-1	Antibcdy=TCF7L2 Cortrol=UCDavis Input Cortrol	USC		wgEncodeEH002071	6/19/2012
DNase-seq	PANC-1	none	UW			6/19/2010
DNase-seq	PANC-1	none	UW	GSM736517	wgEncodeEH000500	6/19/2010
Exon Array	PANC-1	none	UW			6/21/2010
Exon Array	PANC-1	none	UW	GSM472939	wgEncodeEH000373	6/21/2010
Genotype	PANC-1	none	HudsonAlpha	GSM999315	wgEncodeEH001276	10/20/2011
Methyl Array	PANC-1	LabVersion=Methyl450K	HudsonAlpha	GSM999395	wgEncodeEH002227	6/30/2012
Methyl RRBS	PANC-1	none	HudsonAlpha	GSM683866	wgEncodeEH001408	10/6/2011
RNA-seq	PANC-1	RnaExtract=Long PolyA+ RNA	HudsonAlpha	GSM923421	wgEncodeEH001251	5/30/2012
ChIP-seq	Pancreas_OC	Antibody=CTCF	UT-A	GSM1006881	wgEncodeEH003463	4/30/2013
ChIP-seq	Pancreas_OC	Antibody=Input	UT-A		wgEncodeEH003454	4/26/2013
FAIRE-seq	Pancreas_OC	none	UNC	GSM1011129	wgEncodeEH003497	3/19/2013
DNase-seq	PanIsletD	none	Duke	GSM816666	wgEncodeEH001102	7/29/2011
Combined	PanIslets	Composite=wgEncodeOpen ChromSynth	Duke	GSM1002652	wgEncodeEH002261	4/28/2012
DNase-seq	PanIslets	none	Duke			9/17/2010
DNase-seq	PanIslets	none	Duke	GSM816660	wgEncodeEH000575	9/17/2010
FAIRE-seq	PanIslets	none	UNC			7/14/2010
FAIRE-seq	PanIslets	none	UNC	GSM864346	wgEncodeEH000573	7/14/2010
Methyl RRBS	PanIslets	none	HudsonAlpha	GSM683874	wgEncodeEH001373	6/29/2011

IntOGen

At the beginning, IntOGen was a database focusing on the analysis of genes and pathways affected by expression and copy number changes in tumors. Data from public studies was summarized and reanalyzed to identify upregulated, downregulated, lost, or amplified genes and pathways in different tissues. Recently, the analysis have been extended to somatic mutations. The platform contains information about driver genes and pathways from 13 different anatomical sites, including pancreas (214 cases). A list of predicted driver genes in pancreatic cancer with this tool is presented in Figure 5.2(A).

Website: http://www.intogen.org/

The Gene Expression Barcode

The Gene Expression Barcode database contains information about the expressed and unexpressed genes in a tissue. This database not only provides information but also allows the users to process their own data.

Website: http://barcode.luhs.org/index.php?page=intro

The Single-Nucleotide Polymorphism Database

The Single-Nucleotide Polymorphism Database (dbSNP) is the largest database of nucleotide variations. Among the variations included are SNPs, short deletion and insertion polymorphisms, microsatellites (short tandem repeats), multinucleotide polymorphisms, and heterozygous sequences. As of version 138 (available April 2013), dbSNP had amassed more than 40.5 million submissions representing more than 9.5 million distinct variants for human. This database is a useful resource for population genetics, evolutionary relationships, pharmacogenomics, or associations of genetic variation with phenotypic features. In genome–exome sequencing projects, dbSNP is useful to discard potential germline variations in predicted somatic variation lists.

Website: http://www.ncbi.nlm.nih.gov/SNP/snp_summary.cgi

The Catalogue of Somatic Mutations in Cancer

The Catalogue of Somatic Mutations in Cancer (COSMIC) collects genomic somatic variations in human cancers curated from the scientific literature or large-scale projects, such as The Cancer Genome Atlas (TCGA). Release version 66 includes more than 1.5 million somatic variants from more than 900,000 samples. COSMIC can be used to perform gene- or tissue-specific analysis to obtain the distribution of variations across the gene

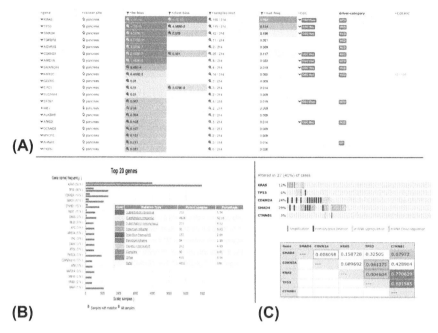

Figure 5.2 *Data Visualization in Different Resources and Databases.* (A) IntOGen view of predicted driver genes in pancreatic cancer. (B) COSMIC top 20 recurrent pancreas mutated genes (left) and total mutations distribution (right). (C) cBioPortal view of the top five recurrent pancreas mutated genes in COSMIC database (up) and co-occurrence analysis (down); Blue→Mutual exclusivity (0 < Odds Ratio < 0.1); Yellow→Tendency toward co-occurrence (2 < Odds Ratio < 10); Orange→Strong tendency toward co-occurrence (Odds Ratio > 10). (For interpretation of the references to color in this figure legend, the reader is referred to the online version of this book.)

or the most frequently mutated genes in a tissue. A summary of 4911 pancreatic tumor mutations included in COSMIC are showed in Figure 5.2(B).

Website: http://cancer.sanger.ac.uk/cancergenome/projects/cosmic/

The cBioPortal for Cancer Genomics

The cBioPortal for Cancer Genomics is a web resource that provides visualization, analysis, and downloads of large-scale cancer genomic data sets. Currently, this database contains 13,106 tumor samples from 43 cancer studies. This tool reduces molecular profiling data from cancer tissues and cell lines into readily understandable genetic, epigenetic, gene expression, and proteomic events. Researchers can explore genetic alterations across samples, tissues, genes, and pathways in an interactive way. When clinical outcomes are available, integrative analysis can be performed. An example of COSMIC data visualization performed in the 66 samples of the pancreatic adenocarcinoma data set with the top five recurrent mutated genes in the pancreas is shown in Figure 5.2(C).

Website: http://www.cbioportal.org/public-portal/index.do

The Cancer Genome Atlas

The TCGA is a large-scale collaborative project to characterize the genomic changes in cancer. TCGA's goal is to advance molecular understanding of cancer to improve diagnosis, treatment, and prevention. For this purpose, all of the data sets and tools that are developed are publicly available to the research community. TCGA collects clinical information, histopathology slide images, and molecular information derived from the samples, such as somatic mutations, RNA/miRNA expression, CNV, and methylation data. The update on September 13, 2013, included 66 samples from pancreatic adenocarcinoma with public access across the TCGA data portal.

Website: http://cancergenome.nih.gov/

The International Cancer Genome Consortium

The ICGC aims to obtain a comprehensive catalogue of genomic, transcriptomic, and epigenomic changes in 50 different tumor types or subtypes and to make the data available to the research community. Five different projects on pancreatic cancer are included in the ICGC. These studies are focused on different pancreatic cancer subtypes (adenocarcinoma, ductal, neuroendocrine, and rare pancreatic exocrine tumors), and raw data from 46 pancreatic adenocarcinoma and 225 ductal adenocarcinomas samples are available across the data portal.

Website: http://icgc.org/#about

The 1000 Genomes Project

The objective of the 1000 Genomes Project is to sequence the genomes of a large number of people and to provide a comprehensive resource on human genetic variation. The goal of this project is to find genetic variants that have frequencies of at least 1% in the populations studied. Although this project is not focused on cancer, the data obtained is useful to filter somatic variants, which could appear in a final list of genome–exome projects, with high frequency in a population.

Website: http://www.1000genomes.org/home

The Cancer Cell Line Encyclopedia

The Cancer Cell Line Encyclopedia (CCLE) project is a detailed genetic and pharmacologic catalogue with a large panel of human cancer cell lines. The CCLE includes 55.7 GB of data, including gene expression, mutations, sample annotations, Affy SNPs, and drug response data. The project server enables researchers to conduct simple analysis or visualization of the available data. The pancreas is represented within 46 cell lines out of 1046 of the total cell lines included.

Website: http://www.broadinstitute.org/ccle/home

The Pancreatic Expression Database

The Pancreatic Expression Database (PED) is the main, specific repository for pancreatic cancer-derived omics data. The database provides an open access tool to mine currently available pancreatic cancer experimental data sets generated by using large-scale transcriptomic, genomic, proteomic, miRNA and methylomic platforms. The website also provides users the opportunity to include their own data set in the database. Currently, the PED includes around 100 manually processed and checked public studies. Moreover, the Pancreatic Expression Landscape tool derived from the Gadaleta et al. [21] (as discussed in the microarrays section), enables researchers to conduct meta-analysis by integrating data from diverse resources.

Website: http://www.pancreasexpression.org/index.html

CONCLUSION AND FUTURE PERSPECTIVES

The technology revolution propelled by the Human Genome Project has made substantial inroads in the field of medicine, especially cancer treatment. Bioinformatics is an integral part of this technology revolution and has become essential in the interpretation of the genomic information. As such, it is a fundamental element in the study of the molecular causes of pancreatic cancer pathophysiology. This chapter provided an overview of the bioinformatics analysis that currently is being applied to genome-wide studies in the field of pancreatic cancer. These bioinformatics methodologies cover a wide range of topics, from data organization to the assessment of sample quality and from the analysis of sequencing data to the prediction of cancer driver genes and processes. The various stages of the bioinformatics analysis, with actual examples taken from pancreatic cancer genome projects, and with descriptions of the available technologies and resources in each case were illustrated. The current limitations in the interpretation of cancer genome data, difficulties in the integration of clinical and genomic data, and challenges in the interpretation of the genomic information in clinical settings also were highlighted. It is anticipated that in the this decade the field will witness major efforts in utilizing these technologies in the diagnosis as well as development of successful therapeutics for the deadly pancreatic cancer.

ACKNOWLEDGEMENTS

This work was partially supported by the Spanish National Bioinformatics Institute (INB) and grants BIO2012-40205, SAF2011-29530 (MINECO, Spain) and COST Action #BM1204: EU_Pancreas (European Cooperation in Science and Technology).

REFERENCES

[1] International Human Genome Sequencing Consortium. Finishing the euchromatic sequence of the human genome. Nature 2004;431:931–45.

[2] Stratton MR, Campbell PJ, Futreal PA. The cancer genome. Nature 2009;458(7239): 719–24.

[3] Nik-Zainal S, Alexandrov LB, Wedge DC, Van Loo P, Greenman CD, Raine K, et al. Mutational processes molding the genomes of 21 breast cancers. Cell 2012;149(5): 979–93.

[4] Nik-Zainal S, Van Loo P, Wedge DC, Alexandrov LB, Greenman CD, Lau KW, et al. The life history of 21 breast cancers. Cell 2012;149(5):994–1007.

[5] Biankin AV, Waddell N, Kassahn KS, Gingras MC, Muthuswamy LB, Johns AL, et al. Pancreatic cancer genomes reveal aberrations in axon guidance pathway genes. Nature 2012;491(7424):399–405.

[6] Quackenbush J. Microarray data normalization and transformation. Nat Genet 2002;32(Suppl.):496–501.

[7] Welsh JB, Sapinoso LM, Su AI, Kern SG, Wang-Rodriguez J, Moskaluk CA, et al. Analysis of gene expression identifies candidate markers and pharmacological targets in prostate cancer. Cancer Res 2001;61:5974–8.

[8] Yu Z, Ford BN, Glickman BW. Identification of genes responsive to BPDE treatment in HeLa cells using cDNA expression assays. Environ Mol Mutagen 2000;36:201–5.

[9] Jiang L, Schlesinger F, Davis CA, Zhang Y, Li R, Salit M, et al. Synthetic spike-in standards for RNA-seq experiments. Genome Res 2011;21:1543–51.

[10] Smyth GK. Limma: linear models for microarray data. In: Gentleman R, Carey V, Dudoit S, Irizarry R, Huber W, editors. Bioinformatics and computational biology solutions using R and bioconductor. New York: Springer; 2005. pp. 397–420.

[11] Carro A, Rico D, Rueda OM, Díaz-Uriarte R, Pisano DG. waviCGH: a web application for the analysis and visualization of genomic copy number alterations. Nucleic Acids Res 2010;38:W182–7.

[12] Crnogorac-Jurcevic T, Missiaglia E, Blaveri E, Gangeswaran R, Jones M, Terris B, et al. Molecular alterations in pancreatic carcinoma: expression profiling shows that dysregulated expression of S100 genes is highly prevalent. J Pathol 2003;201(1):63–74.

[13] Iacobuzio-Donahue CA, Maitra A, Olsen M, Lowe AW, van Heek NT, Rosty C, et al. Exploration of global gene expression patterns in pancreatic adenocarcinoma using cDNA microarrays. Am J Pathol 2003;162(4):1151–62.

[14] Logsdon CD, Simeone DM, Binkley C, Arumugam T, Greenson JK, Giordano TJ, et al.
      Molecular profiling of pancreatic adenocarcinoma and chronic pancreatitis identifies
      multiple genes differentially regulated in pancreatic cancer. Cancer Res 2003;63(10):
      2649–57.
[15] Friess H, Ding J, Kleeff J, Fenkell L, Rosinski JA, Guweidhi A, et al. Microarray-based
      identification of differentially expressed growth- and metastasis-associated genes in
      pancreatic cancer. Cell Mol Life Sci 2003;60(6):1180–99.
[16] Grützmann R, Boriss H, Ammerpohl O, Lüttges J, Kalthoff H, Schackert HK, et al.
      Meta-analysis of microarray data on pancreatic cancer defines a set of commonly dys-
      regulated genes. Oncogene 2005;24(32):5079–88.
[17] Badea L, Herlea V, Dima SO, Dumitrascu T, Popescu I. Combined gene expression
      analysis of whole-tissue and microdissected pancreatic ductal adenocarcinoma identi-
      fies genes specifically overexpressed in tumor epithelia. Hepatogastroenterology
      2008;55(88):2016–27.
[18   Collisson EA, Sadanandam A, Olson P, Gibb WJ, Truitt M, Gu S, et al. Subtypes of
      pancreatic ductal adenocarcinoma and their differing responses to therapy. Nat Med
      2011;17(4):500–3.
[19   Donahue TR, Tran LM, Hill R, Li Y, Kovochich A, Calvopina JH, et al. Integrative
      survival-based molecular profiling of human pancreatic cancer. Clin Cancer Res
      2012;18(5):1352–63.
[20] López-Casas PP, López-Fernández LA. Gene-expression profiling in pancreatic cancer.
      Expert Rev Mol Diagn 2010;10(5):591–601.
[21] Gadaleta E, Cutts RJ, Kelly GP, Crnogorac-Jurcevic T, Kocher HM, Lemoine NR,
      et al. A global insight into a cancer transcriptional space using pancreatic data: impor-
      tance, findings and flaws. Nucleic Acids Res 2011;39(18):7900–7.
[22] Dorrell C, Schug J, Lin CF, Canaday PS, Fox AJ, Smirnova O, et al. Transcriptomes of
      the major human pancreatic cell types. Diabetologia 2011;54(11):2832–44.
[23] Petersen GM, Amundadottir L, Fuchs CS, Kraft P, Stolzenberg-Solomon RZ, Jacobs KB,
      et al. A genome-wide association study identifies pancreatic cancer susceptibility loci on
      chromosomes 13q22.1, 1q32.1 and 5p15.33. Nat Genet 2010;42(3):224–8.
[24] Holmstrom SR, Deering T, Swift GH, Poelwijk FJ, Mangelsdorf DJ, Kliewer SA, et al.
      LRH-1 and PTF1-L coregulate an exocrine pancreas-specific transcriptional network
      for digestive function. Genes Dev 2011;25(16):1674–9.
[25] Tzatsos A, Paskaleva P, Ferrari F, Deshpande V, Stoykova S, Contino G, et al. KDM2B
      promotes pancreatic cancer via Polycomb-dependent and -independent transcriptional
      programs. J Clin Invest 2013;123(2):727–39.
[26] Ho JW, Bishop E, Karchenko PV, Nègre N, White KP, Park PJ. ChIP-chip versus
      ChIP-seq: lessons for experimental design and data analysis. BMC Genomics
      2011;2:134.
[27] Landt SG, Marinov GK, Kundaje A, Kheradpour P, Pauli F, Batzoglou S, et al. ChIP-
      seq guidelines and practices of the ENCODE and modENCODE consortia. Genome
      Res 2012;22(9):1813–31.
[28] http://www.bioinformatics.bbsrc.ac.uk/projects/fastqc.
[29] Hummel M, Bonnin S, Lowy E, Roma G. TEQC: an R package for quality control in
      target capture experiments. Bioinformatics 2011;27(9):1316–7.
[30] Flicek P, Ahmed I, Amode MR, Barrell D, Beal K, Brent S, et al. Ensembl 2013. Nucleic
      Acids Res 2013;41(Database issue):D48–55.
[31] Meyer LR, Zweig AS, Hinrichs AS, Karolchik D, Kuhn RM, Wong M, et al. The
      UCSC Genome Browser database: extensions and updates 2013. Nucleic Acids Res
      2012;41(D1):D64–9.
[32] Kent WJ, Sugnet CW, Furey TS, Roskin KM, Pringle TH, Zahler AM, et al. The human
      genome browser at UCSC. Genome Res 2002;12(6):996–1006.

[33] Li H, Durbin R. Fast and accurate short read alignment with Burrows-Wheeler transform. Bioinformatics 2009;25:1754–60.

[34] Langmead B, Trapnell C, Pop M, Salzberg SL. Ultrafast and memory-efficient alignment of short DNA sequences to the human genome. Genome Biol 2009;10(3):R25.

[35] Homer N, Merriman B, Nelson SF. BFAST: an alignment tool for large scale genome resequencing. PLoS One 2009;4(11):e7767.

[36] Wilbanks EG, Facciotti MT. Evaluation of algorithm performance in ChIP-seq peak detection. PLoS One 2010;5(7):e11471.

[37] Kidder BL, Hu G, Zhao K. ChIP-Seq: technical considerations for obtaining high-quality data. Nat Immunol 2011;12:918–22.

[38] Vega VB, Cheung E, Palanisamy N, Sung WK. Inherent signals in sequencing-based Chromatin-ImmunoPrecipitation control libraries. PLoS One 2009;4(4):e5241.

[39] Teytelman L, Ozaydin B, Zill O, Lefrançois P, Snyder M, Rine J, et al. Impact of chromatin structures on DNA processing for genomic analyses. PLoS One 2009;4(8):e6700.

[40] Laajala TD, Raghav S, Tuomela S, Lahesmaa R, Aittokallio T, Elo LL. A practical comparison of methods for detecting transcription factor binding sites in ChIP-seq experiments. BMC Genomics 2009;10:618.

[41] Micsinai M, Parisi F, Strino F, Asp P, Dynlacht BD, Kluger Y. Picking ChIP-seq peak detectors for analyzing chromatin modification experiments. Nucleic Acids Res 2012;40(9):e70.

[42] Matys V, Kel-Margoulis OV, Fricke E, Liebich I, Land S, Barre-Dirrie A, et al. TRANSFAC and its module TRANSCompel: transcriptional gene regulation in eukaryotes. Nucleic Acids Res 2006;34:D108–10.

[43] Bryne JC, Valen E, Tang MH, Marstrand T, Winther O, da Piedade I, et al. JASPAR, the open access database of transcription factor-binding profiles: new content and tools in the 2008 update. Nucleic Acids Res 2008;36:D102–6.

[44] Bailey TL, Bodén M, Buske FA, Frith M, Grant CE, Clementi L, et al. MEME SUITE: tools for motif discovery and searching. Nucleic Acids Res 2009;37:W202–8.

[45] Salmon-Divon M, Dvinge H, Tammoja K, Bertone P. PeakAnalyzer: genome-wide annotation of chromatin binding and modification loci. BMC Bioinformatics 2010;11:415.

[46] Zhu LJ, Gazin C, Lawson ND, Pagès H, Lin SM, Lapointe DS, et al. ChIPpeakAnno: a Bioconductor package to annotate ChIP-seq and ChIP-chip data. BMC Bioinformatics 2010;11:237.

[47] Huang da W, Sherman BT, Lempicki RA. Systematic and integrative analysis of large gene lists using DAVID bioinformatics resources. Nat Protoc 2009;4(1):44–57.

[48] Liberzon A, Subramanian A, Pinchback R, Thorvaldsdóttir H, Tamayo P, Mesirov JP. Molecular signatures database (MSigDB) 3.0. Bioinformatics 2011;27(12):1739–40.

[49] Hebenstreit D, Gu M, Haider S, Turner DJ, Liò P, Teichmann SA. EpiChIP: gene-by-gene quantification of epigenetic modification levels. Nucleic Acids Res 2011;39(5):e27.

[50] Ye T, Krebs AR, Choukrallah MA, Keime C, Plewniak F, Davidson I, et al. seqMINER: an integrated ChIP-seq data interpretation platform. Nucleic Acids Res 2011;39(6):e35.

[51] Crawford GE, Holt IE, Whittle J, Webb BD, Tai D, Davis S, et al. Genome-wide mapping of DNase hypersensitive sites using massively parallel signature sequencing (MPSS). Genome Res 2006;16(1):123–31.

[52] Giresi PG, Kim J, McDaniell RM, Iyer VR, Lieb JD. FAIRE (Formaldehyde-Assisted Isolation of Regulatory Elements) isolates active regulatory elements from human chromatin. Genome Res 2007;17(6):877–85.

[53] Boyle AP, Guinney J, Crawford GE, Furey TS. F-Seq: a feature density estimator for high-throughput sequence tags. Bioinformatics 2008;24(21):2537–8.

[54] Cui K, Zhao K. Genome-wide approaches to determining nucleosome occupancy in metazoans using MNase-Seq. Methods Mol Biol 2012;833:413–9.

[55] Ernst J, Kellis M. ChromHMM: automating chromatin-state discovery and characterization. Nat Methods 2012;9(3):215–6.

[56] Hoffman MM, Buske OJ, Wang J, Weng Z, Bilmes JA, Noble WS. Unsupervised pattern discovery in human chromatin structure through genomic segmentation. Nat Methods 2012;9(5):473–6.

[57] Nookaew I, Papini M, Pornputtpong N, Scalcinati G, Fagerberg L, Uhlén M, et al. A comprehensive comparison of RNA-Seq-based transcriptome analysis from reads to differential gene expression and cross comparison with microarrays: a case study in *Saccharomyces cerevisiae*. Nucleic Acids Res 2012;40:10084–97.

[58] Marioni JC, Mason CE, Mane SM, Stephens M, Gilad Y. RNA-seq: an assessment of technical reproducibility and comparison with gene expression arrays. Genome Res 2008;18:1509–17.

[59] Mortazavi A, Williams BA, McCue K, Schaeffer L, Wold B. Mapping and quantifying mammalian transcriptomes by RNA-Seq. Nat Methods 2008;5:621–8.

[60] Oshlack A, Wakefield MJ. Transcript length bias in RNA-seq data confounds systems biology. Biol Direct 2009;4:14.

[61] Bullard JH, Purdom EA, Hansen KD, Durinck S, Dudoit S. Statistical inference in mRNA-seq: exploratory data analysis and differential expression. UC Berkeley Division of Biostatistics Working Paper Series 2009;247.

[62] http://encodeproject.org/ENCODE/protocols/dataStandards/RNA_standards_v1_2011_May.pdf.

[63] Toung JM, Morley M, Li M, Cheung VG. RNA-sequence analysis of human B-cells. Genome Res 2011;21(6):991–8.

[64] Trapnell C, Pachter L, Salzberg SL. TopHat: discovering splice junctions with RNA-Seq. Bioinformatics 2009;25(9):1105–11.

[65] Zerbino DR, Birney E. Velvet: algorithms for de novo short read assembly using de Bruijn graphs. Genome Res 2008;18(5):821–9.

[66] Kvam VM, Liu P, Si Y. A comparison of statistical methods for detecting differentially expressed genes from RNA-seq data. Am J Bot 2012;99(2):248–56.

[67] Robles JA, Qureshi SE, Stephen SJ, Wilson SR, Burden CJ, Taylor JM. Efficient experimental design and analysis strategies for the detection of differential expression using RNA-sequencing. BMC Genomics 2012;13:484.

[68] Nookaew I, Papini M, Pornputtpong N, Scalcinati G, Fagerberg L, Uhlén M, et al. A comprehensive comparison of RNA-Seq-based transcriptome analysis from reads to differential gene expression and cross-comparison with microarrays: a case study in *Saccharomyces cerevisiae*. Nucleic Acids Res 2012;14:91.

[69] Pastrello C, Otasek D, Fortney K, Agapito G, Cannataro M, Shirdel E, et al. Visual data mining of biological networks: one size does not fit all. PLoS Comput Biol 2013;9(1):e1002833.

[70] Szklarczyk D, Franceschini A, Kuhn M, Simonovic M, Roth A, Minguez P, et al. The STRING database in 2011: functional interaction networks of proteins, globally integrated and scored. Nucleic Acids Res 2011;39:D561–8.

[71] Ku GM, Kim H, Vaughn IW, Hangauer MJ, Myung Oh C, German MS, et al. Research resource: RNA-Seq reveals unique features of the pancreatic β-cell transcriptome. Mol Endocrinol 2012;26(10):1783–92.

[72] Eizirik DL, Sammeth M, Bouckenooghe T, Bottu G, Sisino G, Igoillo-Esteve M, et al. The human pancreatic islet transcriptome: expression of candidate genes for type 1 diabetes and the impact of pro-inflammatory cytokines. PLoS Genet 2012;8(3):e1002552.

[73] Bramswig NC, Everett LJ, Schug J, Dorrell C, Liu C, Luo Y, et al. Epigenomic plasticity enables human pancreatic α to β cell reprogramming. J Clin Invest 2013;123(3):1275–84.

[74] Morán I, Akerman I, van de Bunt M, Xie R, Benazra M, Nammo T, et al. Human β cell transcriptome analysis uncovers lncRNAs that are tissue-specific, dynamically regulated, and abnormally expressed in type 2 diabetes. Cell Metab 2012;16(4):435–48.

[75] Rodríguez-Seguel E, Mah N, Naumann H, Pongrac IM, Cerdá-Esteban N, Fontaine JF, et al. Mutually exclusive signaling signatures define the hepatic and pancreatic progenitor cell lineage divergence. Genes Dev 2013;27(17):1932–46.

[76] Yu M, Ting DT, Stott SL, Wittner BS, Ozsolak F, Paul S, et al. RNA sequencing of pancreatic circulating tumour cells implicates WNT signalling in metastasis. Nature 2012;487(7408):510–3.

[77] Rubio-Camarillo M, Gómez-López G, Fernández JM, Valencia A, Pisano DG. RUbio-Seq: a suite of parallelized pipelines to automate exome variation and bisulfite-seq analyses. Bioinformatics 2013;29(13):1687–9.

[78] Thorvaldsdóttir H, Robinson JT, Mesirov JP. Integrative Genomics Viewer (IGV): high-performance genomics data visualization and exploration. Brief Bioinform 2013;14(2):178–92.

[79] Kumar P, Henikoff S, Ng PC. Predicting the effects of coding non-synonymous variants on protein function using the SIFT algorithm. Nat Protoc 2009;4(7):1073–81.

[80] Adzhubei IA, Schmidt S, Peshkin L, Ramensky VE, Gerasimova A, Bork P, et al. A method and server for predicting damaging missense mutations. Nat Methods 2010;7(4):248–9.

[81] McLaren W, Pritchard B, Rios D, Chen Y, Flicek P, Cunningham F. Deriving the consequences of genomic variants with the Ensembl API and SNP Effect Predictor. BMC Bioinformatics 2010;26(16):2069–70.

[82] Gonzalez-Perez A, Lopez-Bigas N. Functional impact bias reveals cancer drivers. Nucleic Acids Res 2012;40(21):e169.

[83] Lawrence MS, Stojanov P, Polak P, Kryukov GV, Cibulskis K, Sivachenko A, et al. Mutational heterogeneity in cancer and the search for new cancer-associated genes. Nature 2013 Jul 11;499(7457):214–8.

[84] Punta M, Coggill PC, Eberhardt RY, Mistry J, Tate J, Boursnell C, et al. The Pfam protein families database. Nucleic Acids Res 2012;40:D290–301.

[85] Vazquez M, de la Torre V, Valencia A. Cancer genome analysis. PLoS Comput Biol 2012;8(12):e1002824.

[86] Stephens PJ, Greenman CD, Fu B, Yang F, Bignell GR, Mudie LJ, et al. Massive genomic rearrangement acquired in a single catastrophic event during cancer development. Cell 2011;144(1):27–40.

[87] Villarroel MC, Rajeshkumar NV, Garrido-Laguna I, De Jesus-Acosta A, Jones S, Maitra A, et al. Personalizing cancer treatment in the age of global genomic analyses: PALB2 gene mutations and the response to DNA damaging agents in pancreatic cancer. Mol Cancer Ther 2011;10(1):3–8.

[88] Jones S, Zhang X, Parsons DW, Lin JC, Leary RJ, Angenendt P, et al. Core signaling pathways in human pancreatic cancers revealed by global genomic analyses. Science 2008;321(5897):1801–6.

[89] Jones S, Hruban RH, Kamiyama M, Borges M, Zhang X, Parsons DW, et al. Exomic sequencing identifies PALB2 as a pancreatic cancer susceptibility gene. Science 2009;324(5924):217.

[90] Roberts NJ, Jiao Y, Yu J, Kopelovich L, Petersen GM, Bondy ML, et al. ATM mutations in patients with hereditary pancreatic cancer. Cancer Discov 2012;2(1):41–6.

[91] Wu J, Jiao Y, Dal Molin M, Maitra A, de Wilde RF, Wood LD, et al. Whole-exome sequencing of neoplastic cysts of the pancreas reveals recurrent mutations in components of ubiquitin-dependent pathways. Proc Natl Acad Sci USA 2011;108(52):21188–93.

[92] Furukawa T, Kuboki Y, Tanji E, Yoshida S, Hatori T, Yamamoto M, et al. Whole-exome sequencing uncovers frequent GNAS mutations in intraductal papillary mucinous neoplasms of the pancreas. Sci Rep 2011;1:161.

[93] Yachida S, Jones S, Bozic I, Antal T, Leary R, Fu B, et al. Distant metastasis occurs late during the genetic evolution of pancreatic cancer. Nature 2010;467(7319):1114–7.

[94] Campbell PJ, Yachida S, Mudie LJ, Stephens PJ, Pleasance ED, Stebbings LA, et al. The patterns and dynamics of genomic instability in metastatic pancreatic cancer. Nature 2010;467(7319):1109–13.

[95] Haeno H, Gonen M, Davis MB, Herman JM, Iacobuzio-Donahue CA, Michor F. Computational modeling of pancreatic cancer reveals kinetics of metastasis suggesting optimum treatment strategies. Cell 2012;148(1–2):362–75.

[96] Kalyana-Sundaram S, Kumar-Sinha C, Shankar S, Robinson DR, Wu YM, Cao X, et al. Expressed pseudogenes in the transcriptional landscape of human cancers. Cell 2012;149(7):1622–34.

[97] GTEx Consortium. The Genotype-Tissue Expression (GTEx) project. Nat Genet 2013;45(6):580–5.

[98] Meredith DM, Borromeo MD, Deering TG, Casey BH, Savage TK, Mayer PR, et al. Program specificity for Ptf1a in pancreas versus neural tube development correlates with distinct collaborating cofactors and chromatin accessibility. Mol Cell Biol 2013;33(16):3166–79.

Statistical Analysis of High-Dimensional Data for Pancreatic Cancer

Haijun Gong[1,*], Tong Tong Wu[2,*], Edmund Clarke[3]
[1]Department of Mathematics and Computer Science, Saint Louis University, St. Louis, MO, USA,
[2]Department of Biostatistics and Computational Biology, University of Rochester, Rochester, NY, USA,
[3]Computer Science Department, Carnegie Mellon University, Pittsburgh, PA, USA

Contents

Introduction	133
LASSO Penalized Cox Regression	137
Variable Selection via LASSO Regularized Partial Likelihood	137
Cyclic Coordinate Descent for LASSO Penalized Cox Regression	138
Doubly Regularized Cox Regression	140
Doubly Regularized Cox Regression for Non-Overlap Case	140
Coordinate Descent Algorithm for DrCox Regression	141
DrCox Regression via Coordinate Descent for Overlap Cases	143
Pancreatic Cancer Survival Analysis	144
Microarray Data and Signaling Pathways	144
Data Analysis with LASSO Penalized Cox Regression	145
Data Analysis with Doubly Regularized Cox Regression	145
References	148

INTRODUCTION

Pancreatic ductal adenocarcinoma (PDAC) is the most common type of pancreatic cancer, arising from the lesions that occur in pancreatic ducts. It is one of the leading causes of cancer deaths in the United States due to poor diagnosis in the early stage [1]. Despite extensive research over the past 30 years, the five-year survival rate is still less than 5%, and we are still far from developing effective strategies for the early diagnosis and treatment of this lethal disease [2,3]. PDAC is characterized by early and aggressive metastasis and high resistance to conventional chemotherapy and

---

* Equally contributed first authors.

radiotherapy due to the stromal interaction between the pancreatic cancer cells and fibrous tissue composed of extracellular matrix (ECM) proteins [4]. Tumor signaling is regulated by the complex interactions of thousands of genes and tens or hundreds of signaling pathways. The cross talk between different signaling pathways may be responsible for the pancreatic cancer cell survival even if some pathways are blocked by certain single-gene targeted therapies.

Modern molecular pathologic and genetic technologies have changed the way that we study the complex biological systems. Researchers in the area of pancreatic cancer are able to make genome-wide expression profiling [5,6] within tumors in order to better understand the nature of the disease and eventually design multigene targeted therapy. To analyze those high throughput data, statistical methods are designed and developed specifically to those types of data [7–11]. Due to the high-dimensional nature, two major approaches—feature extraction and feature selection—have been taken to extract the important information from the massive data. The feature extraction approach, for example, principal component analysis (PCA), projects the high-dimensional feature spaces into lower dimensions; while the feature selection approach, for example, least absolute shrinkage and selection operator (LASSO), selects a subset of features from the large number of candidates in the data [10]. The shortcomings associated with the feature extraction approach are well recognized, which include lack of meaningful scientific interpretation. Therefore we focus on the second approach and introduce two statistical methods for high-dimensional data in the chapter. The advantages of the feature selection approach include, but are not limited to, alleviating the effect of the curse of dimensionality, retaining scientific meaning, enhancing generalization capability, improving stability, and accelerating computational speed [12]. This approach can be used in many areas, and, of course, include pancreatic cancer studies.

For different purposes, different statistical models and methods are used to explore novel molecular and epigenetic targets for pancreatic cancer from DNA microarray data and RNA sequencing data. A number of differentially expressed and metastasis-associated genes have been found in pancreatic cancer. For example, recent global genomic analyses [5] identified 69 gene sets and 12 core signaling pathways that are frequently mutated in most pancreatic cancers. Most of those studies focused on the inference and identification of the frequently mutated or metastasis-associated genes. However, an important clinical factor—survival time—has been neglected for a long time. The two methods introduced in this chapter focus on survival analysis in high-dimensional data. Similar ideas can be used in other statistical models (e.g., regression and generalized linear regression) in different studies.

A comprehensive understanding of the genetic signatures and signaling pathways that are directly correlated with pancreatic cancer survival will help cancer researchers to develop effective multigene targeted and personalized therapies for pancreatic cancer patients at different stages of the disease, and improve their survival rates. Stratford et al.'s work [13] analyzed the microarray data of 102 PDAC patients and identified six genetic signatures associated with metastatic pancreatic cancer using a sequence of statistical techniques, including the significance analysis of microarray (SAM) [14], centroid-based predictor [15], Pearson correlation, X-Tile [16], Kaplan–Meier estimator [17], and Cox model [18]. Though the authors applied the Cox model to test whether the six-gene signature is significantly correlated with survival time, the prediction was not based on survival time. These genes could only help discriminate high- and low-risk patients, and they are not directly related to pancreatic cancer survival. The two methods in this chapter are to infer and identify the genetic information that is directly associated with survival time. Both are based on the Cox proportional hazards model [18], which is a classic model used to describe the relationship between survival time and predictor variables.

Survival data differ from the data we usually observe because of the partial missingness. Partial missingness occurs in two forms: censoring and truncation. Right censoring is the most commonly observed type in survival analysis, and we deal with right-censored data here. Ideally, the time when the event of interest happens is observed and collected, but sometimes we only know that the event happens after some time but not exactly when. The former is true survival time and the latter is right-censored survival time. For example, a study is performed to measure the lifetime of cancer patients. If the death of a patient is observed, the lifetime of the patient is known (complete data, as it is safe to assume the birth is known). If the patient is still alive when the study ends, it is only known that the death date is after the study's endpoint (right-censored). Here the event of interest is the survival time of the pancreatic cancer patient, so event/survival time is when the patient dies. Right censoring also occurs for the loss-to-follow-up subjects. With censored observations, the censoring effect has to be considered for unbiased estimation. The Cox proportional hazards model can handle right-censored data with a simple form and easy interpretation. The downside of the Cox model is that it requires the proportionality assumption of the hazards rates, which is strong and not valid in some cases.

In high-dimensional data, the number of features/predictors (genes) far exceeds the number of subjects (patients). The goal of the feature selection approach is to identify a subset of predictors from the large pool of candidates. To this end, one can use the regularization method and penalize the Cox model [8,9,19–21]. For example, a LASSO penalty can be imposed to individual variables to automatically remove unimportant ones by shrinking their regression coefficients to be exactly zero [9]. In this chapter, we first describe a LASSO penalized Cox regression method on individual genes [11]. This model has been applied to analyze the localized and resected PDAC data collected between 1999 and 2007. Twelve signature genes that are directly correlated to the pancreatic cancer survival time are found out of 43,376 probes using this model. Eight of the 12 genes are confirmed to be genetically altered and differentially expressed in the cancer of stomach, colon, ovaries, breast, skin, kidney, lung, and pancreas in in vivo and in vitro experiments [22–27]. As some genes belong to the same pathways and get involved in the same biological processes, it is important to incorporate the pathway information into the analysis. The pathway information is biologically essential to our understanding of gene regulatory network and cancer development [5]. Therefore, we introduce a doubly penalized Cox regression method secondly. By imposing two penalties, one on pathways and the other on individual genes, we can achieve both group and within-group selection for the pancreatic cancer survival analysis. Both models need well-designed computational algorithms for the high-dimensionality data. Cyclic coordinate descent algorithms will also be described in this chapter.

In the next section, we describe the LASSO regularized Cox regression based on the partial likelihood function and the coordinate descent algorithm, which can quickly dismiss irrelevant variables and speed up the estimation of the regression coefficients. Later, we describe the non-overlap and overlap cases of doubly regularized Cox (DrCox) regression model. A modified version of the cyclic coordinate descent algorithms for parameter estimation is also talked about. At last, we apply the two methods to analyze the high-dimensional microarray data of pancreatic cancer patients with localized and resected PDAC collected between 1999 and 2007. The genes and pathways that are found by the two methods are shown in this section.

LASSO PENALIZED COX REGRESSION

The LASSO penalized regression method is a popular variable selection technique used for the analysis of the high-throughput and high-dimensional data. Given high-dimensional microarray data, the LASSO method can identify the most important genes that are related to the phenotype of interest in a fast and effective way. Variable selection and estimation of regression coefficients are performed simultaneously—important variables will have non-zero regression coefficients and unimportant variables will have zero coefficients in the model.

Next, we will describe the general framework for variable selection through regularized partial likelihood of the Cox model first. We then derive the cyclic coordinate descent algorithm, which can estimate the regression coefficients coupled with Newton's method.

Variable Selection via LASSO Regularized Partial Likelihood

Suppose there are n subjects, and each subject has p predictor variables $X = (X_1, \ldots, X_p)^t$. The survival time and the censoring time for the subject i are denoted by T_i and C_i, respectively. We use the triplets $\{(Y_i, \delta_i, X_i), i = 1, \ldots, n\}$ to represent the observed survival data, where $Y_i = \min(T_i, C_i)$ denotes the observed survival time since it might be right-censored, and $\delta_i = I(T_i \leq C_i)$ is a censoring indicator which equals 1 if the actual death is observed and 0 otherwise. The censoring mechanism is assumed to be noninformative. The censoring time C_i and the survival time T_i are assumed to be conditionally independent given the predictor X_i.

The Cox proportional hazards regression model is written as

$$h(t|X) = h_0(t)\exp\left(\sum_{j=1}^{p} \beta_j X_j\right), \tag{6.1}$$

where $h_0(t)$ is the nonparametric baseline hazards function, and β_j is the regression coefficient for X_j. It is reasonable to assume no ties in the observed time when the failure time is continuous. The partial likelihood of the Cox model is

$$L_n(\boldsymbol{\beta}) = \prod_{i \in D} \frac{\exp\left(X_i^t \boldsymbol{\beta}\right)}{\sum_{l \in R_i} \exp\left(X_l^t \boldsymbol{\beta}\right)}$$

where D is the set of indices of uncensored events (i.e., observed deaths), and R_i is the set of the subjects available for the event (i.e., still alive) at time

Y_i. Variable selection can then be conducted by minimizing the negative log-partial likelihood function $l_n(\boldsymbol{\beta}) = \frac{\log\{L_n(\boldsymbol{\beta})\}}{n}$ plus a penalty function $P_\lambda(\boldsymbol{\beta})$ on the coefficients $\boldsymbol{\beta}$:

$$g(\boldsymbol{\beta}) = -l_n(\boldsymbol{\beta}) + P_\lambda(\boldsymbol{\beta}).$$

The penalty function $P_\lambda(\boldsymbol{\beta})$ has to be singular in order to achieve the desired sparsity, hence variable selection. In LASSO penalized method, we penalize the log-partial likelihood by the LASSO penalty $P_\lambda(\boldsymbol{\beta}) = \lambda \sum_{j=1}^{p} |\beta_j|$, which is nondifferentiable at point $\beta_j = 0$, and therefore it is able to eliminate the irrelevant variables and keep the most relevant ones. The objective function is written as

$$g(\boldsymbol{\beta}) = -l_n(\boldsymbol{\beta}) + \lambda \sum_{j=1}^{p} |\beta_j|, \qquad (6.2)$$

where $\lambda > 0$ is a tuning constant, which controls the number of variables included in the final model. The larger λ is, the fewer variables are retained in the model. By minimizing the objective function [2], one can select important predictor variables and estimate regression coefficients simultaneously. The variables with nonzero coefficients will be selected and the rest are eliminated.

Cyclic Coordinate Descent for LASSO Penalized Cox Regression

Since there are usually more predictor variables than subjects ($p > n$) in microarray studies, to tackle the high-dimensionality problem we use a cyclic coordinate descent algorithm. This algorithm has been shown to be computationally efficient [28–32]. Interested readers can refer to [29,30] for more details. The idea of this algorithm is to break a large optimization problem into a sequence of small problems. In other words, instead of estimating all the parameters at the same time, we can update parameters one by one. The advantages of using coordinate descent algorithms include: (1) no matrix operations are involved and only scalar operations are performed, which reduces the computational burden; (2) most updates of the parameters are skipped because of the LASSO penalty; (3) the non-differentiability of the LASSO penalty is well handled; (4) it is numerically robust.

Although the LASSO penalty is nondifferentiable at the origin, its forward and backward directional derivatives exist. We first calculate the forward and backward directional derivatives of β_j along its coordinate direction e_j, which are

$$d_{e_j}g(\boldsymbol{\beta}) = \lim_{t\to 0} \frac{g(\boldsymbol{\beta} + te_j) - g(\boldsymbol{\beta})}{t} = -d_{e_j}l_n(\boldsymbol{\beta}) + \lambda \cdot (-1)^{I(\beta_j < 0)}$$

and

$$d_{-e_j}g(\boldsymbol{\beta}) = \lim_{t\to 0} \frac{g(\boldsymbol{\beta} - te_j) - g(\boldsymbol{\beta})}{t} = -d_{-e_j}l_n(\boldsymbol{\beta}) + \lambda \cdot (-1)^{I(\beta_j > 0)}$$

where $I(\cdot)$ is an indicator function equal to 1 if the condition is true. The directional derivative of $l_n(\boldsymbol{\beta})$ along e_j is equal to its ordinary partial derivatives

$$d_{e_j}l_n(\boldsymbol{\beta}) = \frac{\partial}{\partial \beta_j} l_n(\boldsymbol{\beta}) = \sum_{i \in D} \left\{ x_{ij} - \frac{\sum_{l \in R_i} \exp\left(\boldsymbol{X}_l^t \boldsymbol{\beta}\right) x_{lj}}{\sum_{l \in R_i} \exp\left(\boldsymbol{X}_l^t \boldsymbol{\beta}\right)} \right\}$$

Its directional derivative along $-e_j$ equals $\frac{-\partial l_n(\boldsymbol{\beta})}{\partial \beta_j}$.

Next, we need to decide the direction of the update. If both $d_{e_j}g(\boldsymbol{\beta})$ and $d_{-e_j}g(\boldsymbol{\beta})$ are nonnegative, then the update for β_j is skipped as no improvement can be made. If either directional derivative is negative, then we solve for the minimum along that direction. The two directional derivatives cannot be negative at the same time because of the convexity of $g(\boldsymbol{\beta})$. After determining the direction of updating, Newton's method can be used to solve for the minimum since the objective function is twice differentiable. The update for β_j at the $(m + 1)$th iteration is given by

$$\beta_j^{m+1} = \beta_j^m + \frac{-\frac{\partial}{\partial \beta_j} l_n(\boldsymbol{\beta}^m) + \lambda \cdot (-1)^{I(\beta_j < 0)}}{\frac{\partial^2}{\partial \beta_j^2} l_n(\boldsymbol{\beta}^m)}$$

where $\boldsymbol{\beta}^m$ is the estimate at the mth iteration and

$$
\frac{\partial^2}{\partial \beta_j^2} l_n(\boldsymbol{\beta}^m) = \sum_{i \in D} \left\{ \frac{\left[\sum_{l \in R_i} \exp\left(\boldsymbol{X}_l^t \boldsymbol{\beta} \right) x_{lj} \right]^2}{\left[\sum_{l \in R_i} \exp\left(\boldsymbol{X}_l^t \boldsymbol{\beta} \right) \right]^2} - \frac{\sum_{l \in R_i} \exp\left(\boldsymbol{X}_l^t \boldsymbol{\beta} \right) x_{lj}^2}{\sum_{l \in R_i} \exp\left(\boldsymbol{X}_l^t \boldsymbol{\beta} \right)} \right\}
$$

All parameters should be initiated at the origin.

Unlike the traditional model selection methods, e.g., forward and backward selection, the "threshold" for the LASSO penalized method is not explicitly specified. Instead, the number of selected predictors is controlled by the tuning parameter λ in Eqn (6.2). The bigger is λ, the fewer predictors will be selected. The value of λ can be determined by data-driven methods, for example, k-fold cross validation.

DOUBLY REGULARIZED COX REGRESSION

In the gene regulatory network, genes in the same pathways might get involved in the same biological processes. Therefore, we extend the LASSO method described in the previous section to integrate pathway information and introduce a doubly regularized Cox (DrCox) regression model [21] for the pancreatic cancer survival analysis. We first consider the case where the groups do not overlap, i.e., each gene belongs to only one signaling pathway. Then, we extend to the overlap case, i.e., one gene can belong to multiple groups.

Doubly Regularized Cox Regression for Non-Overlap Case

We assume there are n subjects and p predictor variables (genes) that occur in K groups (pathways). $X_{(k)} = (X_{k1}, \ldots, X_{kp_k})^T$ denotes the p_k predictors in the kth group, and $\beta_{(k)} = (\beta_{k1}, \ldots, \beta_{kp_k})^T$ denotes the corresponding regression coefficients. We further write the predictor variables of the ith subject as $\quad \boldsymbol{X}_i = (X_{i,(1)}^T, \ldots, X_{i,(K)}^T)^T, \quad$ where $\quad \boldsymbol{X}_{i,(k)} = (X_{i,k1}, \ldots, X_{i,kp_k})^T, \quad$ and $i = \{1, \ldots, n\}$. The definition of survival time is the same as before.

The Cox proportional hazards regression model with p genes and K signaling pathways in the non-overlap case is written as

$$
h(t|X) = h_0(t) \exp\left(\sum_{k=1}^{K} \sum_{j=1}^{p_k} \beta_{kj} X_{kj} \right) = h_0(t) \exp\left(\sum_{k=1}^{K} \boldsymbol{X}_{i,(k)}^T \boldsymbol{\beta}_{(k)} \right). \tag{6.3}
$$

The partial likelihood of this Cox model is given by

$$L_n(\boldsymbol{\beta}) = \prod_{i \in D} \frac{\exp\left(\sum_{k=1}^{K} \boldsymbol{X}_{i,(k)}^{T} \boldsymbol{\beta}_{(k)}\right)}{\sum_{l \in R_i} \exp\left(\sum_{k=1}^{K} \boldsymbol{X}_{i,(k)}^{T} \boldsymbol{\beta}_{(k)}\right)}.$$

To achieve the goal of both group and within-group variable selection and retain the convexity property, the doubly regularized Cox (DrCox) regression model imposes a mixture of LASSO penalty and group LASSO penalty to the negative of log-partial likelihood $l_n(\boldsymbol{\beta}) = \frac{\log\{L_n(\boldsymbol{\beta})\}}{n}$. The doubly penalized objective function is

$$
\begin{aligned}
g(\boldsymbol{\beta}) &= -l_n(\boldsymbol{\beta}) + \lambda_1 \sum_{k=1}^{K} \sum_{j=1}^{p_k} |\boldsymbol{\beta}_{kj}| + \lambda_2 \sum_{k=1}^{K} \sqrt{\sum_{j=1}^{p_k} \beta_{kj}^2} \\
&= -l_n(\boldsymbol{\beta}) + \lambda_1 \sum_{k=1}^{K} \left\| \boldsymbol{\beta}_{(k)} \right\|_1 + \lambda_2 \sum_{k=1}^{K} \left\| \boldsymbol{\beta}_{(k)} \right\|_2,
\end{aligned}
\tag{6.4}
$$

where $\|\boldsymbol{\beta}_{(k)}\|_1 = \sum_{j=1}^{p_k} |\boldsymbol{\beta}_{kj}|$ is the LASSO penalty on individual parameters β_{kj} in group k, and $\|\boldsymbol{\beta}_{(k)}\|_2 = \sqrt{\sum_{j=1}^{p_k} \boldsymbol{\beta}_{kj}^2}$ is the group LASSO penalty on kth group of parameters, and λ_1 and λ_2 are two nonnegative tuning constants that control the strength of individual and group selection, which can be determined using data-driven methods (e.g., k-fold cross validation).

Coordinate Descent Algorithm for DrCox Regression

In the non-overlap case, where each variable belongs to only one group, estimation of parameters and selection of important variables can be conducted via the minimization of the Eqn (6.4) iteratively w.r.t. one parameter by one parameter. The first step is to calculate the forward and backward directional derivatives of each parameter. If e_{kj} is the coordinate direction along which β_{kj} varies, then the forward and backward directional derivatives of β_{kj} are

$$d_{e_{kj}}g(\beta) = \lim_{t \to 0} \frac{g(\beta + te_{kj}) - g(\beta)}{t}$$

$$= -\frac{\partial}{\partial \beta_{kj}} l_n(\beta)$$

$$+ \begin{cases} (\lambda_1 + \lambda_2) \cdot (-1)^{I(\beta_{kj} < 0)} & \text{if } \left\| \beta_{(k)} \right\|_2 = 0 \\ \\ \lambda_1 \cdot (-1)^{I(\beta_{kj} < 0)} + \lambda_2 \dfrac{\beta_{kj}}{\left\| \beta_{(k)} \right\|_2} & \text{if } \left\| \beta_{(k)} \right\|_2 > 0 \end{cases}$$

and

$$d_{-e_{kj}}g(\beta) = \lim_{t \to 0} \frac{g(\beta - te_{kj}) - g(\beta)}{t}$$

$$= \frac{\partial}{\partial \beta_{kj}} l_n(\beta)$$

$$+ \begin{cases} (\lambda_1 + \lambda_2) \cdot (-1)^{I(\beta_{kj} > 0)} & \text{if } \left\| \beta_{(k)} \right\|_2 = 0 \\ \\ \lambda_1 \cdot (-1)^{I(\beta_{kj} > 0)} - \lambda_2 \dfrac{\beta_{kj}}{\left\| \beta_{(k)} \right\|_2} & \text{if } \left\| \beta_{(k)} \right\|_2 > 0 \end{cases}$$

where

$$\frac{\partial}{\partial \beta_{kj}} l_n(\beta) = \sum_{i \in D} \left\{ x_{i,kj} - \frac{\sum_{l \in R_i} \exp\left(\sum_{k=1}^{K} X_{i,(k)}^T \beta_{(k)} \right) x_{l,kj}}{\sum_{l \in R_i} \exp\left(\sum_{k=1}^{K} X_{i,(k)}^T \beta_{(k)} \right)} \right\}.$$

If both of the directional derivatives $d_{e_{kj}}g(\beta)$ and $d_{-e_{kj}}g(\beta)$ are non-negative, then the update for β_{kj} is skipped. If either directional derivative is negative, then we can use Newton's method to solve for the minimum along that direction. The update for β_{kj} at iteration $m + 1$ is given by

$$\beta_{kj}^{m+1} = \beta_{kj}^m + \dfrac{-\frac{\partial}{\partial \beta_{kj}} l_n(\boldsymbol{\beta}^m) + \lambda_1 \cdot (-1)^{I\left(\beta_{kj}^m < 0\right)}}{\frac{\partial^2}{\partial \beta_{kj}^2} l_n(\boldsymbol{\beta}^m)}$$

$$+ \dfrac{\lambda_2 \left\{ (-1)^{I\left(\beta_{kj}^m < 0\right)} I_1\left(\beta_{(k)}^m\right) + \frac{\beta_{kj}^m}{\left\| \beta_{(k)}^m \right\|_2} I_2\left(\beta_{(k)}^m\right) \right\}}{\frac{\partial^2}{\partial \beta_{kj}^2} l_n(\boldsymbol{\beta}^m)}$$

where β^m is the estimate at the mth iteration.

DrCox Regression via Coordinate Descent for Overlap Cases

In reality, many different pathways can share one gene. To allow overlapping, we modify the notation and objective function for the non–overlap case. We denote the p variables by $X_1, \ldots, X_p$ with the corresponding regression coefficients $\beta_1, \ldots, \beta_p$. Let $V_k \subseteq \{1, \ldots, p\}$ be the set of indices of variables in the kth group. The objective function designed for the overlap case can be written as

$$g(\boldsymbol{\beta}) = -l_n(\boldsymbol{\beta}) + \lambda_1 \sum_{j=1}^{p} |\beta_j| + \lambda_2 \sum_{k=1}^{K} \sqrt{\sum_{j \in V_k} \beta_j^2}. \tag{6.5}$$

Note one predictor X_j can belong to several pathways but it is only associated with one regression coefficient β_j. The parameter estimation needs to be modified accordingly. If we consider the coordinate direction e_j for β_j, the forward and backward directional derivatives of β_j are

$$d_{e_j} g(\boldsymbol{\beta}) = \lim_{t \to 0} \frac{g(\boldsymbol{\beta} + t e_j) - g(\boldsymbol{\beta})}{t}$$

$$= -d_{e_j} l_n(\boldsymbol{\beta}) + \lambda_1 \cdot (-1)^{I(\beta_j < 0)}$$

$$+ \lambda_2 \sum_{j \in V_k} \left\{ (-1)^{I(\beta_j < 0)} I_1\left(\beta_{(k)}\right) + \frac{\beta_j}{\left\| \beta_{(k)} \right\|_2} I_2\left(\beta_{(k)}\right) \right\}$$

and

$$d_{-e_j}g(\boldsymbol{\beta}) = \lim_{t \to 0} \frac{g(\boldsymbol{\beta} - te_j) - g(\boldsymbol{\beta})}{t}$$

$$= -d_{-e_j}l_n(\boldsymbol{\beta}) + \lambda_1 \cdot (-1)^{I(\beta_j > 0)}$$

$$+ \lambda_2 \sum_{k \in G_j} \left\{ (-1)^{I(\beta_j > 0)} I_1\left(\beta_{(k)}\right) - \frac{\beta_j}{\|\beta_{(k)}\|_2} I_2\left(\beta_{(k)}\right) \right\}$$

where $G_j \subseteq \{1, 2, \ldots, K\}$ are the indices of groups that X_j belongs to. We can update the coefficient by

$$\beta_j^{m+1} = \beta_j^m + \frac{-\frac{\partial}{\partial \beta_j} l_n(\boldsymbol{\beta}^m) + \lambda_1 \cdot (-1)^{I(\beta_j^m < 0)}}{\frac{\partial^2}{\partial \beta_j^2} l_n(\boldsymbol{\beta}^m)}$$

$$+ \frac{\lambda_2 \sum_{k \in G_j} \left\{ (-1)^{I(\beta_j^m < 0)} I_1\left(\beta_{(k)}^m\right) + \frac{\beta_j^m}{\|\beta_{(k)}^m\|_2} I_2\left(\beta_{(k)}^m\right) \right\}}{\frac{\partial^2}{\partial \beta_j^2} l_n(\boldsymbol{\beta}^m)}.$$

PANCREATIC CANCER SURVIVAL ANALYSIS

Microarray Data and Signaling Pathways

The microarray data of pancreatic cancer summarized in Stratford et al.'s work [13] includes 43,376 probes in ROMA platform with 102 samples (PDAC patients), which are publicly available at Gene Expression Omnibus. Among these 102 PDAC patients, 66 died at the end of the study (35% censoring rate). The survival times of these patients range from one month to five years. For each patient, the survival time and the censoring indicator (the patient is still alive or not) were recorded. Additionally, two stage variables, T stage and N stage, were given to describe the stages of pancreatic cancer, where T stage describes the size of the primary tumor ranging from 1 to 4, and N stage describes the spread to nearby (regional) lymph nodes with values 0 or 1. The readers can refer to Stratford et al.'s work for more details.

Jones et al.'s work [5] organized 130 signaling pathway sets that belong to 12 core groups in the pancreatic cancer studies, including the core groups of Wnt/Notch signaling, TGF-beta signaling, Small GTPase-dependent signaling, KRAS signaling, JNK, Integrin signaling, Homophilic cell adhesion, Hedgehhog signaling, DNA damage control, Control of G1/S phase transition, Invasion, and Apoptosis.

In our studies, the whole pancreatic cancer survival dataset of 102 patients is randomly split into the training, validation, and testing sets with equal sizes. The training set is used for model fitting, and the validation set is used for tuning constants selection. The results are then applied to the testing set to examine the model performance.

Data Analysis with LASSO Penalized Cox Regression

We first applied the LASSO penalized Cox regression method [11] to investigate the signature genes that are correlated to the pancreatic cancer survival time. Using the three-fold cross validation, we got the optimal values of $\lambda = 0.3475$. Twelve genes are identified to be associated with the pancreatic cancer survival, and eight of them have been confirmed to be genetically altered and differentially expressed in the cancer of stomach, colon, ovaries, breast, skin, kidney, lung, and pancreas in in vivo and in vitro experiments [22–27,33–40]. These survival-associated genes can be used to grade the stage of PDAC and estimate the survival time of the cancer patients, and help select appropriate therapies for the patients in different stages. These eight genetic signatures and their functions are summarized in Table 6.1. The functions of the rest four genes (SLC22A8, C4orf35, C6orf81, and C6orf58) remain unknown at this point and are worth further investigation.

Data Analysis with Doubly Regularized Cox Regression

Next, we applied the doubly regularized Cox (DrCox) regression model with the cyclic coordinate descent algorithm [21] to the dataset. Different from the analysis using LASSO penalty, this DrCox model can incorporate both genes and pathways information, and simultaneously infer both genetic signatures and important signaling pathways that are related to the pancreatic cancer survival.

Again, we used the three-fold cross validation. We got the optimal tuning constants $\lambda_1 = 0.3$ and $\lambda_2 = 0.1$. The DrCox method inferred four signaling pathways and 15 genes within these pathways from the pool of 12,660 probes of 6910 genes and 130 pathway sets [5] in the pancreatic cancer. The inferred signaling pathways include the four major pathways of "regulation of DNA-dependent transcription" (6 out of 2096 genes are selected), "Ion transport" (7 out of 555 genes are selected), "immune phagocytosis" (1 out of 215 genes is selected), and "TGFβ (spermatogenesis)"

Table 6.1 Eight Genes that are Associated with the Pancreatic Cancer Survival and their Functions Inferred from the LASSO Penalized Cox Regression Model

Genes	Functions
RPS13	Promote cell cycle progression from G1 to S phase. It is frequently mutated or deregulated in colorectal carcinoma, gastric cancer, and pancreatic cancer [22].
PCYT1B	Regulates the phosphatidylcholine biosynthesis. Aberrant choline phospholipid metabolism is associated with the tumors of breast, colon, and ovaries, and gliomas [23,25,33]. It could help to grade the stage of the pancreatic cancer patients.
TREX2	TREX2 is a proapoptotic tumor suppressor that can maintain the genomic integrity under the condition of genotoxic stress. It is downregulated during G2/M phase transition through the cell cycle [26,27].
ZNF233	Zinc finger protein 233 is correlated to the chromosomal abnormality, and it is frequently deregulated in the kidney and pancreatic cancer [5,34].
ATPAF1	ATPAF1 could regulate the oxidative phosphorylation pathway and reduce oxidative stress in tissues. Downregulated ATPAF1 could suppress the mitochondrial biogenesis and G1/S arrest [35,36].
RIMS1	It is a RAS superfamily member that is significantly deregulated in the classical multidrug resistance (MDR) gastric carcinoma [37].
SLC43A2	Regulate the transport of large neutral amino acids across membranes. Its overexpression is associated with the adenocarcinomas and squamous cell carcinoma [38,39].
NRAP	It is one of the top 20 upregulated genes in peripheral and central zones of human pancreatic cancer [40].

(1 out of 268 genes is selected). The selected genes and pathways are summarized in Table 6.2.

Several experimental studies have confirmed that these signaling components are frequently altered in the pancreatic, oral, prostate, colon, breast, and lung cancer [39,41–54], and they could be possible biomarkers of pancreatic cancer survival. Pancreatic cancer patients with these mutated genes and/or deregulated signaling pathways might have a shorter survival time. Especially, the inferred TRP (Ca^{2+}) channel-related genes and KCNK (K^+) channel-related genes in the ion transport pathway could be useful biomarkers for early pancreatic cancer detection, help researchers to grade the cancer stage, and select appropriate therapies to prolong the patients' survival time at different stages.

Table 6.2 Four Signaling Pathways and 15 Genes that are Associated with the Pancreatic Cancer Survival and Their Functions Inferred from the Doubly Regularized Cox Regression Model

Signaling Pathways	Genes	Functions
Regulation of DNA-dependent transcription pathway	DENND4A	DENND4A is a c-myc promoter-binding protein, which mediates signal transduction in the nucleus, regulates the transcription and DNA replication [41].
	KLF13	KLF13 can inhibit the cell growth and neoplastic transformation mediated by K-RAS [42,43].
	ZNF229, ZNF233, ZNF395, ANF432	Some Zinc finger proteins, e.g., ZNF233, are associated with the chromosomal abnormality, and also the kidney and pancreatic cancers [34].
Ion transport pathway	TRP channel and TRPV5, TRPM6	Regulate the calcium-mediated signal transduction. TRPM6 can enhance the secretion of angiogenic factors and promote angiogenesis [44–46].
	KCNK channel and KCNK3, KCNK18	Regulate the potassium (K^+) transport and membrane potential (Vm) in response to different physical and chemical factors [47–49].
	SLC22A8, SLC8A3, SLC24A6	Regulate the transport and excretion of the organic ions, drugs, and toxicants; some genes are cancer-related [39].
Immune phagocytosis pathway	CYBA	The tumor suppressor CYBA regulates the immune system cells, phagocytes, which are involved in autophagy. CYBA's mutation will cause the failure of phagocytosis and immune defects [50–53].
TGFβ signaling pathway (spermatogenesis)	PCYT1B	TGFβ signaling pathway is of importance in the cell growth, cell differentiation, and apoptosis. PCYT1B regulates the choline phospholipid metabolism, which is associated with progression of tumors of breast, colon, and ovaries, and gliomas [23,25,33,54].

ACKNOWLEDGMENTS

TTW and EMC were supported by NSF grants CCF-0926194 and 0926181. HG was supported by the new faculty start-up grant from the Saint Louis University.

REFERENCES

[1] Niederhuber J, Brennan M, Menck H. The National Cancer Data Base report on pancreatic cancer. Cancer 1995;76:1671–7.

[2] Warshaw A, del Castillo CF. Pancreatic carcinoma. N Engl J Med 1992;326:455–65.

[3] Bardeesy N, DePinho RA. Pancreatic cancer biology and genetics. Nat Rev Cancer 2002;2(12):897–909.

[4] Vonlaufen A, Joshi S, Qu C, Phillips PA, Xu Z, Parker NR, et al. Pancreatic stellate cells: partners in crime with pancreatic cancer cells. Cancer Res 2008;68:2085–93.

[5] Jones S, Zhang X, Parsons DW, Lin JC, Leary RJ, Angenendt P, et al. Core signaling pathways in human pancreatic cancers revealed by global genomic analyses. Science 2008;321:1801–6.

[6] Friess H, Ding J, Kleeff J, Fenkell L, Rosinski JA, Guweidhi A, et al. Microarray-based identification of differentially expressed growth- and metastasis-associated genes in pancreatic cancer. Cell Mol Life Sci 2003;60:1180–99.

[7] Ma S, Song X, Huang J. Supervised group LASSO with applications to microarray data analysis. BMC Bioinform 2007;8:60–76.

[8] Sohn I, Kim J, Jung SH, Park C. Gradient LASSO for Cox proportional hazards model. Bioinformatics 2009;25:1775–81.

[9] Tibshirani R. Univariate shrinkage in the Cox model for high dimensional data. Stat Appl Genet Mol Biol 2009;8:21.

[10] Tibshirani R. The LASSO method for variable selection in the Cox model. Stat Med 1997;16:385–95.

[11] Wu TT, Gong H, Clarke EM. A transcriptome analysis by LASSO penalized Cox regression for pancreatic cancer survival. J Bioinform Comput Biol 2011;9:63.

[12] Donoho DL. Aide-memoire. High-dimensional data analysis: the curses and blessings of dimensionality; 2000.

[13] Stratford JK, Bentrem DJ, Anderson JM, Fan C, Volmar KA, Marron JS, et al. A six-gene signature predicts survival of patients with localized pancreatic ductal adenocarcinoma. PLoS Med 2010;7:e1000307.

[14] Tusher VG, Tibshirani R, Chu G. Significance analysis of microarrays applied to the ionizing radiation response. Proc Natl Acad Sci USA 2001;98:5116–21.

[15] Hu Z, Fan C, Oh DS, Marron JS, He X, Qaqish BF, et al. The molecular portraits of breast tumors are conserved across microarray platforms. BMC Genomics 2006;7:96.

[16] Camp RL, Dolled-Filhart M, Rimm DL. X-tile: a new bio-informatics tool for bio-marker assessment and outcome-based cut-point optimization. Clin Cancer Res 2004;10:7252–9.

[17] Kaplan EL, Meier P. Nonparametric estimation from incomplete observations. J Am Stat Assoc 1958;53:457–81.

[18] Cox DR. Regression models and life-tables (with discussion). J Roy Stat Soc B 1972;34:187–220.

[19] Ishwara H, Kogalur UB, Gorodeski E, Minn AJ, Lauer MS. High-dimensional variable selection for survival data. J Am Stat Assoc 2010;105:205–17.

[20] Ma S, Huang J. Additive risk survival model with microarray data. BMC Bioinform 2007;8:192.

[21] Wu TT, Wang S. Doubly regularized Cox regression for high-dimensional survival data with group structures. Stat Interface 2013;6:175–86.

[22] Shi Y, Zhai H, Wang X, Han Z, Liu C, Lan M, et al. Ribosomal proteins S13 and L23 promote multidrug resistance in gastric cancer cells by suppressing drug-induced apoptosis. Exp Cell Res 2004;296:337–46.

[23] Katz-Brull R, Seger D, Rivenson-Segal D, Rushkin E, Degani H. Metabolic markers of breast cancer: enhanced choline metabolism and reduced choline-ether-phospholipid synthesis. Cancer Res 2002;62:1966–70.

[24] Thomas P, Nash G, Aldridge M. Pancreatic acinar cell carcinoma presenting as acute pancreatitis. HPB (Oxford) 2003;5(2):111–3.

[25] Mori N, Delsite R, Natarajan K, Kulawiec M, Bhujwalla Z, Singh K. Loss of p53 function in colon cancer cells results in increased phosphocholine and total choline. Mol Imaging 2004;3:319–23.

[26] Chen MJ, Ma SM, Dumitrache LC, Hasty P. Biochemical and cellular characteristics of the 3′→5′ exonuclease TREX2. Nucleic Acids Res 2007;35:2682–94.

[27] Mazur D, Perrino F. Identification and expression of the TREX1 and TREX2 cDNA sequences encoding mammalian 3′→5′ exonucleases. J Biol Chem 1999;274:19655–60.

[28] Tibshirani R. Regression shrinkage and selection via the LASSO. J Roy Stat Soc B 1996;58:267–88.

[29] Friedman J, Hastie T, Hoefling H, Tibshirani R. Pathwise coordinate optimization. Ann Appl Stat 2007;1:302–32.

[30] Wu TT, Lange K. Coordinate descent algorithms for LASSO penalized regression. Ann Appl Stat 2008;2:224–44.

[31] Wu TT, Chen YF, Hastie T, Sobel E, Lange K. Genomewide association analysis by LASSO penalized logistic regression. Bioinformatics 2009;25(6):714–21.

[32] Tseng P. Convergence of block coordinate descent method for nondifferentiable minimization. J Optim Theory Appl 2001;109:473–92.

[33] Iorio E, Ricci A, Bagnoli M, Pisanu ME, Castellano G, Di Vito M, et al. Activation of phosphatidylcholine-cycle enzymes in human epithelial ovarian cancer cells. Cancer Res 2010;70:2126–35.

[34] Koeman JM, Russell RC, Tan MH, Petillo D, Westphal M, Koelzer K, et al. Somatic pairing of chromosome 19 in renal oncocytoma is associated with deregulated ELGN2-mediated oxygen-sensing response. PLoS Genet 2008;4(9):e1000176.

[35] Wallace D. A mitochondrial paradigm for degenerative diseases and ageing. Novartis Found Symp 2001;235:247–63.

[36] Soung YH, Lee JW, Kim SY, Park WS, Nam SW, Lee JY, et al. Somatic mutations of casp3 gene in human cancers. Hum Genet 2004;115:112–5.

[37] Heim S, Lage H. Transcriptome analysis of different multidrug-resistant gastric carcinoma cells. In Vivo 2005;19:583–90.

[38] Bodoy S, Martín L, Zorzano A, Palacín M, Estévez R, Bertran J. Identification of LAT4, a novel amino acid transporter with system L activity. J Biol Chem 2005;280:12002–11.

[39] Haase C, Bergmann R, Fuechtner F, Hoepping A, Pietzsch J. L-type amino acid transporters LAT1 and LAT4 in cancer: uptake of 3-O-methyl-6-18F-fluoro-L-dopa in human adenocarcinoma and squamous cell carcinoma in vitro and in vivo. J Nucl Med 2007;48:2063–71.

[40] Nakamura T, Kuwai T, Kitadai Y, Sasaki T, Fan D, Coombes KR, et al. Zonal heterogeneity for gene expression in human pancreatic carcinoma. Cancer Res 2007;67:7597–604.

[41] Ray R, Miller D. Cloning and characterization of a human c-myc promoter-binding protein. Mol Cell Biol 1991;11:2154–61.

[42] Fernandez-Zapico ME, Billadeau DD, Urrutia R. Klf13 suppresses the transforming activity of k-Ras by direct downregulation the cyclin B gene. Pancreas 2004;29:360.

[43] Henson B, Gollin S. Overexpression of KLF13 and FGFR3 in oral cancer cells. Cytogenet Genome Res 2010;128:192–8.

[44] Prevarskaya N, Skryma R, Shuba Y. Ion channels and the hallmarks of cancer. Trends Mol Med 2010;16:107–21.

[45] Peng J. TRPV5 and TRPV6 in transcellular Ca(2+) transport: regulation, gene duplication, and polymorphisms in African populations. Adv Exp Med Biol 2011;704:239–75.

[46] Dong H, Shim KN, Li JM, Estrema C, Ornelas TA, Nguyen F, et al. Molecular mechanisms underlying Ca^{2+}-mediated motility of human pancreatic duct cells. Am J Physiol Cell Physiol 2010;299(6):C1493–503.

[47] Goldstein S, Bockenhauer D, O'Kelly I, Zilberberg N. Potassium leak channels and the KCNK family of two-p-domain subunits. Nat Rev Neurosci 2001;2:175–84.

[48] Mu D, Chen L, Zhang X, See LH, Koch CM, Yen C, et al. Genomic amplification and oncogenic properties of the KCNK9 potassium channel gene. Cancer Cell 2003;3: 297–302.

[49] Voloshyna I, Besana A, Castillo M, Matos T, Weinstein IB, Mansukhani M, et al. TREK-1 is a novel molecular target in prostate cancer. Cancer Res 2008;68:1197–203.

[50] Jaiswal S, Chao MP, Majeti R, Weissman IL. Macrophages as mediators of tumor immunosurveillance. Trends Immunol 2010;31:212–9.

[51] Chao MP, Majeti R, Weissman IL. Programmed cell removal: a new obstacle in the road to developing cancer. Nat Rev Cancer 2011;12(1):58–67.

[52] Chao MP, Weissman IL, Majeti R. The CD47-SIRPalpha pathway in cancer immune evasion and potential therapeutic implications. Curr Opin Immunol 2012;24:225–32.

[53] Nakano Y, Longo-Guess CM, Bergstrom DE, Nauseef WM, Jones SM, Bánfi B. Mutation of the Cyba gene encoding p22phox causes vestibular and immune defects in mice. J Clin Invest 2008;118:1176–85.

[54] Righi V, Roda JM, Paz J, Mucci A, Tugnoli V, Rodriguez-Tarduchy G, et al. 1H HR-MAS and genomic analysis of human tumor biopsies discriminate between high and low grade astrocytomas. NMR Biomed 2009;22:629–37.

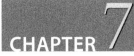

CHAPTER 7

Gene Expression Profiling in Pancreatic Cancer

Christian Pilarsky, Robert Grützmann
Department of Visceral-, Thoracic- and Vascular Surgery, Medizinische Universität Carl Gustav Carus, TU Dresden, Dresden, Germany

Contents

Introduction	151
Summary	164
References	165

INTRODUCTION

In recent years omics technologies have generated a wealth of information regarding differences between normal and tumor cells. Therefore these technologies have slowly become an integral part of modern cancer research. Their use has led to the identification of new targets in several cancers; however, in pancreatic cancer most of the efforts have remained futile. The lack of the implementation of omics technologies, coupled with no clear diagnostic markers or effective therapies, has blocked any progress against pancreatic cancer, which is still associated with a poor survival rate.

Gene expression analysis is based on the analysis of the amount of RNA molecules in a given sample and on the comparison of samples generated from different states of a given tissue or cell line. This leads to two main focus points for such an analysis: (1) the composition of the tissue/cell line, and (2) the quality of the RNA prepared from such samples. Expression profiling can be performed on several types of specimen. Whereas cell lines, xenograft tumors, and tissues from genetically engineered mice models can be obtained fresh and in a standardized fashion, obtaining material from human tumors and/or body fluids is a rather laborious task that might result in only a small amount of usable tissue [1–4]. Collection of a large number of tissue samples is therefore needed to generate a usable tissue bank for further analysis.

Often times tissue sampling is performed by individual members of different parts of a hospital in an unorganized fashion. This leads to the collection of an inadequate number of samples, double collection, and inappropriate handling of samples. Collections of such a type also lack usability since

151

project descriptions submitted to the institutional review boards (IRB) are usually highly specific and therefore the tissue cannot be used for other investigations. This unorganized approach leads also to the absence of standard operating procedures (SOP), which are important to standardize tissue quality. Finally, these efforts result in a lack of specimens from control groups. To produce highly reliable expression data, selection of the right control group is crucial.

The successful model that has been established in recent years is banking of tissues and body fluids from a large number of probands, and a large number of tissue repositories have been established that are seeking the collaboration of other academic groups in different scientific fields. There are even efforts to establish tissue banks on national and international levels [5]. The advantage of this model is multiple. In a tissue bank, SOP should exist to obtain the sample in a reproducible manner, the tissue can be used in different projects after additional application at the local IRB, and quickly after the establishment of a tissue bank a large number of samples are available for analysis. Comprehensive tissue bank approaches allow for the integration of various tissue samples from one subject, i.e., frozen and paraffin-embedded tissue. Such tissue banks are usually established by large organizations, which are also able to integrate clinical metadata into such a bank, enhancing the intrinsic value of the sample for cooperation and analysis. As an example, in pancreatic cancer it is very interesting to know the special subtype of a given sample and other clinical pathological data, which enable the researcher to find new markers for those subtypes [6].

The best practice for a pancreatic cancer expression–profiling project today would be to obtain the tissue from a tissue bank with all clinically relevant data. The researchers should also strive to obtain all the different tissue types (frozen, paraffin-embedded tissue, serum, plasma, other) not only for the patients to be analyzed but also from a larger number of benign controls.

Solid tumor samples consist of a variety of tissues, of which the tumor cells might comprise only a small part [7]. The adjacent additional tissues might contain surrounding stromal and endothelial cells but at least in clinical samples also normal tissue. Depending on the tissue of interest, microdissection might be needed to delineate the true expression changes between the tumor cell and their normal counterpart. In pancreatic cancer, due to its high content of stromal tissue, this is usually the case. Microdissection can be performed either manually or by the aid of a laser-based system. Both methods differ in their resolution. Manual microdissection might only lead to an enrichment of the tumor tissue to about 90%, whereas with a laser-based system, pure tumor cells can be obtained. Manual microdissection enables the researcher to produce samples much faster with superior quality, which is needed for gene expression profiling [8]. If laser assisted microdissection is used, the selection of instruments can be crucial for the success of the project, but individual cells can be picked and investigated [9]. However, manual microdissection performed by educated researchers is a cheap technology, since laser-based microdissection needs special equipment and consumables. The key to a successful experiment is not dependent on the used technology but is associated with the knowledge of the individual performing the isolation procedure. In pancreatic cancer, the distinction between benign and tumor epithelial tissue is difficult, therefore pathologists experienced with the pancreatic cancer histology should be involved in such a project. Microdissection is also the technique of choice if other tissue in a tumor should be analyzed. If microdissection is employed, usually only low amounts of RNA can be obtained. Therefore, RNA amplification has to be performed. The standard technique is the linear amplification based on T7 RNA polymerase initiated by a T7 promoter sequence, which is generated during first strand synthesis. If the resulting amount of RNA is still not adequate, a second RNA amplification can be used. Amplification of RNA is an integral part of the sample preparation in Affymetrix 3'IVT microarray, making Affymetrix microarray the technology of choice for samples with small RNA amounts since the RNA amplification can be started from amounts as low as 1 ng of total RNA. However, it can also be used in RNA-Seq, but the inherent loss of 5' sequences during amplification will diminish the return of RNA-Seq information if splicing or chimeras are to be analyzed. For those scientific questions, unamplified high quality total RNA should be used.

In recent years it has become clear that the surrounding stromal tissue is of great importance in the growth of the pancreatic tumors and that eliminating stromal tissue might be a feasible way to treat it successfully [10]. However, not always pure cancer tissue needs to be obtained. In those cases the cancer tissue in question should be sectioned, stained, and screened for tumor content by qualified pathologists. Care should be taken in those cases that the tissue composition between the different sample groups is comparable.

Today preparation of RNA from tissues has become mainstream technology. It is advisable that in modern expression analysis approaches kits should be used from reliable suppliers, and they should be the same during the whole experiment. Isolation of ribonucleic acid with such a system should also result in the preparation of miRNA as a component of the total RNA. Such systems enable the researchers to investigate the miRNA expression by a separate array or by RNA-Seq from the same sample from which other expression profiles are generated. The second important step in expression profiling, beside identification of the right tissue compartment, is the quality control of the obtained RNA. An industry standard like the Bioanalyzer System from Agilent should be used. As a result, from such an analysis, not only the amount of RNA but also the quality determined by the RNA integrity number (RIN) can be obtained (Figure 7.1). RNA with a RIN number below 4 should not be used in any gene expression profiling experiment. For some RNA-Seq procedures (as the analysis of alternative splicing and chimera detection) the RIN should be at least 8. Most of the gene expression profiling experiments employ at least one step of reverse transcription. This step is crucial for the success of the experiment. It should always be performed with the same reagents and carefully controlled.

The best practice is to use kits from commercial sources for RNA preparation and following enzymatic manipulation. The quality of the RNA should be monitored with an Agilent Bioanalyzer and finally within in an

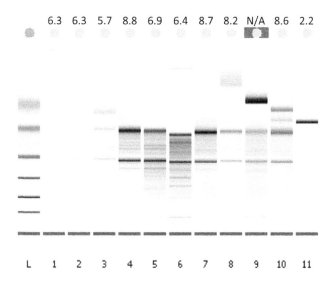

Figure 7.1 *Example of the Result from Agilent Bioanalyzer 2100 Assay.* The numbers above the lanes indicate the RNA integrity number (RIN), an estimate for the quality of the prepared RNA. On the outer most left lane the molecular weight marker is displayed. N/A: RIN is not accessible, typically shown if the assay failed or the RIN is too low. (For color version of this figure, the reader is referred to the online version of this book.)

experimental set up. The supplier of the components should not be changed and the lot numbers should be documented.

Within the omics technologies, expression profiling is one of the oldest areas of research. Whereas the beginning of expression profiling could be dated to the invention of the northern blot, gene expression profiling took stage with the invention of TaqMan PCR systems and came to fruition with reverse hybridization techniques during the late 1990s and 2000. Nowadays three major types of expression profiling are performed in the lab. Quantitative RT-PCR (qRT-PCR) enables the researcher to analyze the expression of genes fast in a high number of samples, but is usually restricted to a gene number in the low hundreds if special adapted technologies are used. Based on the nature of PCR, only a very small amount of RNA is needed to successfully complete an assay. Due to these reasons, quantitative PCR is also used in the routine clinical chemistry workup with standardized expression assay like Oncotype DX in breast cancer [11].

Quantitative real-time polymerase chain reaction (qRT-PCR) is a well-established tool for the quantification of gene expression [12,13]. It is based on the polymerase chain reaction (PCR) developed by Mullis et al. in the 1980s [14]. QRT-PCR allows quantifying the amount of template, usually the gene of interest, and an amplification control called housekeeping gene in the original sample. QRT-PCR systems detect and quantify a fluorescent reporter signal, which increases in proportion to the amount of PCR product in a reaction. To generate comparable data, the fluorescence is collected at each cycle, making it possible to monitor the PCR during the exponential amplification phase. The most common methods for detecting target templates include the 5′ nuclease (TaqMan) and the SYBR green assays. The TaqMan assay uses an oligonucleotide probe, which specifically anneals to a complementary sequence in the amplicon [15]. To generate and detect fluorescence the oligonucleotide probe carries a fluorescein group at 5′ end and a quencher. When the oligonucleotide probe is intact, the proximity of the reporter dye to the quencher dye results in suppression of the reporter fluorescence. As the Taq DNA polymerase extends the PCR primer, the 5′ exonuclease activity of the polymerase will degrade the oligonucleotide probe. As a result, the reporter dye gets separated from the quencher dye, resulting in increased fluorescence of the reporter. Since the fluorescent signal is generated only if the oligonucleotide probe hybridizes with its complementary target, nonspecific amplification is not detected. In contrast to the TaqMan assay, the SYBR green assay uses the unique feature of SYBR green to emit light only if the substance is bound to double-stranded

DNA, therefore the generated fluorescence signal is a measure of the total dsDNA amount in the reaction at the end of each cycle [16]. SYBR green assays can be performed fast and cheap for a lot of different genes but are highly sensitive to amplification artifacts. Therefore, during the establishment of a qRT-PCR assay using SYBR green, a quality control step has to be introduced assuring that the PCR product is free of contaminants. This can be achieved by a combination of agarose gel electrophoresis and melting point analysis. Multiple options are available for quantitation of the resulting PCR products. For gene expression analysis relative quantitation is commonly used for quantitative measurement. Within a sample a comparison is made between the gene of interest to that of a control gene, and it is based on the cycle threshold (Ct) value. This value is calculated based on the numbers of PCR cycles at which the reporter fluorescence emission increases beyond a threshold level. The Ct value is correlated to the level of starting mRNA. The higher the starting mRNA amounts, the lower the Ct value, as less PCR cycles are required for the reporter fluorescence emission intensity to reach the threshold [17]. In relative quantitation the Ct of the control gene is subtracted from the Ct of the gene of interest. The resulting difference in cycle number (ΔCt) is the exponent of the base 2 (due to the doubling function of PCR), representing the fold difference of template for these two genes. A prerequisite for the application of the relative quantitation method is that the genes analyzed have similar abundance in the tissue analyzed and PCR efficiencies [18].

The best practice is to perform reverse transcription with random primer with a well-established commercially obtainable enzyme and qRT-PCR with SYBR green assays for a large number of genes of interest with optimized primer combinations (obtainable from various commercial resources) using the appropriate control gene or set of control genes. If the number of genes has been reduced, a repetition of the experiments using TaqMan assays might be reasonable.

In the field of high-throughput analysis of gene expression, either microarrays or next-generation sequencing technologies are used. The most common microarray technology now is the Affymetrix platform, enabling the researcher to quickly analyze gene expression in a sample of interest based on a standardized array product with defined performance. As a result of the advent of massive parallel sequencing technology, sequencing of RNA molecules has been become one of the central analysis technologies for cancer researchers. Both technologies have their advantages. Microarrays represent a stable technology with well-understood limitations. The bioinformatics analysis is due to a number of freeware programs that are straightforward and can be performed without specialized bioinformatics know-how on basic computer hardware. Streamlined analysis pipelines are available for larger experiments. In recent years microarray platforms have become cheaper, enabling more researchers to perform gene expression analysis during their experiments.

Microarray technologies for gene expression profiling have clearly derived from the northern blotting method dating back to the mid-1970s [19]. To measure the gene expression profile of a given sample, one crucial invention was to reverse the direction of the blotting in reverse Northern blot approaches for the identification of cDNAs in cloning [20]. The large-scale expressed sequence tag (EST) projects generated cDNA clones and made clone libraries freely available to researchers [21]. Therefore, early arrays for expression profiling were made of cDNA clones spotted in order for hybridization with RNA or cDNA. Additional miniaturization and the use of a rigid surface instead of the membranes used for classic blotting systems led to the technology that is now known as cDNA microarrays in the 1990s [22,23]. cDNA microarray platforms have been used in many laboratories but have failed to generate substantial commercial interest. This was due in part to the lack of standardization and quality control. Since the individual cDNA clones used to generate the arrays could be different between laboratories, the results from the hybridization might be different as well. cDNA microarrays were almost exclusively used as two-color analysis array, and the data generated were based on the ratio of the fluorescence generated. Since the type of reference RNA used for analysis varied between the laboratories, those ratios varied as well, making comparison of the data between sets of experiments performed in different laboratories difficult. Most of the cDNA microarrays were produced in house in academic research centers, making it difficult to control the quality of each array, leading to dropouts and other artifacts and resulting in difficult-to-interpret data. Taken together, spotted cDNA microarray performed in an inferior manner compared to other gene expression platforms and is therefore currently only used in a minor fraction of experiments if other means of gene expression profiling are not available [24].

During the years when cDNA microarrays were invented, other scientists worked on a different technology using in situ–synthesized oligonucleotide microarrays for gene expression profiling [25,26]. The arrays are produced by generating 25 sequences directly onto a planar array surface, using light-directed chemical synthesis of nucleic acids and technologies, borrowed from semiconductor manufacturing. Photolithographic synthesis uses a chemically activated silica substrate, and light-sensitive masking agents construct the sequence one nucleotide at a time across the entire array [26]. A different concept underlies the so-called bead arrays. For those, an optical "imaging" fiber is etched such that a bead can fit into etched wells right on the tip of the fiber. Different oligonucleotide sequences are attached to each bead, and thousands of beads can be self-assembled onto the fiber bundle. A subsequent decoding process is carried out to determine which bead occupies which well. Complementary oligonucleotides present in the sample bind to the beads, and bound oligonucleotides are measured by using a fluorescent label [27].

Oligonucleotide and bead arrays usually are so-called "single-channel" or "one-color" microarrays. In contrast to most of the cDNA microarrays, the results represent an estimate of the absolute levels of gene expression. These values of gene expression may be compared to other genes within the same sample or to the same gene across a large panel of array experiments. This format of data can easily be normalized and compared to other arrays from other sources. Thanks to the large amount of data generated by the international academic research community based on those platforms, comparability is one of the major advantages. A PubMed literature search showed that most of the different cancers have been profiled and that the daunting task at hand is to integrate those data into the more complex picture of genetic changes during pancreatic cancer development.

The large amount of data generated a need for standardization, which was addressed by a number of academic efforts, prior to the flood of data from expression profiling experiments [28]. The results of these efforts have since been adopted by many journals as a minimal requirement for the submission of papers incorporating microarray results, leading to the publication of "raw" data from a huge number of experiments. The data are stored in large public data repositories, such as NCBI gene expression omnibus (GEO) and EBI ArrayExpress. Also meta-databases have been established to provide the researcher a picture of the expression of a gene of interest in a diverse set of cancer-related tissues, such as Oncomine or the Pancreas expression database (Table 7.1) [29].

As the field of gene expression profiling progressed and the black spots on the map of molecular biology were filled, great hopes developed for the further use of microarrays in molecular classification in cancer. This would have introduced the field of gene expression profiling into the clinical

Table 7.1 Collection of Web Links for Databases and Software for Gene Expression Profiling

Cloud services for RNA sequencing data analysis
http://nimbusinformatics.com
http://www.lcsciences.com
https://igor.sbgenomics.com
https://dnanexus.com
Software repository for R packages
http://www.bioconductor.org
Software for statistical analysis of microarrays
http://www.hsph.harvard.edu/cli/complab/dchip/
http://www-stat.stanford.edu/~tibs/SAM/
Data repositories
http://www.ebi.ac.uk/arrayexpress/
http://www.ncbi.nlm.nih.gov/geo/
http://dcc.icgc.org/projects
https://tcga-data.nci.nih.gov/tcga/tcgaHome2.jsp
Packages for the detection of gene expression signatures
http://www.broadinstitute.org/cancer/software/genepattern/
http://tnasas.bioinfo.cnio.es
Software for the functional annotation of gene sets
http://david.abcc.ncifcrf.gov
http://akt.ucsf.edu/EGAN/
Database for cancer-related gene expression data
https://www.oncomine.org/
http://pancreasexpression.org/

workup of patient tumors, perhaps leading to new measures for the improvement of cancer patient survival. Several studies in this field generated signatures for various stages of the disease [30]; as well, pancreatic cancer signatures to determine the postoperative survival time of patients could be determined [31]. However this field sustained a serious setback after it was shown by the MAQC-II study that the extraction of signatures with current software packages is not feasible [32].

Existing microarray data have been proven to be a reliable source for the extraction of genes of interest for further analysis. The use of highly controlled input material, preferably from microdissected tissue, led to an improved understanding of the different pathways that are involved in the subtypes of ampullary carcinoma [6]. Gene expression analysis has also been helpful in understanding the crucial changes between normal and cancerous epithelia as well as benign and tumor-associated stroma [33–40,40–45].

As with other technologies, the use of DNA sequencing for gene expression profiling has its roots in the early days of the omics revolution. The first approaches employed the sequencing of cDNA libraries to generate small bits of genetic information to understand which part of the genome is actually transcribed—the so-called expressed sequence tags [46]. Using the results from these efforts, databases were created allowing for expression profiling in the computer for the identification of candidate genes in pancreatic cancer [47]. With the advent of next-generation sequencing instruments, large-scale sequencing of RNA regained focus in the science community. A typical sample goes through billions of fragmented DNAs (reads) simultaneously in a highly parallel way (massively parallel sequencing). The occurring sequencing errors in reading numerous bases are compensated by reading multiple (30–40x) DNA fragments for an accurate determination of the sequence, thereby determining somatic mutations and allelic status of polymorphisms. Typically around 90 Gb of sequence representing 30-fold coverage is obtained to call 99% of all variant alleles [48,49]. High coverage with multiple reads are needed to identify mutations that may exist only in low allele frequencies in many situations since cancer samples from patients are "contaminated" with normal tissues. Multiple tumor subclones with different genetic alterations within a tumor, comprising intratumor heterogeneity, exist, aggravating the need for even more coverage [50]. The pathogenesis of cancer is heterogeneous in terms of the spectrum of gene mutations within the same histology subtype. Therefore, sequencing of many different tumor samples is necessary to understand the full spectrum of causative mutations. Several ongoing projects are analyzing large numbers of cancer specimens, in the Cancer Genome Atlas (TCGA) initiated by NIH/NCI in the United States and the International Cancer Genome Consortium (ICGC), a network of institutes from multiple nations [51] (Table 7.1).

RNA-Seq can be used to overcome major shortcomings of whole exome sequencing. It can detect somatic mutations, and the importance to monitor recurrent mutations in cancer has been shown in ovarian cancer [52]. RNA-Seq can be used for gene expression profiling with possible higher sensitivity than microarrays, since the detection rate of transcripts is only limited by the number of reads produced. This has to be countered by the intrinsic problems of RNA-Seq. Since every available RNA molecule is sequenced, the gene expression profiling is biased to highly expressed genes. In contrast, microarrays tend to limit the signal of highly expressed genes and therefore generate expression profiles that overrepresent genes with intermediate expression [53,54]. RNA-Seq starts to replace microarray analysis for gene expression profiling for different reasons, but the major reason is that RNA-Seq acts as a one-stop shop for the determination of mutations, allele frequency, gene expression (mRNA, but also non-coding RNA), and most importantly for the detection of chimeric RNA molecule, differential splicing events, and identification of unknown classes of RNA molecules. The detection of chimeric RNA molecules enabled researchers for the very first time to identify translocation candidates for further analysis. Translocations are notoriously difficult to identify, since the partners are unknown and conventional cytogenetic analysis lacks the resolution. However, the current limits of RNA-Seq limit the usable samples with large amounts of high-quality RNA typically found in cell lines and tumor xenografts [55]. Moreover, next-generation sequencing is a converging technology like the smartphone. By its ability to integrate the different technologies relevant to cancer research (mutation detection, copy number assignment, gene expression profiling, and others), it frees the researcher from specific challenges of each technological platform, leading to new scientific questions. Advancements in molecular biology of pancreatic cancer have led to an already interesting picture. The resulting picture from gene expression profiles and other investigations demonstrates a number of changes. This leads to questions about which cells in the cancer are associated with these type of changes, making it worthwhile to analyze not just whole tumors but also parts of the cancer [56].

During the early days of gene expression profiling with microarray, the bioinformatics challenge was to isolate the data, estimate the experimental (technical and biological) error, and assign a gene expression value to a given gene. These merely technical issues have been solved so that new challenges can be tackled. In case of a gene expression analysis with Affymetrix microarrays, for the non-bioinformatician the program dChip (see Table 7.1) is a good starting point to begin the analysis. It is easy to use, fast, the workflow is very well streamlined, and it is also able to handle non-Affymetrix data.

However, the best software for non-bioinformaticians for RNA-Seq still has to emerge. The major challenge in working with RNA-Seq data is the huge amount of data produced. Handling the data is mostly out of the scope of biologists, therefore collaboration with a bioinformatician or the use of turnkey Web applications is advised (Table 7.1).

The real challenge for scientists working on gene expression data still is the assignment of biological information to their resulting list of genes of interest. Databases connecting biological information from other sources are available but often presented so they are difficult to use. However, in recent years some packages, like DAVID or EGAN (Table 7.1), have evolved that enable the researcher to analyze the biologic relevance of differentially expressed genes using networks of genes. As with all other software in this field, they rely on the computerized analysis of natural language, therefore their output has to be scrutinized before proceeding with additional experiments. Additionally, after performing such analysis, many genes are unconnected to other parts and remain single in a biologic network. This is inherent to such software and shows the amount of effort that still has to be put into the assignment of function to a huge number of genes. Therefore, it remains obligatory for scientist in this field to search on their own in literature databases for their highest-ranking genes. As with interpreting biological information into gene expression data, the analysis of gene expression signatures software has evolved to help the scientist to identify those genes. GenePattern and TNASAS are the best examples (see Table 7.1).

This is especially true in the comparison of tumor to normal tissue. The identification of differential expressed genes leads to a long list of potential candidate genes. After the annotation of those genes to different classes of molecular function of cellular organization, the scientist can investigate if there is a constant pattern in the expression profiling data. Grützmann et al. reported a comparison between ductal adenocarcinoma tissue and normal ductal tissue of the pancreas leading to several hundred candidate genes [37]. More detailed analysis of different classes of proteins showed a distinct pattern in protein kinases. Interestingly, in ductal adenocarcinoma, protein kinases associated with the cell cycle are highly overexpressed, whereas the expression of proteins in the class of receptor tyrosine kinases is lost in the cancer (Figure 7.2).

Another area to analyze the genes of interest from gene expression experiments, which is still an open research area, is the comparison of gene expression experiments. Data collection is done in two central databases (GEO and ArrayExpress, Table 7.1), but they do not enable the researchers to obtain the big picture of the gene expression of a given gene throughout the vast number of experiments performed. Curated databases like Oncomine (Table 7.1) are better suited for this purpose but lack the latest experiments due to the fact that all the data must be reanalyzed and prepared for integration.

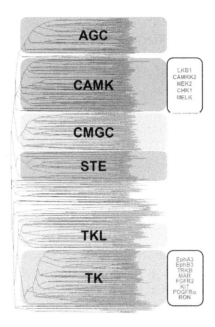

Figure 7.2 *Expression of Different Protein Kinases in Pancreatic Ductal Adenocarcinoma.* The human kinome was grouped in functional classes and the differential expressed kinases annotated. Red: overexpressed in tumors; green: underexpressed (CAMK: Ca^{2+}/calmodulin-dependent protein kinase; TK: tyrosine kinase). The expression of the well-known tumor suppressor gene LKB1/STK11 associated with the Peutz-Jeghers syndrome is lost in pancreatic cancer, indicating a fundamental role of this protein in the development of sporadic pancreatic ductal adenocarcinoma. (For interpretation of the references to color in this figure legend, the reader is referred to the web version of this book.)

Several groups have described expression data. Since the comparison of data is difficult, evaluation of these data has to be performed on the basis of each experiment. The lack of reproducibility of gene expression data is mainly due to the fact that the number of analyzed tumors remains small compared to the number of genes analyzed. Whereas statistical concerns can be addressed in post hoc investigations, the mere fact that each group decided to analyze only a minute fraction of naturally occurring pancreas cancers might lead to different results. Inclusion of published data might on the other hand enable the researcher to find new insights into pancreatic cancer as was demonstrated elegantly by Collisson et al. [57]. By a combination of internal and external data they were able to show that pancreatic cancer might consist of three different subtypes, warranting the further analysis of those for different therapeutic approaches. Gene expression analysis in pancreatic cancer also includes the analysis of miRNA expression. As in gene expression profiling, using mRNA differential expression of various miRNA molecules is reported [58,59]. Since the number of miRNAs is still growing, important miRNAs might still be discovered. MiRNA analysis displays also the advantage of RNA-Seq. With RNA-Seq every molecule might be discovered, which might be dependent only on the technical expertise of the scientist. MiRNA analysis with arrays lead to a skewed picture since only those miRNAs can be analyzed that are known at the date of array design. With all gene expression data, additional validation is needed to demonstrate the clinical relevance of a given gene. The technology of choice is high-throughput tissue microarray (TMA) analysis, enabling the investigation of protein expression in a large number of cases of pancreatic cancer [31,60]. From the results, the relevance of a protein for the treatment of patients might be deduced by associating the gene expression with parameters like postoperative survival. TMAs switch the problem of large-scale gene expression analysis from small number of samples—large number of genes into large number of samples—to small number of genes. Successful analysis of TMA data relies on the availability of the associated clinical data (and of course their quality) and the suitability of the technology used for the detection of a gene or protein. TMAs are usually produced from formalin-fixed paraffin-embedded (FFPE) tissue. This results in the availability of large sets of patient samples with a long follow-up time, but also in the restriction of available standard technologies to use such a class of tissues. Immunohistochemistry is the method of choice to investigate the protein expression of a given gene. Unfortunately, results for only the minority of protein antibodies that can be used with FFPE tissue are available, restricting the possible investigative space considerably.

SUMMARY

Since the inception of molecular biology beginning in the 1970s, gene expression profiling of RNA, structural and sequence analysis of DNA, and the delineation of the proteome have provided a powerful insight in the aberrations of cancer tissue, leading to the first drugs that attack those changes. In the future, technological progress will enable researchers to understand crucial changes even better, and gene expression profiling will aid in the successful evaluation of pancreatic tumors that may lead to the establishment of superior biomarkers and therapeutic targets.

REFERENCES

[1] Bell WC, Sexton KC, Grizzle WE. How to efficiently obtain human tissues to support specific biomedical research projects. Cancer Epidemiol Biomarkers Prev Publ Am Assoc Cancer Res Cosponsored Am Soc Prev Oncol 2009;18:1676–9.

[2] Bell WC, Sexton KC, Grizzle WE. Organizational issues in providing high-quality human tissues and clinical information for the support of biomedical research. Methods Mol Biol 2010;576:1–30.

[3] Grizzle W, Grody WW, Noll WW, Sobel ME, Stass SA, Trainer T, et al. Recommended policies for uses of human tissue in research, education, and quality control. Ad Hoc Committee on Stored Tissue, College of American Pathologists. Arch Pathol Lab Med 1999;123:296–300.

[4] Grizzle WE, Bell WC, Sexton KC. Issues in collecting, processing and storing human tissues and associated information to support biomedical research. Cancer Biomarkers Sect Dis Markers 2010;9:531–49.

[5] Beele H, van Wijk MJ, Parker R, Sánchez-Ibáñez J, Brubaker SA, Wulff B, et al. Report of the clinical donor case workshop of the European Association of Tissue Banks annual meeting 2012. Cell Tissue Bank 2013.

[6] Ehehalt F, Rümmele P, Kersting S, Lang-Schwarz C, Rückert F, Hartmann A, et al. Hepatocyte nuclear factor (HNF) 4α expression distinguishes ampullary cancer subtypes and prognosis after resection. Ann Surg 2011;254:302–10.

[7] Hanahan D, Weinberg RA. Hallmarks of cancer: the next generation. Cell 2011;144:646–74.

[8] Kristiansen G. Manual microdissection. Methods Mol Biol 2010;576:31–8.

[9] Vandewoestyne M, Goossens K, Burvenich C, Van Soom A, Peelman L, Deforce D. Laser capture microdissection: should an ultraviolet or infrared laser be used? Anal Biochem 2013;439:88–98.

[10] Olive KP, Jacobetz MA, Davidson CJ, Gopinathan A, McIntyre D, Honess D, et al. Inhibition of Hedgehog signaling enhances delivery of chemotherapy in a mouse model of pancreatic cancer. Science 2009;324:1457–61.

[11] Yorozuya K, Takeuchi T, Yoshida M, Mouri Y, Kousaka J, Fujii K, et al. Evaluation of Oncotype DX Recurrence Score as a prognostic factor in Japanese women with estrogen receptor-positive, node-negative primary stage I or IIA breast cancer. J Cancer Res Clin Oncol 2010;136:939–44.

[12] Gibson UE, Heid CA, Williams PM. A novel method for real time quantitative RT-PCR. Genome Res 1996;6:995–1001.

[13] Higuchi R, Fockler C, Dollinger G, Watson R. Kinetic PCR analysis: real-time monitoring of DNA amplification reactions. Biotechnol Nat Publ Co 1993;11:1026–30.

[14] Mullis KB, Faloona FA. Specific synthesis of DNA in vitro via a polymerase-catalyzed chain reaction. Methods Enzymol 1987;155:335–50.

[15] Holland PM, Abramson RD, Watson R, Gelfand DH. Detection of specific polymerase chain reaction product by utilizing the 5′–3′ exonuclease activity of Thermus aquaticus DNA polymerase. Proc Natl Acad Sci USA 1991;88:7276–80.

[16] Schneeberger C, Speiser P, Kury F, Zeillinger R. Quantitative detection of reverse transcriptase-PCR products by means of a novel and sensitive DNA stain. PCR Methods Appl 1995;4:234–8.

[17] Winer J, Jung CK, Shackel I, Williams PM. Development and validation of real-time quantitative reverse transcriptase-polymerase chain reaction for monitoring gene expression in cardiac myocytes in vitro. Anal Biochem 1999;270:41–9.

[18] Pfaffl MW. Quantification strategies in real-time PCR. AZ Quant PCR 2004;1:89–113.

[19] Alwine JC, Kemp DJ, Stark GR. Method for detection of specific RNAs in agarose gels by transfer to diazobenzyloxymethyl-paper and hybridization with DNA probes. Proc Natl Acad Sci USA 1977;74:5350–4.

[20] Simon MP, Besmond C, Cottreau D, Weber A, Chaumet-Riffaud P, Dreyfus JC, et al. Molecular cloning of cDNA for rat L-type pyruvate kinase and aldolase B. J Biol Chem 1983;258:14576–84.

[21] White O, Dunning T, Sutton G, Adams M, Venter JC, Fields C. A quality control algorithm for DNA sequencing projects. Nucleic Acids Res 1993;21:3829–38.

[22] DeRisi J, Penland L, Brown PO, Bittner ML, Meltzer PS, Ray M, et al. Use of a cDNA microarray to analyse gene expression patterns in human cancer. Nat Genet 1996;14:457–60.

[23] Schena M, Shalon D, Davis RW, Brown PO. Quantitative monitoring of gene expression patterns with a complementary DNA microarray. Science 1995;270:467–70.

[24] MAQC Consortium, Shi L, Reid LH, Jones WD, Shippy R, Warrington JA, et al. The MicroArray Quality Control (MAQC) project shows inter- and intraplatform reproducibility of gene expression measurements. Nat Biotechnol 2006;24:1151–61.

[25] Lipshutz RJ, Morris D, Chee M, Hubbell E, Kozal MJ, Shah N, et al. Using oligonucleotide probe arrays to access genetic diversity. BioTechniques 1995;19:442–7.

[26] Pease AC, Solas D, Sullivan EJ, Cronin MT, Holmes CP, Fodor SP. Light-generated oligonucleotide arrays for rapid DNA sequence analysis. Proc Natl Acad Sci USA 1994;91:5022–6.

[27] Bibikova M, Lin Z, Zhou L, Chudin E, Garcia EW, Wu B, et al. High-throughput DNA methylation profiling using universal bead arrays. Genome Res 2006;16:383–93.

[28] Brazma A, Hingamp P, Quackenbush J, Sherlock G, Spellman P, Stoeckert C, et al. Minimum information about a microarray experiment (MIAME)-toward standards for microarray data. Nat Genet 2001;29:365–71.

[29] Rhodes DR, Yu J, Shanker K, Deshpande N, Varambally R, Ghosh D, et al. ONCOMINE: a cancer microarray database and integrated data-mining platform. Neoplasia 2004;6:1–6.

[30] Arpino G, Generali D, Sapino A, Lucia DM, Frassoldati A, de Laurentis M, et al. Gene expression profiling in breast cancer: a clinical perspective. Breast 2013;22:109–20.

[31] Winter C, Kristiansen G, Kersting S, Roy J, Aust D, Knösel T, et al. Google goes cancer: improving outcome prediction for cancer patients by network-based ranking of marker genes. PLoS Comput Biol 2012;8:e1002511.

[32] Shi L, Campbell G, Jones WD, Campagne F, Wen Z, Walker SJ, et al. The MicroArray Quality Control (MAQC)-II study of common practices for the development and validation of microarray-based predictive models. Nat Biotechnol 2010;28:827–38.

[33] Brandt R, Grützmann R, Bauer A, Jesnowski R, Ringel J, Löhr M, et al. DNA microarray analysis of pancreatic malignancies. Pancreatology 2004;4:587–97.

[34] Broadhead ML, Clark JCM, Dass CR, Choong PFM. Microarray: an instrument for cancer surgeons of the future? ANZ J Surg 2010;80:531–6.

[35] Feldmann G, Maitra A. Molecular genetics of pancreatic ductal adenocarcinomas and recent implications for translational efforts. J Mol Diagn 2008;10:111–22.

[36] Goonetilleke KS, Siriwardena AK. Current status of gene expression profiling of pancreatic cancer. Int J Surg 2008;6:81–3.

[37] Grützmann R, Pilarsky C, Ammerpohl O, Lüttges J, Böhme A, Sipos B, et al. Gene expression profiling of microdissected pancreatic ductal carcinomas using high-density DNA microarrays. Neoplasia 2004;6:611–22.

[38] Grützmann R, Saeger HD, Lüttges J, Schackert HK, Kalthoff H, Klöppel G, et al. Microarray-based gene expression profiling in pancreatic ductal carcinoma: status quo and perspectives. Int J Colorectal Dis 2004;19:401–13.

[39] Grützmann R, Boriss H, Ammerpohl O, Lüttges J, Kalthoff H, Schackert HK, et al. Meta-analysis of microarray data on pancreatic cancer defines a set of commonly dysregulated genes. Oncogene 2005;24:5079–88.

[40] Harada T, Chelala C, Crnogorac-Jurcevic T, Lemoine NR. Genome-wide analysis of pancreatic cancer using microarray-based techniques. Pancreatology 2009;9:13–24.

[41] Harsha HC, Kandasamy K, Ranganathan P, Rani S, Ramabadran S, Gollapudi S, et al. A compendium of potential biomarkers of pancreatic cancer. PLoS Med 2009;6:e1000046.
[42] López-Casas PP, López-Fernández LA. Gene-expression profiling in pancreatic cancer. Expert Rev Mol Diagn 2010;10:591–601.
[43] Matthaei H, Dal Molin M, Maitra A. Identification and analysis of precursors to invasive pancreatic cancer. Methods Mol Biol 2013;980:1–12.
[44] Pilarsky C, Ammerpohl O, Sipos B, Dahl E, Hartmann A, Wellmann A, et al. Activation of Wnt signalling in stroma from pancreatic cancer identified by gene expression profiling. J Cell Mol Med 2008;12:2823–35.
[45] Yeh JJ. Prognostic signature for pancreatic cancer: are we close? Future Oncol 2009;5:313–21.
[46] Adams MD, Dubnick M, Kerlavage AR, Moreno R, Kelley JM, Utterback TR, et al. Sequence identification of 2,375 human brain genes. Nature 1992;355:632–4.
[47] Grützmann R, Pilarsky C, Staub E, Schmitt AO, Foerder M, Specht T, et al. Systematic isolation of genes differentially expressed in normal and cancerous tissue of the pancreas. Pancreatology 2003;3:169–78.
[48] Li H, Ruan J, Durbin R. Mapping short DNA sequencing reads and calling variants using mapping quality scores. Genome Res 2008;18:1851–8.
[49] Yoshida K, Sanada M, Ogawa S. Deep sequencing in cancer research. Jpn J Clin Oncol 2013;43:110–5.
[50] Martinez P, Birkbak NJ, Gerlinger M, McGranahan N, Burrell RA, Rowan AJ, et al. Parallel evolution of tumour subclones mimics diversity between tumours. J Pathol 2013;230:356–64.
[51] Cancer Genome Atlas Research Network, Genome Characterization Center, Chang K, Creighton CJ, Davis C, Donehower L, et al. The Cancer Genome Atlas Pan-Cancer analysis project. Nat Genet 2013;45:1113–20.
[52] Shah SP, Köbel M, Senz J, Morin RD, Clarke BA, Wiegand KC, et al. Mutation of FOXL2 in granulosa-cell tumors of the ovary. N Engl J Med 2009;360:2719–29.
[53] Mastrokolias A, den Dunnen JT, van Ommen GB, 't Hoen PA, van Roon-Mom WM. Increased sensitivity of next generation sequencing-based expression profiling after globin reduction in human blood RNA. BMC Genomics 2012;13:28.
[54] Mooney M, Bond J, Monks N, Eugster E, Cherba D, Berlinski P, et al. Comparative RNA-Seq and microarray analysis of gene expression changes in B-cell lymphomas of Canis familiaris. PLoS One 2013;8:e61088.
[55] Edgren H, Murumagi A, Kangaspeska S, Nicorici D, Hongisto V, Kleivi K, et al. Identification of fusion genes in breast cancer by paired-end RNA-sequencing. Genome Biol 2011;12:R6.
[56] Gerlinger M, Rowan AJ, Horswell S, Larkin J, Endesfelder D, Gronroos E, et al. Intra-tumor heterogeneity and branched evolution revealed by multiregion sequencing. N Engl J Med 2012;366:883–92.
[57] Collisson EA, Sadanandam A, Olson P, Gibb WJ, Truitt M, Gu S, et al. Subtypes of pancreatic ductal adenocarcinoma and their differing responses to therapy. Nat Med 2011;17:500–3.
[58] Lee EJ, Gusev Y, Jiang J, Nuovo GJ, Lerner MR, Frankel WL, et al. Expression profiling identifies microRNA signature in pancreatic cancer. Int J Cancer 2007;120:1046–54.
[59] Volinia S, Calin GA, Liu C-G, Ambs S, Cimmino A, Petrocca F, et al. A microRNA expression signature of human solid tumors defines cancer gene targets. Proc Natl Acad Sci USA 2006;103:2257–61.
[60] Pérez-Mancera PA, Rust AG, van der Weyden L, Kristiansen G, Li A, Sarver AL, et al. The deubiquitinase USP9X suppresses pancreatic ductal adenocarcinoma. Nature 2012;486:266–70.

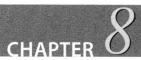

CHAPTER 8

Genetic Susceptibility and Risk of Pancreatic Cancer

Jason Hoskins, Jinping Jia, Laufey T. Amundadottir

Laboratory of Translational Genomics, Division of Cancer Epidemiology and Genetics, National Cancer Institute, National Institutes of Health, Bethesda, MD, USA

Contents

Introduction	169
Familial Risk of Pancreatic Cancer	170
Rare, High-Risk Pancreatic Cancer Susceptibility Genes and Multicancer Syndromes	171
Common, Low-Risk Pancreatic Cancer Susceptibility Loci	174
Common Pancreatic Cancer Risk Loci in Non-European Populations	179
Pathway Analyses of Pancreatic Cancer GWAS Data Sets	181
Future GWAS and Gene Mapping Approaches	186
Websites	188
References	188

INTRODUCTION

This year in the United States, an estimated 45,220 people will be diagnosed with pancreatic cancer and 38,460 will die from the disease [1]. Although pancreatic cancer is the 10th most commonly diagnosed cancer in the United States, it is the 4th most common cause of cancer death in both sexes [1]. The best chance for survival is early detection when the tumor can be removed surgically. Most pancreatic cancers are asymptomatic at early stages, however, and by the time they are diagnosed, the majority of patients present with distant metastases. Only about 15–20% of pancreatic adenocarcinoma (PDAC) cases are diagnosed early enough for surgery [1]. Survival is correlated to stage: patients who present with distant metastases at diagnosis have dismal 5-year survival rates of only 2%, whereas patients diagnosed at an early stage exceed 20%, indicating the potential benefit of early detection [2]. These rates are still bleak, however, and call out for new and better strategies for prevention, early diagnosis, and treatment of pancreatic cancer to reduce the burden of this disease.

Molecular Diagnostics and Treatment of Pancreatic Cancer   Published by Elsevier Inc.

Known risk factors for pancreatic cancer include smoking, diabetes, obesity, chronic pancreatitis, heavy alcohol consumption, age, and a family history of the disease [3–12]. A small proportion of the familial aggregation of pancreatic cancer can be explained by hereditary cancer syndromes and inherited forms of pancreatitis, caused by rare high-risk inherited mutations [13–21]. The genetic basis for the majority of familial aggregation of pancreatic cancer has yet to be explained. The search for common and rare germline variants that influence risk of pancreatic cancer through genome-wide association studies (GWAS) and high-throughput sequencing based studies is under way, and this search holds the promise of increasing our knowledge of variants and genes that play a role in inherited susceptibility of this devastating disease.

FAMILIAL RISK OF PANCREATIC CANCER

Epidemiological studies have shown that individuals with a family history of pancreatic cancer are at an increased risk of developing pancreatic cancer. One of the largest studies reported to date was conducted within the Pancreatic Cancer Cohort consortium (PanScan) and included 11 studies (10 cohort and 1 case–control studies) with 1183 cases and 1205 controls. A family history of pancreatic cancer in a first-degree relative was associated with an increased risk of pancreatic cancer with an odds ratio (OR) of 1.76 (95% confidence interval, CI 1.19–2.61). Individuals with two or more first-degree relatives diagnosed with pancreatic cancer, although not common, were at even greater risk (OR = 4.26, 95% CI 0.48–37.79) [11]. Results from other large studies have described similar increases. A cancer registry–based analysis conducted within the Swedish Family-Cancer Database reported a 1.73-fold increase in the incidence of pancreatic cancer (standardized incidence ratio, SIR = 1.73, 95% CI 1.13–2.54) among offspring of patients diagnosed with PDAC [22].

A study linking the Utah Cancer Registry to the Utah Population Database, showed a significant familial clustering for pancreatic cancer, both in first-degree (RR = 1.84; 95% CI 1.47–2.29; $P < 0.0001$) and second-degree (RR = 1.59; 95% CI 1.31–2.91; $P < 0.0001$) relatives of individuals with pancreatic cancer [23]. A population-based study in Iceland, linking cancer registry information, including all pancreatic cancer patients diagnosed in the country from 1955 to 2002 ($n = 930$) with a population-wide genealogy database, reported somewhat higher risk to first-degree relatives (RR = 2.33, 90% CI 1.83–2.96) [24].

RARE, HIGH-RISK PANCREATIC CANCER SUSCEPTIBILITY GENES AND MULTICANCER SYNDROMES

Up to 10% of pancreatic cancer cases in the United States occur in the context of a familial pattern [25–27]. Many cases of inherited pancreatic cancer are attributable to inherited chronic inflammatory conditions like hereditary pancreatitis (HP) and cystic fibrosis (CF), or familial multi-cancer syndromes like Peutz–Jeghers syndrome (PJS), Familial Atypical Multiple Mole Melanoma (FAMMM), or Lynch syndrome. Hereditary pancreatic cancer cases containing ≥2 afflicted first-degree family members, and not attributed to such predefined syndromes, are classified as familial pancreatic cancer (FPC) syndrome [26]. Because only ~20% of these FPC cases have been associated with specific mutations, the hereditary basis for FPC remains largely unclear.

HP is characterized by recurrent bouts of acute pancreatitis (inflammation of the pancreas) in childhood or early adolescence that eventually develops into chronic pancreatitis [27,28]. The most common mutation found in HP cases is in the cationic trypsinogen gene *PRSS1*, although mutations also have been observed in *SPINK1* (encoding a serine protease inhibitor), *PRSS2* (encoding anionic trypsinogen), and *CTRC* (encoding chymotrypsin C). These mutations lead to inappropriate protease activity within the pancreatic parenchyma, causing autodigestive injury and inflammation. Patients with HP have a 26- to 60-fold increased risk of pancreatic cancer depending on the etiology, with a lifetime risk of up to 40% [26–28]. This lifetime risk is increased to 75% with onset typically 20 years earlier for smokers with HP. Chronic pancreatitis is a PDAC risk factor even without a genetic basis, and in each case, persistent inflammation appears to promote this effect. Pancreatic acinar cells display surprising resistance to robust oncogenic insults in mouse models (including heterozygous expression of $Kras^{G12V}$ or conditional *TP53* or *Cdkn2a* knockouts), but induction of pancreatitis greatly accelerates PanIN and PDAC development in $Kras^{G12V}$-expressing mice [29,30]. This protumorigenic effect may work by abrogating oncogene-induced senescence [29].

Consistent with the important role of inflammation in pancreatic tumor progression, CF patients have a PDAC risk ratio of 5.3 [26,28,31]. CF is caused by an autosomal recessive mutation in the *CFTR* gene, which encodes a cyclic AMP (cAMP)-mediated chloride channel. The pancreatic pathology of CF stems from obstruction of pancreatic ducts by excessively thick mucus secretions, which can lead to chronic inflammation and fibrosis. Interestingly, a study of young onset pancreatic cancer cases found that 8.4% were heterozygous carriers of the *CFTR* mutation, compared with the 4.1% frequency in controls, despite the lack of CF symptoms in carriers [32].

PJS is associated with monoallelic mutations in the *STK11* gene (also called *LKB1*), resulting in haplo-insufficient tumor suppressor activity. This leads to benign gastrointestinal polyps and a greatly increased lifetime risk of breast, gynecologic, and gastrointestinal cancers [33]. Individuals with PJS have a 132-fold increased risk of developing pancreatic cancer, making *STK11* one of the most penetrant susceptibility genes identified thus far for inherited pancreatic cancer [26]. *STK11* encodes a serine–threonine kinase involved in the regulation of diverse processes, such as cell growth, cell polarity, energy metabolism, and apoptosis [33]. Many of these effects are mediated through AMP-activated protein kinase and mammalian target of rapamycin signaling, although *STK11* directly regulates other pathways as well. Although *STK11* knockout in murine pancreatic epithelium does result in ductal metaplasia and cystadenomas, there is no progression to PanINs or PDAC without additional mutations like oncogenic *KRAS*, suggesting that *STK11* mutations support, rather than drive, tumorigenesis [33].

FAMMM syndrome commonly is caused by inactivating mutations of the *p16INK4A* tumor suppressor, which increases PDAC risk 13- to 20-fold [25,34–36]. The *p16INK4A* and *p19ARF* tumor suppressors overlap in the *CDKN2A* gene, although they are encoded by distinct first exons and shared downstream exons with alternative reading frames. In several PDAC cases, however, germline and sporadic mutations were identified that alter *p16INK4A* without affecting *p19ARF*, strongly suggesting that changes in p16INK4A activity are the source of heritable risk [25,37–39]. Expression of *p16INK4A* is induced by environmental stresses, age, and aberrant proliferation, leading to inhibition of CDK4/6-mediated RB phosphorylation, ultimately blocking S-phase entry [25,40–42]. This senescence effect must be overcome for full progression of pancreatic neoplasias to PDAC, and germline mutations in one allele puts carriers at a much higher risk of total loss of *p16INK4A* function.

Lynch syndrome results from germline mutations in mismatch repair (MMR) genes (e.g., *MSH2, MSH6, MLH1, PMS1,* or *PMS2*) [26–28]. Upon biallelic deficiency of an MMR gene, genomic instability rises, which is manifest in microsatellite-instable tumors of the colon. Lynch syndrome patients are at extremely high risk of colon cancer, but risks for some extracolonic cancers are increased as well. This includes pancreatic cancer, for which up to an ~8.6-fold increased risk has been reported [27]. Microsatellite instability testing in pancreatic and breast tumors from 15 patients afflicted with Lynch syndrome showed minor instability in only one tumor, and no biallelic deficiency was revealed by genotyping or immunohistochemistry of relevant MMR genes in any case [43]. Furthermore, microsatellite instability was identified in only 1 of 338 sporadic PDAC tumors, which was due to apparent epigenetic downregulation of *MLH1* [44]. These results raise the possibility that at least some proportion of Lynch syndrome–related pancreas tumors could be promoted through mechanisms independent of MMR impairment.

Familial adenomatous polyposis (FAP) syndrome results from autosomal dominant germline mutations in *APC*, which encodes a scaffold protein that forms a complex with Axin, *GSK3*, and β-catenin [28]. Wnt signaling disrupts this interaction, causing release and accumulation of β-catenin, thus activating transcription of the protumor factors c-Myc, c-Jun, and cyclin D1. Mutations in *APC* causing FAP lead to constitutive activation of the Wnt signaling cascade. FAP syndrome presents with early onset colonic or gastric polyps that can progress to carcinomas. Additionally, FAP causes a 4.6-fold increased risk of developing PDAC [26,28].

Pancreatic cancer is also part of the broad multicancer spectrum of Li–Fraumeni syndrome, which is caused by germline mutations in the *TP53* tumor suppressor gene [26,28]. *TP53* encodes p53, whose transcriptional activity is greatly induced in response to a wide range of cellular stresses, including DNA damage, hypoxia, nutrient deprivation, or oncogene activation [25,28]. Induction results largely from stabilization of p53 and can lead to cell-cycle arrest, apoptosis, senescence, modulation of nutrient consumption, or changes in reactive oxygen species production, depending on various post-translational modifications [45]. Given the well-established role of p53 in tumor suppression, along with observed somatic *TP53* mutations in >50% of PDAC tumors, it is not surprising that pancreatic cancer is part of the Li-Fraumeni spectrum of cancers. It is estimated that ~1.3% of Li-Fraumeni cases develop PDAC, making it a relatively minor genetic risk factor [26,28].

Hereditary breast and ovarian cancer (HBOC) syndrome features high risk of early onset familial breast or gynecologic cancers and modestly increased risk of prostate and pancreatic cancer [26,27,46,47]. Germline mutations in *BRCA1* or *BRCA2*, identified nearly 20 years ago, are responsible for ~90% of HBOC cases. Both *BRCA1* and *BRCA2* are important in homologous repair and double-strand break repair of DNA, and *BRCA1* also plays a role in cell-cycle regulation. Although well established as a cause of HBOC, the relevance of *BRCA1* to pancreatic cancer risk is murky. Studies have found 0 to 2.56-fold increased pancreatic cancer risk in

BRCA1 mutation carriers. In contrast, up to 16% of cases from FPC kindreds reportedly carried *BRCA2* mutations, and a large study of *BRCA2*-mutated HBOC cases estimated a 3.5-fold increased risk of PDAC. Some germline *BRCA2* mutations have been identified in sporadic or familial pancreatic cancer cases with no reported family history of breast or ovarian cancer, or in some cases, any cancer at all [27,47]. For this reason, *BRCA2* mutations often are associated with FPC syndrome in addition to HBOC.

Because of the large proportion of unexplained FPC cases, whole genome sequencing (WGS) and exome sequencing (ES) of FPC kindreds recently were performed to identify causal mutations. This led to the discovery of germline deleterious mutations in the *PALB2* and *ATM* genes in ~3.1 and ~2.4% of tested FPC cases, respectively [16,48]. *ATM* encodes a serine–threonine kinase involved in initiating DNA double-strand break repair by phosphorylating downstream effectors, including *BRCA1* [46,48]. *PALB2* encodes a protein scaffold for *BRCA1* and *BRCA2* and promotes intranuclear localization and stabilization of *BRCA2*. It is an interesting coincidence that *BRCA2*, *ATM*, and *PALB2* are all involved in the same double-strand break and homologous DNA repair pathway. A germline missense mutation of the *PALLD* gene was identified in all affected members of one FPC family; however, mutations in this gene have not been found in any other families tested, suggesting it is not a common cause of FPC [28].

COMMON, LOW-RISK PANCREATIC CANCER SUSCEPTIBILITY LOCI

Many common diseases are known to cluster in families and are believed to be influenced by both genetic and environmental factors. As discussed, pancreatic cancer is no exception. It most likely is influenced by environmental interactions with multiple germline variants with a wide range in allele frequencies and effect sizes. Until a few years ago, family-based linkage studies were the main approach to map genes for disease, including pancreatic cancer. The strength of linkage analysis is in finding high-risk, mostly uncommon, germline variants in families with a high concentration of cases with a specific disease. The linkage approach was quite successful for Mendelian disorders, but it has limited power and low resolution for variants of small effects that probably explain much of the inherited susceptibility to complex diseases.

GWAS have now become an important addition to the linkage approach. The identification of genetic variants that contribute to the risk of common diseases has become possible in the last several years, through the generation of the human genome sequence and annotation of human genetic variation by the HapMap and 1000G consortia [49–52]. These advances, coupled with improvements in technology, allowed the construction of so-called single-nucleotide polymorphism (SNP) chips or SNP arrays that enable genome-wide interrogation of germline variants with relative ease. These brought on the GWAS era, which has been tremendously successful for a multitude of complex diseases, including various cancers and traits associated with a risk of cancer (e.g., body mass index (BMI), diabetes, and smoking) in identifying approximately 2000 associations for more than 300 complex diseases and traits [53,54]. Genotyping arrays used for GWAS are designed to identify common susceptibility alleles in an agnostic manner, and for the first few years, assessed hundreds of thousands of SNPs in thousands of individuals. Newer arrays assess even higher numbers of SNPs (up to 5 million) and thereby can target both common and less common variants.

Although the first GWAS for pancreatic cancer was not published until 2009, these studies now have been performed in individuals of both European and Asian ancestry. The first pancreatic cancer GWAS studies were performed by PanScan, conducted within the framework of the National Cancer Institute–sponsored Cohort Consortium, with the aim of identifying susceptibility markers for this deadly disease. Two phases of the GWAS have been reported, PanScan I and II [55,56]. East phase consisted of 12 nested case–control studies within prospective cohort studies and 8 case–control studies. The total number of subjects included 3851 patients diagnosed with PDAC and 3934 control subjects, of which ~95% were of European ancestry [55,56]. A combined analysis identified four genome-wide significant pancreatic cancer risk loci marked by common variants with small effect sizes: chromosome 9q34.2 marked by SNP rs505922 in the *ABO* blood group gene ($P = 5.37 \times 10^{-8}$, $OR_{Allele} = 1.20$), chr1q32.1 in the *NR5A2* gene (rs3790844; $P = 2.5 \times 10^{-10}$; $OR_{Allele} = 0.77$); chr5p15.33 in the *CLPTM1L-TERT* gene region (rs401681; $P = 3.7 \times 10^{-7}$; $OR_{Allele} = 1.19$); and chr13q22.1 in a non-genic region (rs9543325; $P = 3.3 \times 10^{-11}$; $OR_{Allele} = 1.26$). Common variants in the *CLPTM1L-TERT* locus have been associated with multiple cancers, through a number of GWAS, including lung, bladder, prostate, breast, melanoma, glioma, ovarian, testicular, and basal cell cancer, whereas the other three loci appear to be pancreatic cancer specific [57–68].

Two additional pancreatic cancer GWAS are ongoing in subjects of European ancestry. One study is the third phase of PanScan (PanScan III), which includes a GWAS of ~2000 pancreatic cancer cases and ~5000 control subjects with replication of top findings in ~2500 case and ~3500 control subjects. In addition, the Pancreatic Cancer Case Control Consortium (PanC4) is conducting a GWAS that includes ~4000 case–control pairs. These two studies will bring the total number of subjects with GWAS data to ~10,000 pancreatic cancer cases and ~13,000 controls, leading to much improved statistical power and presumably the discovery of additional PDAC risk loci.

The main risk SNPs on 9q34.2 in the *ABO* gene (rs505922, $OR_{Allele} = 1.20$, $P = 5.37 \times 10^{-8}$) reportedly have been associated with risk for venous thrombosis, stroke, ulcer, and Grave's disease, as well as with circulating tumor necrosis factor (TNF)α, soluble intercellular adhesion molecule (sICAM), and alkaline-phosphatase levels through GWAS [69–74]. The protective allele of rs505922 is in complete linkage disequilibrium (LD) with the O allele of the *ABO* locus ($r^2 = 1$). The *ABO* gene encodes a glycosyltransferase (histo-blood group ABO system transferase) that catalyzes the transfer of carbohydrates to the H antigen, forming the structure of the ABO blood groups first described by Karl Landsteiner in 1900. Small studies published in the 1950 and 1960s reported an association between ABO blood type and gastrointestinal cancers, both gastric and pancreatic cancer, consistent with the results from PanScan [75,76].

The discovery of the ABO risk locus reawakened interest in the blood groups and risk of pancreatic cancer. Using PanScan I GWAS data, individual ABO alleles were inferred and their association with pancreatic cancer risk determined [77]. Individuals with inferred A (AA and AO), AB, and B (BB and BO) blood groups had an increased risk of pancreatic cancer as compared with the O group: 1.38 (95% CI 1.18–1.62), 1.47 (95% CI 1.07–2.02), and 1.53 (95% CI 1.21–1.92), respectively, indicating that ABO genotypes are risk alleles for pancreatic cancer [77]. Extending this study to investigate whether glycosyltransferase activity influences pancreatic cancer risk, genotypes were established in a similar manner to mark the A1 and A2 alleles, as the former has higher glycosyltransferase activity than the latter [78]. The A1 alleles conferred an increased risk of pancreatic cancer (OR = 1.38, 95% CI 1.20–1.58), whereas A2 alleles did not (OR = 0.96, 95% CI 0.77–1.20) [79]. A significant difference was not seen between the two nonfunctional O variants (O-01 and O-02) or by secretor status as characterized by alleles at rs601338 in the *FUT2* gene on 19q13.33 [79]. This gene encodes galactoside 2-alpha-ʟ-fucosyltransferase 2 (the H antigen), and an A allele at rs601338 introduces a stop codon at amino acid 154 (W154X). Individuals homozygous for this allele do not express an intact H antigen and do not produce ABO antigens in body fluids [80]. Although more work is needed to solve the mechanism of action at 9q34.2, an increased glycosyl-transferase activity, either toward the H antigen or other proteins glycosyl-ated by the protein product of the *ABO* gene, may explain the risk.

Studies investigating the underlying mechanism for the link between blood groups and pancreatic cancer risk suggested a possible mechanistic link to gastric infection by *Helicobacter pylori*, as both non-O blood groups and gastric colonization by *H. pylori* are risk factors for pancreatic cancer [55,81]. In this study, an increased risk of pancreatic cancer was associated with non-O blood groups (OR = 1.37, 95% CI 1.02–1.83, $P = 0.034$) and seropositivity for CagA-negative *H. pylori* (OR = 1.68, 95% CI 1.07–2.66, $P = 0.025$). Furthermore, the association between pancreatic cancer risk and seropositivity for CagA-negative *H. pylori* was found in individuals with non-O blood types (OR = 2.78, 95% CI 1.49–5.20, $P = 0.0014$), but not in those with the O blood type (OR = 1.28, 95% CI 0.62–2.64, $P = 0.51$), suggesting that the presence of A and B blood group antigens may influence how the bacteria binds to the gastric mucosa [82].

The most significant SNP on chr1q32.1 maps to the first intron of the *NR5A2* gene (rs3790844, $OR_{Allele} = 0.77$, $P = 2.5 \times 10^{-10}$). This gene encodes an orphan nuclear receptor subfamily 5 group A member 2 and is a plausible candidate gene for the action of risk variants on chr1q32.1. *NR5A2* (sometimes referred to as liver receptor homolog-1) is a transcription factor that plays vital roles in early development, cholesterol synthesis, bile acid homeostasis, and steroidogenesis [83]. *NR5A2* can replace octamer-binding protein 4 (Oct-4) during the reprogramming of somatic mouse cells to induce pluripotent stem cells, indicating an important role in regulating stemness, probably in part through its interaction with DAX1 and transcriptional activation of the *OCT4* gene [84,85]. It activates expression of cyclin E1, cyclin D1, and c-Myc by directly binding the *CCNE1* promoter but indirectly binding the *CCND1* and *MYC* promoters. In the former case, β-catenin acts as a coactivator for promoter-bound NR5A2, but in the latter cases, the roles are reversed and NR5A2 acts as a coactivator for promoter-bound β-catenin [86]. In the adult pancreas, *NR5A2* is an important regulator of exocrine pancreatic function where it cooperates with pancreas-specific transcription factor 1 to directly bind and activate a series of acinar specific genes [87].

Mice heterozygous for *NR5A2* exhibit increased rates of acinar to ductal metaplasia and impaired recovery after caerulein-induced acute pancreatitis [30]. Furthermore, *NR5A2* haploinsufficiency cooperates with pancreatitis in a pancreatic cancer mouse model driven by oncogenic *KRAS*, increasing the number of preneoplastic PanIN lesions and driving their progression toward PDAC [30]. Likewise, in mouse models, caerulein-induced pancreatitis leads to a transient downregulation of multiple acinar and endocrine genes, including *NR5A2*, *HNF1A*, and pancreas–duodenum homeobox protein 1 (*PDX1*). This effect correlates with increased proliferation of acinar cells [88]. HNF-1A was shown to bind the promoter and to regulate expression of the *NR5A2* gene [88]. Thus, reduced expression of *NR5A2* and other acinar genes may contribute to increased proliferation and faster progression of PanINs in mouse pancreatic cancer models. Although the mechanism of NR5A2's apparent tumor suppressive effects are still unclear, they may be related to the functional action of the risk variants on chr1q32.1.

The most significant pancreatic cancer GWAS SNP on chr5p15.33 was rs401681 ($P = 3.7 \times 10^{-7}$, $OR_{Allele} = 1.19$, 95% CI 1.11–1.27) located in a multi–cancer-risk locus containing two genes, *TERT* and *CLPTM1L* [89]. *TERT* encodes the catalytic subunit of telomerase, which is well known for its essential role in maintaining telomere ends and increased telomerase activity commonly seen in human cancers [90–92]. Telomerase also has telomere-independent functions, including in the regulation of gene expression, cell survival, epithelial to mesenchymal transition, and mitochondrial function [93]. The function of *CLPTM1L* is not as clear, although its encoded protein, cleft lip and palate-associated transmembrane 1-like protein, has been proposed to be a survival factor in lung cancer in which case it protects cancer cells from apoptosis after treatment with DNA-damaging agents [94,95]. A gain of chromosome 5p is one of the most recurrent chromosomal abnormalities in human cancers, including pancreatic cancer [96]. In many tumors, the amplified region includes the *TERT* gene but not *CLPTM1L*. This is reversed, however, in many tumors in which only *CLPTM1L* is amplified and overexpressed, indicating that *TERT* may not be the only gene in this region important for cancer [97,98].

Haplotype analysis based on the PanScan GWAS data indicated that 5p15.33 was the only one of the four susceptibility loci with more significant haplotypes as compared with the individual SNPs (by three orders of magnitude) [56]. Intriguingly, the T allele of rs401681 has been associated with increased risk of pancreatic cancer and melanoma [56,63,67] while also having been associated with decreased risk of lung, prostate, bladder, and basal cell carcinoma [58,59,63,67]. It is not clear how the same locus can confer increased or decreased risk depending on the cancer type, but this suggests that more than one mechanism may be at play.

The top-ranked GWAS SNP on chr13q22.1, rs9543325 ($P = 3.27 \times 10^{-11}$, $OR_{Allele} = 1.26$, 95% CI 1.18–1.35), is found in a 600 kb nongenic region [56]. The lack of transcription near the risk locus suggests that the functional variant could affect a putative regulatory element in an allele-specific manner. This regulatory element could affect gene expression at great distance through intra- or interchromosomal interactions. The chr13q22.1 risk locus is flanked by two genes encoding transcription factors of the Kruppel-like family: *KLF5* and *KLF12* [99]. Both genes play a role in regulating cell growth and transformation [100,101] and *KLF5* is upregulated in pancreatic cancer [102]. Other genes in the region include *PIBF1*, *DIS3*, *BORA*, and *MZT1*, all of which are located upstream of *KLF5*. *PIBF1* is overexpressed in a number of malignant tumor types, and it is thought to play a role in progesterone-dependent immunomodulation [103,104]. *DIS3* encodes a ubiquitously expressed nuclear 3′–5′ riboexonuclease broadly involved in RNA processing and surveillance [105,106]. Mutations in *DIS3* have been identified in acute myeloid leukemia and multiple myeloma, and its expression correlated with metastatic potential in colorectal cancer [107–109]. *BORA* is a cofactor of aurora kinase A, which regulates cell proliferation and frequently is amplified in tumors [110]. *MZT1* is a member of the gamma-tubulin ring complex that is involved in mitotic spindle organization [111]. Although to date *MZT1* has not been associated with any cancers, its role in mitosis and chromosomal segregation suggests possible relevance to tumor progression. Any of these distantly neighboring genes could be functionally relevant to the mechanism by which the chr13q22.1 GWAS locus confers risk of PDAC.

COMMON PANCREATIC CANCER RISK LOCI IN NON-EUROPEAN POPULATIONS

In fully interrogating risk loci for any disease, it is important to conduct GWAS across multiple populations. In addition to the PanScan GWAS, in which the majority of subjects were of European ancestry, GWAS have now been performed in case–control studies from China and Japan. Additional studies of Asian ancestry are needed to increase the power for detection. Hopefully these will continue to grow, as well as those for other ethnicities like populations of West Asian, African, South American, and Middle Eastern ancestry, for whom pancreatic cancer GWAS have not been reported.

The Japanese GWAS was performed with 991 cases diagnosed with advanced pancreatic ductal adenocarcinoma and 5209 control subjects. This study identified three loci with GWAS significance on chromosomes 6p25.3/*FOXQ1* (rs9502893: $OR_{Allelic} = 1.29$, $P = 3.30 \times 10^{-7}$), 12p11.21/*BICD1* (rs708224: $OR_{Allelic} = 1.32$, $P = 3.3 \times 10^{-7}$) and 7q36.2/*DPP6* (rs6464375: $OR_{Recessive} = 3.73$, $P = 4.4 \times 10^{-7}$) [112]. Risk loci previously discovered in Europeans (PanScan) showed moderate (chr13q22.1: rs9543325, $P_{Allelic} = 1.69 \times 10^{-4}$) or weak (chr9q34.2: rs505922, $P_{Allelic} = 0.0369$; 1q32.1: rs3790844, $P_{Allelic} = 0.0124$) association in the Japanese study population [112].

In the Chinese scan (ChinaPC), a two-phased approach was performed with a GWAS of 981 pancreatic cancer cases and 1991 control subjects in the discovery phase and a replication in 2603 cases and 2877 controls. Five risk loci were noted: chr21q21.3/*BACH1* (rs372883: $OR = 0.79$ $P = 2.24 \times 10^{-13}$), chr21q22.3/*TFF1* (rs1547374: $OR = 0.79$, $P = 3.71 \times 10^{-13}$), chr10q26.11/*PRLHR* gene (rs12413624: $OR = 1.23$, $P = 5.12 \times 10^{-11}$), chr22q13.32/*FAM19A5* (rs5768709: $OR = 1.25$, $P = 1.41 \times 10^{-10}$), and chr5p13.1/*DAB2* gene (rs2255280: $OR = 0.81$, $P = 4.18 \times 10^{-10}$) [113]. This group also replicated the chr13q22.1 locus initially discovered in PanScan (through a perfectly correlated SNP, rs4885093, $P = 1.57 \times 10^{-12}$), and noted loci on chr1q32.1 (rs3790843, $P = 0.0106$) and chr5p15.33 (rs401681, $P = 7.35 \times 10^{-5}$), albeit at lower significance. On the other hand, SNPs marking 9q34.2 (rs505922) in the European scan and those marking 6p25.3 (rs9502893), 12p11.21 (rs708224), and 7q36.2 (rs6464375) in the Japanese scan were not nominally significant in the Chinese scan [113].

A replication of the Chinese and Japanese pancreatic cancer risk loci recently was attempted in 1299 PDAC cases and 2884 controls from the European PANcreatic Disease ReseArch (PANDoRA) case–control consortium. None of the seven pancreatic cancer susceptibility loci identified in the two Asian populations were associated significantly with the risk of pancreatic cancer in Europeans, although one SNP was monomorphic in Europeans [114].

We are slowly filling in the landscape for inherited susceptibility variants that influence risk of pancreatic cancer (Figure 8.1). Even as this picture evolves, however, each risk locus uncovered requires significant functional exploration. All pancreatic cancer risk loci identified to date through GWAS are nonprotein coding. Because our understanding of the nongenic regions of the genome is limited, this task may be even more arduous than the identification of the risk variant themselves. It involves the identification of target genes influenced by risk variants and the mechanism by which they mediate

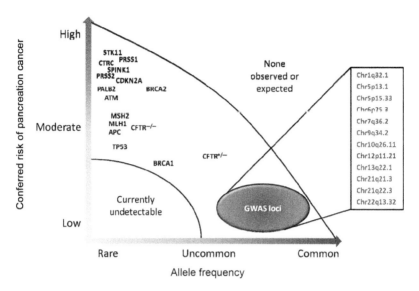

Figure 8.1 *The Current Picture for Inherited Pancreatic Cancer Risk.* Allele frequencies ranging from rare to common are shown on the *x*-axis, and effect sizes ranging from low to high are shown on the *y*-axis. GWAS loci are color coded by population (European = blue; Chinese = red; Japanese = purple). (For interpretation of the references to color in this figure legend, the reader is referred to the online version of this book.)

altered risk in people with different genotypes. The marker SNPs identified in the GWAS is in most cases a proxy for the functional variant; therefore, fine-mapping efforts followed by genomic and functional analysis of multiple highly correlated tag SNPs are the next steps after a GWAS identifies a risk locus for a specific disease or trait. These efforts involve genomic and functional approaches, such as investigating gene expression levels, splicing, promoter or enhancer strength, DNA methylation, protein to DNA binding, and chromosome conformation, to link risk genotypes to differences in specific molecular phenotypes to establish the underlying mechanism at each locus.

PATHWAY ANALYSES OF PANCREATIC CANCER GWAS DATA SETS

GWAS interrogate the association between hundreds of thousands or even millions of genetic variants and a phenotype of interest. Since their launch approximately 8 years ago, studies of the genetic underpinnings of disease have entered a new era and led to the identification of a large number of risk loci for multiple diseases, including pancreatic cancer as described previously. Although extremely successful, the GWAS approach does have limitations. Because of its agnostic methodology, every SNP on a given genotyping platform is examined in an identical manner, without prior knowledge of a biological function or known functional impact. In one sense this is a great plus, as we are not always "smart" enough to pinpoint the genes most likely to be associated with a phenotype, as numerous unsuccessful candidate gene association studies in the past have shown [115]. To utilize the benefits of the GWAS approach while reducing false-positive signals from testing large numbers of hypotheses, stringent thresholds are used for significance in GWAS [116]. Through the large numbers of cases and controls used in a typical GWAS, a number of significant risk loci usually are discovered, and the list typically grows with increased sample sets and additional phases and meta-analyses of each study. Extremely large data sets are required to assess variants with small effects, and the risk loci usually do not explain a large fraction of the heritability of the trait under investigation [115]. Some genes or loci therefore may be truly associated with disease but may not reach the stringent threshold of "genome-wide significance" due to limited power. Because of these limitations, approaches have been pursued that can complement the standard single-marker GWAS approach. One of these is pathway-based analysis of GWAS data [117]. Genes and their encoded proteins do not function in isolation, but rather they interact with other genes and proteins to perform specific tasks, or mediate signals that result in specific outcomes (i.e., gene expression, signal transduction, altered metabolic rates, etc.). The analysis of groups of related genes therefore can be a complementary approach to GWAS, using biological insight to reduce the space of genes tested from that of the whole genome to a much smaller set of genes. Pathway analyses thus aim at combining weak signals from a number of SNPs located within genes that lie in the same pathway.

Genes in a pathway can either be coparticipants in specific biological pathways or networks, or each can act in a similar functional manner. The GWAS pathway approach investigates whether test statistics for markers in a group of genes are associated consistently with a phenotype, above what can be expected by chance. The association can be detected from investigating the joint effect of multiple SNPs in a single gene or from groups of genes that are related because they are members of the same pathway. Two main approaches to pathway-based analysis of GWAS data exist: one is an SNP P-value enrichment approach, and the other uses individual SNP genotypes to derive test statistics for each gene. The former uses P-values as input, whereas the latter requires genotype data to derive gene- and pathway-level significance through permutations. The latter thus can use more than one marker per gene for significance tests. Enrichment scores for pathways are derived from gene P-values using resampling procedures to assess statistical significance. This can be achieved by comparing genes in a pathway to genes that are not associated (self-contained methods) or to all other genes in the genome (competitive methods).

Most pathway studies use a single association signal for each gene. This is commonly the SNP with the lowest P-value (min$P$) within each gene, which—after adjustment for multiple comparisons—is assigned as the gene level P-value. A drawback to this approach is that it may miss additive effects among SNPs within a gene. Other methods apply a supervised principal component analysis to extract independent signals within a gene [118,119]. This method examines joint effects of genes with a phenotype while accounting for the LD between correlated SNPs. Another option is to use resample-based procedures to correct for biases introduced by differences in gene lengths and regional LD, such as the SNP ratio test [120], the set-based analysis in PLINK [121], and the adaptive rank truncated product (ARTP) method [122,123]. Numerous curated pathway annotation databases, including Kyoto Encyclopedia of Genes and Genomes (KEGG), Gene Ontology, BioCarta, and many others are valuable sources for pathway-based GWAS (for review see [117] and [124]).

For pancreatic cancer, four individual pathway-based studies have taken slightly different approaches to analyze pancreatic cancer GWAS data from the PanScan consortium [55,56]. These studies nicely highlight different strategies that can be undertaken to mine GWAS data by (1) using a narrow set of specific pathways that are thought to be involved in pancreatic cancer, (2) an agnostic pathway-based approach using a comprehensive set of known pathways, (3) interrogating risk variants for diseases other than pancreatic cancer, and (4) using external data sets, such as protein–protein interaction networks, to enrich for genes that are important for specific functions within cells. In the first study, 23 biological pathways and gene sets hypothesized to be relevant for pancreatic cancer, based on pathway database and literature searches, were tested for pathway-based association using an adaptive combination of P-values in the ARTP method [122,123]. SNPs from the two GWAS (PanScan I and II) were selected in each gene with a boundary of 20 kb upstream to 10 kb downstream of each gene. Of the 23 pathways, a nominally significant association was noted for five pathways: pancreatic development, *H. pylori* infection, hedgehog signaling, allergies related to Th1/Th2 immune response, and apoptosis (Table 8.1). After

Table 8.1 Pathways and Genes Noted through Pathway-Based Analyses of Pancreatic Cancer GWAS Data Sets

Approach	Pathway	Most significant genes
ARTP	Pancreatic development	*NR5A2, HNF1A, HNF4G, PDX1, HNF1B*
	Helicobacter pylori infection	*ABO*
	Hedgehog signaling	*SHH, BTRC, HHIP*
	Th1/Th2 immune response	*TGFBR2, CCL18, IL13RA2*
	Apoptosis	*MAPK8, BCL2L11, FAS, FASLG, CASP7*
Pleiotropy scan		*HNF1A*
GRASS	Neuroactive ligand–receptor interaction	*ABO, HNF1A,* and *SHH*
	Olfactory transduction	*OR13C4*
DMS/PPI	Myc-mediated apoptosis signaling, Neuregulin signaling, ERK/MAPK signaling, FAK signaling, PTEN signaling	*EGFR, ATF7IP, GRB2, NCK1, ESR1, ACTB, RAC1, MEPCE, STAT3, FASLG, SRC, EP300, ATXN1, BCAR1, MYC, LCK, FAS, DLG2, DOCK1*

excluding genes identified in the original pancreatic cancer GWAS [55,56] (*NR5A2, ABO,* and *SHH*), only the pancreatic development pathway remained significant ($P=8.3\times10^{-5}$). The most significant genes in this pathway were *NR5A2* ($P=1.0\times10^{-6}$), *HNF1A* ($P=1.4\times10^{-4}$), *HNF4G* ($P=4.8\times10^{-4}$), *PDX1* ($P=0.0079$), and *HNF1B* ($P=0.019$) [123]. These five genes encode important components of the transcriptional networks that govern embryonic development of the pancreas and maintain homeostasis in adults [125,126]. The earliest steps of exocrine pancreatic development are regulated by *PDX1* (encoding *PDX1*), which is a direct regulator of *NR5A2* in this process [127,128]. *HNF1A* and *HNF1B* encode hepatocyte nuclear factors 1 alpha and beta (*HNF1A* and *HNF1B*) also known as transcription factors 1 and 2 (TCF1 and TCF2), respectively. *HNF1A* primarily is known to regulate the growth and function of islet cells, and *HNF1B* plays an essential role in controlling pancreatic organogenesis and differentiation [125]. Heterozygous compound knockout mouse models have shown that *PDX1, NR5A2, HNF1A,* and *HNF1B* act in a tightly regulated feedback circuit in regulating pancreas development and homeostasis [128,129]. Furthermore, mutations in *HNF1A, PDX1,* and *HNF1B* are responsible for maturity onset diabetes of the young (MODY) types 3, 4, and 5, respectively [130–132]. Both mutations and common variants in *HNF1A* and *HNF1B* have been associated with risk of type II diabetes [133–135]. SNPs in the *HNF1B* gene also have been associated with prostate and endometrial cancer [136–138]. These results suggest possible functional interrelationships between inherited variation in genes important for pancreatic development and cancer risk.

The second approach was an agnostic search that analyzed a large set of predefined pathways from the KEGG database using the gene set ridge regression in association studies (GRASS) method [139]. Of the 197 pathways analyzed, 2 were associated significantly with the risk of pancreatic cancer after adjusting for multiple testing: neuroactive ligand–receptor interaction ($P = 0.00,002$) and olfactory transduction ($P = 0.0001$) (Table 8.1) [140]. Using a logistic kernel machine test, four genes were deemed to significantly contribute to these two pathways after Bonferroni correction: *ABO*, *HNF1A*, *OR13C4*, and *SHH* [140]. The third approach analyzed PanScan data for associations between pancreatic cancer risk and the full catalog of published GWAS SNPs from the National Human Genome Research Institute (NHGRI) [141]. The authors termed their method "pleiotropy scan" as it restricted the association analysis to variants putatively influencing multiple phenotypes. This approach used a two phased strategy, by first analyzing PanScan I and then using PanScan II for replication. This study also identified SNPs in the *HNF1A* gene as being important for pancreatic cancer risk (Table 8.1), but no additional loci were significant [142].

Biologically meaningful information can be extracted from GWAS data by integration with additional high-throughput data sets, such as transcriptome, epigenome, or protein–protein interaction data sets. This layered approach also aims to reduce the amount of hypotheses tested, but instead of using predefined pathways, it seeks to apply functionally relevant data sets. The goal is to examine whether association signals from GWAS are enriched within the space of biologically relevant data that can include (1) potentially active genomic regions (using epigenome data that define histone modification marks, DNase hypersensitivity region, and DNA methylation), (2) genes or gene sets that are either coexpressed or differentially expressed in normal and tumor-derived pancreatic samples (transcriptome data sets), or (3) genes known to encode proteins that interact with each other or lie in specific protein networks.

An illustration of the last example is a recent study that used dense module searching to look for genes or pathways within human protein–protein interaction (PPI) modules and networks that were enriched in significant association signals from pancreatic cancer GWAS data [143]. SNPs from PanScan I were mapped to genes if they were located within 20 kb upstream or downstream of the gene body; the most significant SNP in each gene was then selected to represent that gene, followed by integration with PPI networks. This approach yielded 93 significantly enriched modules, containing 159 unique genes. These were combined and used to construct a PPI subnetwork for pancreatic cancer. The genes showing the highest degree if interaction in this network (degree ≥6) were *EGFR, ATF7IP, GRB2, NCK1, ESR1, ACTB, RAC1, MEPCE, STAT3, FASLG, SRC, EP300, ATXN1, BCAR1, MYC, LCK, FAS, DLG2,* and *DOCK1* (Table 8.1). Pathway analysis for these genes indicated enrichment in Myc-mediated apoptosis signaling $(P=1.70\times10^{-7})$, Neuregulin signaling $(P=2.82\times10^{-7})$, extracellular signal-regulated kinase/mitogen activated protein kinase (ERK/MAPK) signaling $(P=1.62\times10^{-6})$, FAK signaling $(P=2.51\times10^{-6})$, and PTEN signaling $(P=3.24\times10^{-6})$. The epidermal growth factor receptor (EGFR) was the most connected protein in the pancreatic cancer subnetwork. EGFR is a plasma membrane growth factor receptor located directly upstream of RAS. As *KRAS* mutations are extremely frequent in pancreatic cancer, one might believe that an active EGFR would not augment signals from an already mutated *KRAS*. However, overexpression of TGF-alpha, one of the EGFR ligands, dramatically increases the progression of PanIN lesions to metastatic pancreatic cancer in transgenic $KRAS^{G12D}$ mouse models, indicating that activation of the EGFR indeed can cooperate with an enhanced *KRAS*-mediated transformation in the pancreas [144].

A limiting factor to pathway approaches in general is that it involves mapping SNPs from GWAS to genes; for pragmatic reasons, this usually is the closest gene (gene body and 10–20 kb up- and downstream of the start and stop codon of each gene). One must keep in mind, however, that the SNP(s) in question may or may not functionally influence the gene they reside in or lie close to. Many examples of long-range interactions within and between chromosomes that regulate gene expression are missed by this approach. A second caveat is that the results from GWAS are preliminary, and in many cases, fine-mapping yields much improved association signals. The latter caveat can be overcome by imputation before pathway analysis.

FUTURE GWAS AND GENE MAPPING APPROACHES

GWAS has yielded enormously helpful insight into the etiology of pancreatic cancer. As compared with more common cancers, the GWAS approach is at a relatively early stage for pancreatic cancer and more can be expected as increased sample sets and additional populations are analyzed. The reasons for this are twofold: First, pancreatic cancer is not common, ranking number 10 in incidence in the United States and number 13 worldwide [1,145]. Second, pancreatic cancer is highly lethal [145,146], and patients often have passed away before they can be recruited to participate in studies. Furthermore, only a subset of pancreatic cancer patients undergoes surgery, resulting in low recruitment rates. This disproportionally affects hospital-based case–control studies versus cohort-based studies and can lead to biased estimates for risk loci if they are correlated with severity or survival of pancreatic cancer. The GWAS approach has led to the identification of 67 risk loci for breast cancer [147] and 77 for prostate cancer [148]. Together, these loci explain approximately 30% of the familial risk of prostate cancer and 28% for breast cancer [147,148]. For pancreatic cancer, 18 risk loci have been identified to date through GWAS (10 in Europeans and 8 in Asians) albeit with limited replication between European and Asian populations.

Additional GWAS continue to become available, and as sample sizes grow, statistical power will increase and additional loci likely will be identified. Imputation and meta-analyses of existing and new GWAS data sets are bound to uncover even more loci. Efforts in pancreatic cancer GWAS outside of main effects likely will expand by investigations of susceptibility variants for survival, pharmacologic responses as well as gene–gene and gene–environmental interactions [149–151]. For other diseases, however, susceptibility loci identified through GWAS are not likely to explain the majority of inherited risk for pancreatic cancer. With the emergence of next-generation sequencing, these efforts will grow in use for gene mapping. The recent identification of mutations in the *ATM* and *PALB2* genes in pancreatic cancer kindreds with unknown etiology nicely demonstrated this use of next-generation sequencing [16,48]. ES and WGS also likely will be undertaken in sporadic cases as well as in cases with specific phenotypes, such as an early age of onset and epidemiologic risk factors (e.g., BMI, smoking, pancreatitis). ES and WGS are well suited for the discovery of less common risk variants, with low to intermediate effects, in contrast to linkage or GWAS approaches. As population-based sequencing studies already have shown, the number of uncommon and rare polymorphic variants in the human genome, although underrepresented in public databases to date, is very high [152], and may explain a substantial portion of germline risk for disease. Furthermore, high-throughput sequencing approaches will enable the assessment of variants not captured on GWAS platforms, such as indels and copy number variants. We therefore enter another exciting era of genome mapping in the discovery of susceptibility variants for destructive diseases like pancreatic cancer.

WEBSITES

The Pancreatic Cancer Cohort Consortium (PanScan), http://epi.grants.cancer.gov/PanScan/

The Pancreatic Cancer Case Control Consortium (PanC4), http://panc4.org/

NHGRI Catalog of Published Genome-Wide Association Studies, http://www.genome.gov/gwastudies/

REFERENCES

[1] Siegel R, Naishadham D, Jemal A. Cancer statistics, 2013. CA Cancer J Clin 2013;63(1):11–30.
[2] Howlader N, Noone AM, Krapcho M, Neyman N, Aminou R, Waldron W, et al, editors. SEER cancer statistics review, 1975–2008. Bethesda (MD): National Cancer Institute; 2011 [http://seer.cancer.gov/csr/1975_2008/, based on November 2010 SEER data submission, posted to the SEER web site.].
[3] Lynch SM, et al. Cigarette smoking and pancreatic cancer: a pooled analysis from the pancreatic cancer cohort consortium. Am J Epidemiol 2009;170(4):403–13.
[4] Huxley R, Ansary-Moghaddam A, Berrington de Gonzalez A, Barzi F, Woodward M. Type-II diabetes and pancreatic cancer: a meta-analysis of 36 studies. Br J Cancer 2005;92(11):2076–83.
[5] Arslan AA, et al. Anthropometric measures, body mass index, and pancreatic cancer: a pooled analysis from the Pancreatic Cancer Cohort Consortium (PanScan). Arch Intern Med 2010;170(9):791–802.
[6] Raimondi S, Lowenfels AB, Morselli-Labate AM, Maisonneuve P, Pezzilli R. Pancreatic cancer in chronic pancreatitis; aetiology, incidence, and early detection. Best Pract Res Clin Gastroenterol 2010;24(3):349–58.
[7] Michaud DS, et al. Alcohol intake and pancreatic cancer: a pooled analysis from the pancreatic cancer cohort consortium (PanScan). Cancer Causes Control 2010;21(8):1213–25.
[8] Iodice S, Gandini S, Maisonneuve P, Lowenfels AB. Tobacco and the risk of pancreatic cancer: a review and meta-analysis. Langenbecks Arch Surg 2008;393(4):535–45.
[9] Jiao L, et al. Body mass index, effect modifiers, and risk of pancreatic cancer: a pooled study of seven prospective cohorts. Cancer Causes Control 2010;21(8):1305–14.
[10] Everhart J, Wright D. Diabetes mellitus as a risk factor for pancreatic cancer. A meta-analysis. JAMA 1995;273(20):1605–9.
[11] Jacobs EJ, et al. Family history of cancer and risk of pancreatic cancer: a pooled analysis from the Pancreatic Cancer Cohort Consortium (PanScan). Int J Cancer 2010;127(6):1421–8.
[12] Hruban RH, Canto MI, Goggins M, Schulick R, Klein AP. Update on familial pancreatic cancer. Adv Surg 2010;44:293–311.
[13] Goldstein AM, et al. High-risk melanoma susceptibility genes and pancreatic cancer, neural system tumors, and uveal melanoma across GenoMEL. Cancer Res 2006;66(20):9818–28.

[14] Lynch HT, Fusaro RM, Lynch JF, Brand R. Pancreatic cancer and the FAMMM syndrome. Fam Cancer 2008;7(1):103–12.

[15] van Lier MG, et al. High cancer risk in Peutz–Jeghers syndrome: a systematic review and surveillance recommendations. Am J Gastroenterol 2010;105(6):1258–64. author reply 1265.

[16] Jones S, et al. Exomic sequencing identifies PALB2 as a pancreatic cancer susceptibility gene. Science 2009;324(5924):217.

[17] Kastrinos F, et al. Risk of pancreatic cancer in families with Lynch syndrome. JAMA 2009;302(16):1790–5.

[18] Consortium. TBCL. Cancer risks in BRCA2 mutation carriers. The Breast Cancer Linkage Consortium J Natl Cancer Inst 1999;91(15):1310–6.

[19] Lowenfels AB, et al. Hereditary pancreatitis and the risk of pancreatic cancer. International Hereditary Pancreatitis Study Group. J Natl Cancer Inst 1997;89(6):442–6.

[20] Howes N, et al. Clinical and genetic characteristics of hereditary pancreatitis in Europe. Clin Gastroenterol Hepatol 2004;2(3):252–61.

[21] Witt H, et al. Mutations in the gene encoding the serine protease inhibitor, Kazal type 1 are associated with chronic pancreatitis. Nat Genet 2000;25(2):213–6.

[22] Hemminki K, Li X. Familial and second primary pancreatic cancers: a nationwide epidemiologic study from Sweden. Int J Cancer 2003;103(4):525–30.

[23] Shirts BH, Burt RW, Mulvihill SJ, Cannon-Albright LA. A population-based description of familial clustering of pancreatic cancer. Clin Gastroenterol Hepatol 2010;8(9):812–6.

[24] Amundadottir LT, et al. Cancer as a complex phenotype: pattern of cancer distribution within and beyond the nuclear family. PLoS Med 2004;1(3):e65.

[25] Hezel AF, Kimmelman AC, Stanger BZ, Bardeesy N, Depinho RA. Genetics and biology of pancreatic ductal adenocarcinoma. Genes Dev 2006;20(10):1218–49.

[26] Bartsch DK, Gress TM, Langer P. Familial pancreatic cancer–current knowledge. Nat Rev Gastroenterol Hepatol 2012;9(8):445–53.

[27] Klein AP. Genetic susceptibility to pancreatic cancer. Mol Carcinog 2012;51(1): 14–24.

[28] Landi S. Genetic predisposition and environmental risk factors to pancreatic cancer: a review of the literature. Mutat Res 2009;681(2–3):299–307.

[29] Guerra C, et al. Pancreatitis-induced inflammation contributes to pancreatic cancer by inhibiting oncogene-induced senescence. Cancer Cell 2011;19(6):728–39.

[30] Flandez M, et al. Nr5a2 heterozygosity sensitises to, and cooperates with, inflammation in KRasG12V-driven pancreatic tumourigenesis. Gut 2013.

[31] Maisonneuve P, Marshall BC, Lowenfels AB. Risk of pancreatic cancer in patients with cystic fibrosis. Gut 2007;56(9):1327–8.

[32] McWilliams R, et al. Cystic fibrosis transmembrane regulator gene carrier status is a risk factor for young onset pancreatic adenocarcinoma. Gut 2005;54(11): 1661–2.

[33] Korsse SE, Peppelenbosch MP, van Veelen W. Targeting LKB1 signaling in cancer. Biochim Biophys Acta 2013;1835(2):194–210.

[34] Whelan AJ, Bartsch D, Goodfellow PJ. Brief report: a familial syndrome of pancreatic cancer and melanoma with a mutation in the CDKN2 tumor-suppressor gene. N Engl J Med 1995;333(15):975–7.

[35] Bergman W, Watson P, de Jong J, Lynch HT, Fusaro RM. Systemic cancer and the FAMMM syndrome. Br J Cancer 1990;61(6):932–6.

[36] Vasen HF, et al. Risk of developing pancreatic cancer in families with familial atypical multiple mole melanoma associated with a specific 19 deletion of p16 (p16-Leiden). Int J Cancer 2000;87(6):809–11.

[37] Rozenblum E, et al. Tumor-suppressive pathways in pancreatic carcinoma. Cancer Res 1997;57(9):1731–4.

[38] Liu L, et al. Mutation of the CDKN2A 5' UTR creates an aberrant initiation codon and predisposes to melanoma. Nat Genet 1999;21(1):128–32.

[39] Lal G, et al. Patients with both pancreatic adenocarcinoma and melanoma may harbor germline CDKN2A mutations. Genes Chromosomes Cancer 2000;27(4):358–61.

[40] Nielsen GP, et al. Immunohistochemical survey of p16INK4A expression in normal human adult and infant tissues. Lab Invest 1999;79(9):1137–43.

[41] Krishnamurthy J, et al. Ink4a/Arf expression is a biomarker of aging. J Clin Invest 2004;114(9):1299–307.

[42] Sherr CJ. The INK4a/ARF network in tumour suppression. Nat Rev Mol Cell Biol 2001;2(10):731–7.

[43] Grandval P, et al. Is the controversy on breast cancer as part of the Lynch-related tumor spectrum still open? Fam Cancer 2012;11(4):681–3.

[44] Laghi L, et al. Irrelevance of microsatellite instability in the epidemiology of sporadic pancreatic ductal adenocarcinoma. PLoS One 2012;7(9):e46002.

[45] Li T, et al. Tumor suppression in the absence of p53-mediated cell-cycle arrest, apoptosis, and senescence. Cell 2012;149(6):1269–83.

[46] Foulkes WD, Shuen AY. In brief: BRCA1 and BRCA2. J Pathol 2013;230(4):347–9.

[47] Foulkes WD. Inherited susceptibility to common cancers. N Engl J Med 2008;359(20):2143–53.

[48] Roberts NJ, et al. ATM mutations in patients with hereditary pancreatic cancer. Cancer Discov 2012;2(1):41–6.

[49] Lander ES, et al. Initial sequencing and analysis of the human genome. Nature 2001;409(6822):860–921.

[50] Venter JC, et al. The sequence of the human genome. Science 2001;291(5507):1304–51.

[51] Consortium IH. The International HapMap Project. Nature 2003;426(6968):789–96.

[52] Genomes. A map of human genome variation from population-scale sequencing. Nature 2010;467(7319):1061–73.

[53] Hindorff LA, et al. A Catalog of Published Genome-Wide Association Studies. Available at: www.genome.gov/gwastudies.

[54] Manolio TA. Bringing genome-wide association findings into clinical use. Nat Rev Genet 2013;14(8):549–58.

[55] Amundadottir L, et al. Genome-wide association study identifies variants in the ABO locus associated with susceptibility to pancreatic cancer. Nat Genet 2009;41(9):986–90.

[56] Petersen GM, et al. A genome-wide association study identifies pancreatic cancer susceptibility loci on chromosomes 13q22.1, 1q32.1 and 5p15.33. Nat Genet 2010;42(3):224–8.

[57] Landi MT, et al. A genome-wide association study of lung cancer identifies a region of chromosome 5p15 associated with risk for adenocarcinoma. Am J Hum Genet 2009;85(5):679–91.

[58] McKay JD, et al. Lung cancer susceptibility locus at 5p15.33. Nat Genet 2008;40(12):1404–6.

[59] Amos CI, et al. Genome-wide association scan of tag SNPs identifies a susceptibility locus for lung cancer at 15q25.1. Nat Genet 2008;40(5):616–22.

[60] Broderick P, et al. Deciphering the impact of common genetic variation on lung cancer risk: a genome-wide association study. Cancer Res 2009;69(16):6633–41.

[61] Hsiung CA, et al. The 5p15.33 locus is associated with risk of lung adenocarcinoma in never-smoking females in Asia. PLoS Genet 2010;6(8).

[62] Kote-Jarai Z, et al. Seven prostate cancer susceptibility loci identified by a multi-stage genome-wide association study. Nat Genet 2011;43(8):785–91.

[63] Rafnar T, et al. Sequence variants at the TERT-CLPTM1L locus associate with many cancer types. Nat Genet 2009;41(2):221–7.

[64] Chung CC, et al. Fine mapping of a region of chromosome 11q13 reveals multiple independent loci associated with risk of prostate cancer. Hum Mol Genet 2011;20(14):2869–78.

[65] Shete S, et al. Genome-wide association study identifies five susceptibility loci for glioma. Nat Genet 2009;41(8):899–904.

[66] Turnbull C, et al. Variants near DMRT1, TERT and ATF7IP are associated with testicular germ cell cancer. Nat Genet 2010;42(7):604–7.

[67] Stacey SN, et al. New common variants affecting susceptibility to basal cell carcinoma. Nat Genet 2009;41(8):909–14.

[68] Barrett JH, et al. Genome-wide association study identifies three new melanoma susceptibility loci. Nat Genet 2011;43(11):1108–13.

[69] Pare G, et al. Novel association of ABO histo-blood group antigen with soluble ICAM-1: results of a genome-wide association study of 6,578 women. PLoS Genet 2008;4(7):e1000118.

[70] Chu X, et al. A genome-wide association study identifies two new risk loci for Graves' disease. Nat Genet 2011;43(9):897–901.

[71] Melzer D, et al. A genome-wide association study identifies protein quantitative trait loci (pQTLs). PLoS Genet 2008;4(5):e1000072.

[72] Germain M, et al. Genetics of venous thrombosis: insights from a new genome wide association study. PLoS One 2011;6(9):e25581.

[73] Williams FM, et al. Ischemic stroke is associated with the ABO locus: the EuroCLOT study. Ann Neurol 2013;73(1):16–31.

[74] Tanikawa C, et al. A genome-wide association study identifies two susceptibility loci for duodenal ulcer in the Japanese population. Nat Genet 2012;44(4):430–4. S431–432.

[75] Marcus DM. The ABO and Lewis blood-group system. Immunochemistry, genetics and relation to human disease. N Engl J Med 1969;280(18):994–1006.

[76] Aird I, Bentall HH, Roberts JA. A relationship between cancer of stomach and the ABO blood groups. Br Med J 1953;1(4814):799–801.

[77] Wolpin BM, et al. Pancreatic cancer risk and ABO blood group alleles: results from the pancreatic cancer cohort consortium. Cancer Res 2010;70(3):1015–23.

[78] Yamamoto F, McNeill PD, Hakomori S. Human histo-blood group A2 transferase coded by A2 allele, one of the A subtypes, is characterized by a single base deletion in the coding sequence, which results in an additional domain at the carboxyl terminal. Biochem Biophys Res Commun 1992;187(1):366–74.

[79] Wolpin BM, et al. Variant ABO blood group alleles, secretor status, and risk of pancreatic cancer: results from the pancreatic cancer cohort consortium. Cancer Epidemiol Biomarkers Prev 2010;19(12):3140–9.

[80] Ferrer-Admetlla A, et al. A natural history of FUT2 polymorphism in humans. Mol Biol Evol 2009;26(9):1993–2003.

[81] Michaud DS. Role of bacterial infections in pancreatic cancer. Carcinogenesis 2013;34(10):2193–7.

[82] Risch HA, Yu H, Lu L, Kidd MS. ABO blood group, *Helicobacter pylori* seropositivity, and risk of pancreatic cancer: a case-control study. J Natl Cancer Inst 2010;102(7):502–5.

[83] Fayard E, Auwerx J, Schoonjans K. LRH-1: an orphan nuclear receptor involved in development, metabolism and steroidogenesis. Trends Cell Biol 2004;14(5):250–60.

[84] Kelly VR, Xu B, Kuick R, Koenig RJ, Hammer GD. Dax1 up-regulates Oct4 expression in mouse embryonic stem cells via LRH-1 and SRA. Mol Endocrinol 2010;24(12):2281–91.

[85] Heng JC, et al. The nuclear receptor Nr5a2 can replace Oct4 in the reprogramming of murine somatic cells to pluripotent cells. Cell Stem Cell 2010;6(2):167–74.

[86] Botrugno OA, et al. Synergy between LRH-1 and beta-catenin induces G1 cyclin-mediated cell proliferation. Mol Cell 2004;15(4):499–509.

[87] Holmstrom SR, et al. LRH-1 and PTF1-L coregulate an exocrine pancreas-specific transcriptional network for digestive function. Genes Dev 2011;25(16):1674–9.

[88] Molero X, et al. Gene expression dynamics after murine pancreatitis unveils novel roles for Hnf1alpha in acinar cell homeostasis. Gut 2012;61(8):1187–96.

[89] Chung CC, Chanock SJ. Current status of genome-wide association studies in cancer. Hum Genet 2011;130(1):59–78.

[90] Bodnar AG, et al. Extension of life-span by introduction of telomerase into normal human cells. Science 1998;279(5349):349–52.

[91] Hahn WC, et al. Creation of human tumour cells with defined genetic elements. Nature 1999;400(6743):464–8.

[92] Kim NW, et al. Specific association of human telomerase activity with immortal cells and cancer. Science 1994;266(5193):2011–5.

[93] Ding D, Zhou J, Wang M, Cong YS. Implications of telomere-independent activities of telomerase reverse transcriptase in human cancer. FEBS J 2013;280(14): 3205–11.

[94] Yamamoto K, Okamoto A, Isonishi S, Ochiai K, Ohtake Y. A novel gene, CRR9, which was up-regulated in CDDP-resistant ovarian tumor cell line, was associated with apoptosis. Biochem Biophys Res Commun 2001;280(4):1148–54.

[95] James MA, et al. Functional characterization of CLPTM1L as a lung cancer risk candidate gene in the 5p15.33 locus. PLoS One 2012;7(6):e36116.

[96] Baudis M. Genomic imbalances in 5918 malignant epithelial tumors: an explorative meta-analysis of chromosomal CGH data. BMC Cancer 2007;7:226.

[97] Vazquez-Mena O, et al. Amplified genes may be overexpressed, unchanged, or down-regulated in cervical cancer cell lines. PLoS One 2012;7(3):e32667.

[98] Lando M, et al. Gene dosage, expression, and ontology analysis identifies driver genes in the carcinogenesis and chemoradioresistance of cervical cancer. PLoS Genet 2009;5(11):e1000719.

[99] McConnell BB, Yang VW. Mammalian Kruppel-like factors in health and diseases. Physiol Rev 2010;90(4):1337–81.

[100] Dong JT, Chen C. Essential role of KLF5 transcription factor in cell proliferation and differentiation and its implications for human diseases. Cell Mol Life Sci 2009;66(16):2691–706.

[101] Nakamura Y, et al. Kruppel-like factor 12 plays a significant role in poorly differentiated gastric cancer progression. Int J Cancer 2009;125(8):1859–67.

[102] Mori A, et al. Up-regulation of Kruppel-like factor 5 in pancreatic cancer is promoted by interleukin-1beta signaling and hypoxia-inducible factor-1alpha. Mol Cancer Res 2009;7(8):1390–8.

[103] Lachmann M, et al. PIBF (progesterone induced blocking factor) is overexpressed in highly proliferating cells and associated with the centrosome. Int J Cancer 2004;112(1):51–60.

[104] Srivastava MD, Thomas A, Srivastava BI, Check JH. Expression and modulation of progesterone induced blocking factor (PIBF) and innate immune factors in human leukemia cell lines by progesterone and mifepristone. Leuk Lymphoma 2007; 48(8):1610–7.

[105] Houseley J, LaCava J, Tollervey D. RNA-quality control by the exosome. Nat Rev Mol Cell Biol 2006;7(7):529–39.

[106] Tomecki R, et al. The human core exosome interacts with differentially localized processive RNases: hDIS3 and hDIS3L. EMBO J 2010;29(14):2342–57.

[107] Ding L, et al. Clonal evolution in relapsed acute myeloid leukaemia revealed by whole-genome sequencing. Nature 2012;481(7382):506–10.

[108] Walker BA, et al. Intraclonal heterogeneity and distinct molecular mechanisms characterize the development of t(4;14) and t(11;14) myeloma. Blood 2012;120(5): 1077–86.

[109] Lim J, et al. Isolation of murine and human homologues of the fission-yeast dis3+ gene encoding a mitotic-control protein and its overexpression in cancer cells with progressive phenotype. Cancer Res 1997;57(5):921–5.

[110] Macurek L, Lindqvist A, Medema RH. Aurora-A and hBora join the game of Polo. Cancer Res 2009;69(11):4555–8.

[111] Hutchins JR, et al. Systematic analysis of human protein complexes identifies chromosome segregation proteins. Science 2010;328(5978):593–9.

[112] Low SK, et al. Genome-wide association study of pancreatic cancer in Japanese population. PLoS One 2010;5(7):e11824.

[113] Wu C, et al. Genome-wide association study identifies five loci associated with susceptibility to pancreatic cancer in Chinese populations. Nat Genet 2012;44(1): 62–6.

[114] Campa D, et al. Lack of replication of seven pancreatic cancer susceptibility loci identified in two Asian populations. Cancer Epidemiol Biomarkers Prev 2013;22(2):320–3.

[115] Manolio TA, et al. Finding the missing heritability of complex diseases. Nature 2009;461(7265):747–53.

[116] Chanock SJ, et al. Replicating genotype-phenotype associations. Nature 2007;447(7145):655–60.

[117] Wang K, Li M, Hakonarson H. Analysing biological pathways in genome-wide association studies. Nat Rev Genet 2010;11(12):843–54.

[118] Chen X, et al. Pathway-based analysis for genome-wide association studies using supervised principal components. Genet Epidemiol 2010;34(7):716–24.

[119] Zaykin DV, Zhivotovsky LA, Westfall PH, Weir BS. Truncated product method for combining P-values. Genet Epidemiol 2002;22(2):170–85.

[120] O'Dushlaine C, et al. The SNP ratio test: pathway analysis of genome-wide association datasets. Bioinformatics 2009;25(20):2762–3.

[121] Purcell S, et al. PLINK: a tool set for whole-genome association and population-based linkage analyses. Am J Hum Genet 2007;81(3):559–75.

[122] Yu K, et al. Pathway analysis by adaptive combination of P-values. Genet Epidemiol 2009;33(8):700–9.

[123] Li D, et al. Pathway analysis of genome-wide association study data highlights pancreatic development genes as susceptibility factors for pancreatic cancer. Carcinogenesis 2012;33(7):1384–90.

[124] Ramanan VK, Shen L, Moore JH, Saykin AJ. Pathway analysis of genomic data: concepts, methods, and prospects for future development. Trends Genet 2012;28(7):323–32.

[125] Maestro MA, et al. Distinct roles of HNF1beta, HNF1alpha, and HNF4alpha in regulating pancreas development, beta-cell function and growth. Endocr Dev 2007;12:33–45.

[126] Martin M, Hauer V, Messmer M, Orvain C, Gradwohl G. Transcription factors in pancreatic development. Animal models. Endocr Dev 2007;12:24–32.

[127] Kaneto H, et al. PDX-1 functions as a master factor in the pancreas. Front Biosci 2008;13:6406–20.

[128] Annicotte JS, et al. Pancreatic-duodenal homeobox 1 regulates expression of liver receptor homolog 1 during pancreas development. Mol Cell Biol 2003;23(19):6713–24.

[129] Haumaitre C, et al. Lack of TCF2/vHNF1 in mice leads to pancreas agenesis. Proc Natl Acad Sci USA 2005;102(5):1490–5.

[130] Glucksmann MA, et al. Novel mutations and a mutational hotspot in the MODY3 gene. Diabetes 1997;46(6):1081–6.

[131] Carette C, et al. Exonic duplication of the hepatocyte nuclear factor-1beta gene (transcription factor 2, hepatic) as a cause of maturity onset diabetes of the young type 5. J Clin Endocrinol Metab 2007;92(7):2844–7.

[132] Yamagata K, et al. Mutations in the hepatocyte nuclear factor-1alpha gene in maturity-onset diabetes of the young (MODY3). Nature 1996;384(6608):455–8.

[133] Voight BF, et al. Twelve type 2 diabetes susceptibility loci identified through large-scale association analysis. Nat Genet 2010;42(7):579–89.

[134] Furuta H, et al. Nonsense and missense mutations in the human hepatocyte nuclear factor-1 beta gene (TCF2) and their relation to type 2 diabetes in Japanese. J Clin Endocrinol Metab 2002;87(8):3859–63.

[135] Holmkvist J, et al. Common variants in HNF-1 alpha and risk of type 2 diabetes. Diabetologia 2006;49(12):2882–91.

[136] Thomas G, et al. Multiple loci identified in a genome-wide association study of prostate cancer. Nat Genet 2008;40(3):310–5.

[137] Spurdle AB, et al. Genome-wide association study identifies a common variant associated with risk of endometrial cancer. Nat Genet 2011;43(5):451–4.

[138] Eeles RA, et al. Multiple newly identified loci associated with prostate cancer susceptibility. Nat Genet 2008;40(3):316–21.

[139] Chen LS, et al. Insights into colon cancer etiology via a regularized approach to gene set analysis of GWAS data. Am J Hum Genet 2010;86(6):860–71.

[140] Wei P, Tang H, Li D. Insights into pancreatic cancer etiology from pathway analysis of genome-wide association study data. PLoS One 2012;7(10):e46887.

[141] Hindorff LA, et al. Potential etiologic and functional implications of genome-wide association loci for human diseases and traits. Proc Natl Acad Sci USA 2009; 106(23):9362–7.

[142] Pierce BL, Ahsan H. Genome-wide "pleiotropy scan" identifies HNF1A region as a novel pancreatic cancer susceptibility locus. Cancer Res 2011;71(13):4352–8.

[143] Jia P, Zheng S, Long J, Zheng W, Zhao Z. dmGWAS: dense module searching for genome-wide association studies in protein-protein interaction networks. Bioinformatics 2011;27(1):95–102.

[144] Siveke JT, et al. Concomitant pancreatic activation of Kras(G12D) and Tgfa results in cystic papillary neoplasms reminiscent of human IPMN. Cancer Cell 2007;12(3):266–79.

[145] Ferlay J, et al. Estimates of worldwide burden of cancer in 2008: GLOBOCAN 2008. Int J Cancer 2010;127(12):2893–917.

[146] Hidalgo M. Pancreatic cancer. N Engl J Med 2010;362(17):1605–17.

[147] Garcia-Closas M, et al. Genome-wide association studies identify four ER negative-specific breast cancer risk loci. Nat Genet 2013;45(4):392–8. 398e391-392.

[148] Eeles RA, et al. Identification of 23 new prostate cancer susceptibility loci using the iCOGS custom genotyping array. Nat Genet 2013;45(4):385–91. 391e381-382.

[149] Wu C, et al. Genome-wide association study of survival in patients with pancreatic adenocarcinoma. Gut 2014;63(1):152–60.

[150] Willis JA, et al. A replication study and genome-wide scan of single-nucleotide polymorphisms associated with pancreatic cancer risk and overall survival. Clin Cancer Res 2012;18(14):3942–51.

[151] Innocenti F, et al. A genome-wide association study of overall survival in pancreatic cancer patients treated with gemcitabine in CALGB 80303. Clin Cancer Res 2012;18(2):577–84.

[152] Marth GT, et al. The functional spectrum of low-frequency coding variation. Genome Biol 2011;12(9):R84.

Pancreatic Cancer Proteomics

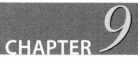

CHAPTER *9*

Proteomics in Pancreatic Cancer Translational Research

Sheng Pan, Ru Chen, Teresa A. Brentnall

Department of Medicine, University of Washington, Seattle, WA, USA

Contents

Introduction	198
Overview of Proteomics Technologies	198
Separation of Proteins and Peptides	199
Quantitative Methods for Global Protein Profiling	200
Mass Spectrometry	201
Bioinformatics for Protein/Peptide Analysis	201
Targeted Proteomics	202
Proteomics Study of Pancreatic Tissue	202
Pancreatic Ductal Adenocarcinoma	202
Pancreatic Intraepithelial Neoplasia	203
Chronic Pancreatitis	204
Analysis of Isolated Cells	204
Blood Biomarker Discovery	205
Global Profiling of Plasma/Serum	205
Targeted Proteomics for Protein Biomarker Detection	206
Analysis of Pancreatic Juice and Cyst Fluid	207
Pancreatic Juice	207
Pancreatic Cyst Fluid	208
Functional and Hypothesis-Driven Proteomic Studies	209
Targeted Interrogation of KRAS Proteins	209
Identification of Protein Receptors	210
Determination of Protein Activities	210
Investigation of Cancer-Associated Cell Invasiveness	210
Post-translational Modifications	211
Phosphorylation	211
Glycosylation	212
Summary	213
Acknowledgment	213
References	214

INTRODUCTION

Despite advances in our understanding of pancreatic cancer development in the past decade, the disease remains the fourth most common cause of cancer death in the United States [1,2]. Unfortunately, its 5-year survival rate has not been improved significantly in the past 30 years. The major reason for this poor prognosis is that the majority of pancreatic cancer patients are diagnosed at a late stage with metastatic, inoperable disease, in which no effective treatments are currently available. Even for the small group of patients diagnosed with resectable cancer and who do undergo surgical resection, the 5-year survival rate approximates 15–40% [3,4]. Methods for earlier detection and more effective therapeutic treatments are much needed to improve the clinical outcome of pancreatic cancer.

Proteins are the essential molecules that regulate and participate in biological functions. Proteome alterations that are associated with diseases may include changes in protein expression, post-translational modifications (PTMs) and protein–protein interactions, which may all lead to malfunction of cellular biological processes. Identification and quantification of protein abnormalities associated with pancreatic cancer pathways, thus, may supply molecular information that provides new disease surrogates for diagnosis or novel therapeutic targets. In some cases, identification of a key regulatory protein could provide information for both diagnostics and treatment, known as theranostics.

Over the past decade, researchers have looked beyond the scope of genomics to explore protein-driven functional changes that are associated with pancreatic tumorigenesis. Advances in proteomics, especially quantitative proteomics, enables systematic investigation of malignancy-related proteome alterations that affect cellular physiology and function. This type of information can provide for new hypotheses bridging the gap between basic biological understanding and translational research. As illustrated in Figure 9.1, clinical specimens for proteomics investigation can include pancreatic tissues, plasma/serum, pancreatic juice, and cyst fluids, as well as isolated cells, from individuals who are in good health and those with cancer or other pancreatic diseases. Such samples are investigated to identify signaling pathways and molecular events underlying pancreatic tumorigenesis—laying a foundation for translational exploration of key proteins to improve patient care.

OVERVIEW OF PROTEOMICS TECHNOLOGIES

A major challenge in proteomics analysis arises from the enormous complexity of protein constituents and the vast dynamic range in protein abundance in biological samples. Comprehensive interrogation of a protein profile,

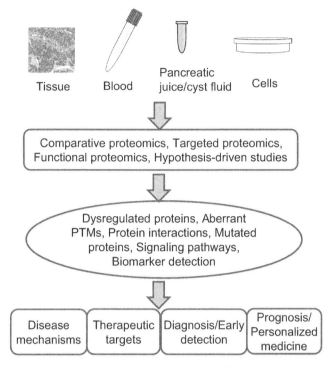

Figure 9.1 *Proteomics in Pancreatic Cancer Studies.* (For color version of this figure, the reader is referred to the online version of this book.)

particularly of low-abundant proteins in a complex biological system that may consist of thousands or more protein species with the addition of their iso-forms, PTMs, mutations, and polymorphisms is a dedicated task and requires a concerted approach drawn from different techniques. A typical proteomics pipeline requires four technical modules, including sample preparation, pro-tein/peptide separation, mass spectrometric analysis, and bioinformatics. In addition, shotgun proteomics-based quantitative analysis entails a variety of stable isotope-labeling methodologies that can be used to introduce differen-tial mass tags on proteins or peptides to facilitate the quantitative analysis.

Separation of Proteins and Peptides

In large-scale proteomics profiling experiments, effective fractionation and separation of proteins and peptides before mass spectrometric analysis enhances the analytical range and capacity. The nature of the biological specimens and experimental design can influence the approach used to prepare proteins for analysis. For gel-based quantitative analysis, two-dimensional electrophoresis (2-DE) is the most common way to separate proteins in a complex biological sample, and the staining intensities of proteins are used to achieve comparative quantification [5]. The identification of selected protein spots is accomplished through mass spectrometric analysis, typically via in-gel digestion of proteins. Alternatively, shotgun proteomics-based approaches rely on analysis and assignment of peptides for protein identification. Because mass spectrometric analysis at the peptide level provides substantially better analytical sensitivity and mass accuracy compared with direct protein analysis, shotgun proteomics permits sophisticated amino acid sequence identification using an automatic database search. Digestion of a vast number of proteins in a biological sample, however, can generate numerous peptide species with significant dynamic differences in abundance, unavoidably multiplying the complexity of the sample for analysis. In such a setting, a variety of separation techniques have been utilized to effectively separate or fractionate a complex biological sample at either the protein or peptide level before the mass spectrometric interrogation. Typically, orthogonal mechanisms are coupled to maximize the separation efficiency. Proteins can be separated using electrophoresis, liquid chromatography (LC), or size exclusion before enzymatic digestion, whereas at the peptide level, 2D LC is commonly used for peptide fractionation with the combination of ion chromatography and reverse-phase LC, such as is used in the multi-dimensional protein identification technology (MudPIT) [6].

Quantitative Methods for Global Protein Profiling

Differential stable isotopic labeling is the most common and versatile approach for quantitative proteomics analysis. This technique provides mass tags, which allow mass spectrometry to distinguish peptides with identical sequence but from different sample origins (e.g., diseased cases versus healthy controls) for quantitative comparison. There are different ways to incorporate stable isotope labeling onto proteins or peptides, including chemical derivatization and metabolic and enzymatic labeling [7,8]. Chemical derivatization is the most widely used methodology for stable isotope labeling and can be categorized into two types, isotopic and isobaric, based on how the isotopic signals are generated in mass spectrometric analysis. Isotopic-type stable isotope labeling methods, such as isotope-coded affinity tags (ICAT) [9] and isotope-coded protein label (ICPL) [10], quantify peptides at the MS level, while isobaric types, such as isobaric tags for relative and absolute quantitation (iTRAQ) [11] and tandem mass tags (TMT) [12], allow the mass spectrometer to generate and acquire differential isotopic reporting peaks at the tandem mass spectrometry (MS/MS) level after collision-induced dissociation (CID). Chemical derivatization approaches are post protein isolation methods that are well suited for analyzing almost any sample types, including clinical specimens such as tumor tissue, plasma/serum, and pancreatic juice. Metabolic incorporation of stable isotope labeling, such as stable isotope labeling by amino acids in cell culture (SILAC) [13,14], utilizes cell culturing to introduce isotopic tags on proteins by supplementing stable isotopic-labeled amino acid in cell culture medium and is particularly suitable for cell model studies. The enzymatic method, such as O^{18} labeling [15], takes a different route to introduce isotopic labeling on peptides by enzymatic digestion of proteins in an O^{18}-enriched buffer. Last, with advances in high-resolution mass spectrometric instrument and bioinformatics, label-free-based quantitative proteomics, based on spectral count or signal intensity, also have been applied in a variety of studies [16,17].

Mass Spectrometry

Mass spectrometer is the center of proteomics analysis, and its major components consist of the ion source, mass analyzer, and detection unit. Ion plume is produced and introduced into mass spectrometer through ion source; the ions are then separated in mass analyzer under an ultra-high vacuum based on their mass-to-charge value and recorded by a detector. The most commonly used ion source techniques are electrospray ionization (ESI) and matrix-assisted laser desorption/ionization (MALDI), both of which are used widely in proteomics analysis [7]. Several types of mass analyzers are available, including ion trap, orbitrap, time-of-flight (TOF), and quadrupole. These mass analyzers can be used independently or can be combined to achieve a tandem analysis. Recently, an ion mobility technique has been introduced, providing an additional dimension for resolving a complex biological sample within a mass spectrometer. In MS/MS analysis, peptides are fragmented in a collision cell and the fragmentation pattern of each of the peptide is used for sequence identification. In addition to the most commonly used CID mechanism, other soft ionization methods, including electron-transfer dissociation (ETD) and electron-capture dissociation (ECD) have been developed to facilitate protein PTM analysis [18].

Bioinformatics for Protein/Peptide Analysis

The last module of a proteomics pipeline is bioinformatics data processing, which includes a series of integrated software, from data format conversion to peptide/protein sequence assignment, statistical validation, and quantitative analysis. The MS/MS spectra generated are searched against a protein database for peptide/protein sequence identification using database searching algorithms, such as SQUEST [19], MASCOT [20], and X!tandem [21], followed by statistical validation and false discovery assessment. For quantitative experiments, based on peptide/protein registry, analytical software is used to compare the differential signal intensities between the sample and the control to obtain quantitative information reflecting peptide/protein relative abundance in the samples compared.

Targeted Proteomics

In addition to nonbias quantitative proteomics methods for global protein profiling, targeted proteomics utilizes the concept of isotope dilution and provides highly specific and sensitive detection of candidate analytes in a complex biological sample. This approach is increasingly applied in translational and biomarker studies [22,23]. The most widely used mass spectrometry technique for targeted proteomics analysis is the triple quadrupole-based selected (or multiple) reaction monitoring (SRM or MRM) technique. The development of targeted proteomics technology has opened a new avenue for quantitative detection of targeted proteins, peptides, or even specific forms of PTMs in a complex biological system, carrying great promise to facilitate biomarker development for pancreatic cancer and other diseases.

PROTEOMICS STUDY OF PANCREATIC TISSUE

Pancreatic Ductal Adenocarcinoma

A variety of proteomics approaches have been applied to investigate the proteome of pancreatic tumor tissue in comparison to noncancerous tissue. These studies include 2-DE based [24,25], ICAT-based [26,27], iTRAQ-based [28], and label-free-based [29] quantitative proteomics, identifying a group of valuable proteins associated with PDAC progression and metastasis. Although much work remains to be done to fully characterize the translational value of these protein candidates, some of the overexpressed proteins in PDAC have been further studied for their potential value for a variety of clinical applications. Galectin-1 (LGALS1) [25,26,28,29] was characterized as a functional receptor of tissue plasminogen activator (tPA, PLAT) and has been implicated in pancreatic cancer progression [30] and survival [31]; its expression, which is associated with dampening of the immune response, is negatively associated with long-term survival in resectable PDAC patients [31]. Gelsolin (GSN) [26,29] and lumican (LUM) [26,28,29] were further evaluated in plasma using SRM-based targeted proteomics as biomarker candidates to distinguish early stage PDAC (stages I and II) from chronic pancreatitis and healthy controls [32]. Plectin-1 (PLEC), another pancreatic cancer–associated protein [26,29] has been developed into a molecular imaging agent for the identification of primary and metastatic pancreatic cancer [33,34]. Annexin II (ANXA2) [26,28,29] and cofilin (CFL1) [26,28] are significantly associated with chemoresistance in patients with resected pancreatic cancer [35–37]. 14-3-3 sigma (SFN) [26] was found upregulated in the malignant epithelia of lymph node metastases [38] and was also involved with the resistance of pancreatic cancer cells to cisplatinum–induced apoptosis [39]. Moesin (MSN) [28] was characterized to be associated with lymph node metastases along with c14orf166 and radixin [40]. Tissue proteomics studies of pancreatic cancer have revealed that protein-driven stromal–epithelial interactions regulate neoplastic cell expansion, migration, invasion, and immunologic escape. The secretion of growth factors and cytokines by tumor cells and the surrounding stromal cells further induce cancer-associated angiogenesis and suppress the immune response [41,42].

Pancreatic Intraepithelial Neoplasia

Pancreative intraepithelial neoplasia (PanIN) represents the precancerous lesions of pancreatic adenocarcinoma and is grade 1–3. PanIN 3 is believed to be the most clinically relevant stage for early detection of pancreatic cancer when intervention and cure is possible. Quantitative proteomics using ICAT and iTRAQ labeling techniques was applied to investigate the tissue proteome of PanIN 3 lesions using PDAC, chronic pancreatitis, and normal pancreas as comparisons [28]. Over 200 differentially expressed proteins were identified in PanIN 3 tissues with many of them concurrently expressed in pancreatic cancer tissue, suggesting that proteome dysregulation in PanIN 3 lesion may start before cancer invasion. Some of the cancer-associated proteins that were overexpressed in PanIN 3 lesions included laminin beta 1 (LAMB1), 14-3-3 theta (YWHAQ), decorin (DCN), LGALS1, vimentin (VIM), and actinin 4 (ACTN4). On the basis of the immunohistochemistry (IHC) analysis, LAMB1 was highly expressed in stroma adjacent to both PanIN lesion and cancerous tissue; ACTN4 showed increased expression in both the epithelial and stromal elements of advanced PanIN lesions (75%) and tumor tissues (76%); LGALS1 expressed strongly in stroma of advanced PanIN lesions (70%) and tumor tissues (95%). Functional clustering and network analysis of the differentially expressed proteins in PanIN 3 lesions reveals that many of the key proteins are involved in cell mobility and inflammatory response; myc proto-oncogene protein (c-MYC) was an important regulatory protein in these PanIN 3 lesions [28]. The dysregulations of proteome in PanIN 3 lesion before cellular invasion of cancer was also observed in an engineered mouse model of pancreatic cancer [43].

Chronic Pancreatitis

As a chronic inflammatory disorder of pancreas, chronic pancreatitis is a risk factor for pancreatic cancer and the two diseases share many common clinical and molecular features [44–46]. A tissue proteomics study observed that many differentially expressed proteins in chronic pancreatitis were frequently involved in PDAC [27]. Using clinically well-characterized formalin-fixed paraffin embedded (FFPE) tissues and a label-free quantitative proteomics, it was observed that in comparison with normal pancreas the number of proteins differentially expressed in the tissues of mild chronic pancreatitis, severe chronic pancreatitis, and PDAC increased as the disease severity increased [29]. Similarities in proteome alterations between severe chronic pancreatitis and PDAC included a decrease of digestive enzymes and an increase of extracellular matrix (ECM) proteins, glycoproteins, and inflammatory proteins. Although several molecular events, including activation of acute phase response, prothrombin activation, and pancreatic fibrosis, were commonly shared between chronic pancreatitis and PDAC, metabolic changes were significantly associated with PDAC only. Validation of protein expression using IHC or Western blot confirmed that ANXA2 and insulin-like growth factor binding protein 2 (IGFBP2) were overexpressed in cancer but not in chronic pancreatitis, whereas cathepsin D (CTSD), integrin beta-1 (ITGB1), plasminogen (PLG), versican (VCAN), LUM, and collagen alpha-1(XIV) chain (Col14A1) were overexpressed in both diseases [27,29]. Overall, the studies suggested that more than 50% of the differential proteins in chronic pancreatitis were expressed concurrently in PDAC tissue.

Analysis of Isolated Cells

Proteomics and mass spectrometry were also applied to study isolated cells from pancreatic cancerous tissue using laser capture microdissection. The studies of isolated pancreatic neoplastic cells using 2-DE have identified the overexpression of S100A6 in malignant epithelial cells [47] and S100P and SFN in lymph node metastatic malignant epithelial cells [38]. Stromal cells play an important role in pancreatic tumorigenesis. Using a similar approach, S100A8 and S100A9 were found to be overexpressed in isolated stromal cells surrounding malignant pancreatic ductal cells [48]. A subpopulation of pancreatic tumor cells with cell surface markers $CD44^+CD24^+ESA^+$ has been identified as pancreatic cancer stem cells [49]. Using capillary isoelectric focusing and LC MS/MS, 169 differential proteins were identified in pancreatic cancer stem cells isolated from human xenograft tumors in mice using noncancerous cells as a comparison [50]. Signaling pathway analysis suggested that molecular events related to apoptosis, cell proliferation, inflammation, and metastasis were involved significantly in the pancreatic cancer stem cells.

BLOOD BIOMARKER DISCOVERY
Global Profiling of Plasma/Serum

Early detection of pancreatic cancer when it is curable would significantly improve the survival rate of this highly lethal disease. The current clinically used blood biomarker for pancreatic cancer, CA19-9, does not provide sufficient accuracy for early detection of pancreatic cancer. New blood tests that afford better specificity and sensitivity for diagnosis or prognosis are much needed. Proteomics provides a unique and powerful approach for blood biomarker discovery, allowing systematic profiling of hundreds and thousands of proteins in plasma or serum in a high-throughput fashion. Comparison of blood specimens obtained from pancreatic cancer patients versus diseased and healthy controls, renders a nonbiased approach to identify significant proteins or signature peptides that may be quantitatively associated with the presence and progression of pancreatic cancer.

The proteome of human plasma or serum is highly complicated, comprising tens of thousands of proteins with a dynamic range in concentrations exceeding 10-orders of magnitude [51,52]. In addition to the functional proteins that are endogenous to the circulatory system, a large number of tissue proteins can shed into the blood, including proteins that are secreted from tumor cells. Several studies have reported global profiling of plasma or serum from patients with PDAC, attempting to identify novel surrogate biomarkers to improve current pancreatic cancer detection [53–59]. Plasma profiling studies using 2-DE [53,55] identified leucine-rich alpha-2-glycoprotein (LRG) as an upregulated protein in the plasma from patients with pancreatic cancer. Since the origin and function of plasma LRG remains unclear, its clinical value as a blood biomarker for pancreatic cancer detection requires additional validation. More recently, shotgun proteomics-based large-scale quantitative protein profiling experiments were carried out to systematically study the proteomics alterations associated with pancreatic cancer. One study used genetically engineered mouse models to investigate the proteome of plasma from tumor-bearing mice at early and late stage of pancreatic cancer and identified more than 1400 proteins in the mouse plasma [54]. Using enzyme-linked immunosorbent assay (ELISA), a subset of mouse model-based protein candidates were tested in human sera, suggesting that the measurement of ALCAM protein (ALCAM), intercellular adhesion molecule 1 (ICAM1), neutrophil gelatinase-associated lipocalin (LCN2), tissue inhibitor of metalloproteinase 1 (TIMP1), lithostathine 1 (REG1A), regenerating islet-derived protein 3 (REG3), and insulin-like growth factor-binding protein 4 (IGFBP4), as a panel, was able to outperform CA19-9 in distinguishing pancreatic cancer patients from the matched controls (healthy and chronic pancreatitis). In a different investigation in human plasma, large-scale quantitative proteomics experiments were conducted to profile the proteome of plasma from patients with PDAC in comparison with chronic pancreatitis and healthy controls [56]. More than 1300 proteins, across eight orders of magnitude in plasma concentration, were identified using stringent identification criteria. Among these proteins, 76% and 6% of them were also identified in pancreatic tissues and pancreatic juice, respectively, suggesting the feasibility of detecting tumor-associated signals in blood. Many differential proteins in pancreatic tumor tissue and pancreatic juice were also found concurrently expressed in pancreatic cancer plasma, including neutrophil defensin 1 (DEFA1), pancreatic secretory trypsin inhibitor (SPINK1) thrombospondin-1 (THBS1), TIMP1, ICAM1, LUM, flavin reductase (BLVRB), collagen alpha-1(I) chain (COL1A1), EGF-containing fibulin-like extracellular matrix protein 1 (EFEMP1), L-lactate dehydrogenase B chain (LDHB), transforming growth factor beta-1 (TGFB1), IGFBP2, Ig mu chain C region (IGHM), glutathione peroxidase 3 (GPX3), immunoglobulin J chain (IGJ), and ZYX protein (ZYX), just to name a few. Using an independent plasma cohort, ELISA validation showed that a biomarker panel of TIMP1 and ICAM1 provided better sensitivity and specificity compared to CA19-9 in identifying pancreatic cancer patients from the diseased and healthy matched controls.

Targeted Proteomics for Protein Biomarker Detection

Although large-scale quantitative proteomics profiling studies can identify differentially expressed proteins in pancreatic cancer specimens, the specificity and sensitivity of each individual protein associated with pancreatic cancer needs to be further evaluated for their value in clinical application, regardless of whether these proteins are discovered in pancreatic cancer tissue, PanIN lesions, or body fluids. This is particularly the case in developing blood-based biomarkers for pancreatic cancer detection. For instance, the blood concentration of a dysregulated tissue protein discovered in pancreatic tumor may or may not quantitatively correspond to its tissue expression, depending on its function, origin, cellular location, abundance, and other factors. With mass spectrometry-based targeted proteomics, the plasma/serum concentration of a large number of protein candidates can be measured accurately without the dependence on an ELISA assay for each targeted protein. Using a clinically well-characterized plasma cohort, including patients with early stage PDAC, chronic pancreatitis and healthy control, five pancreatic cancer–associated proteins that are overexpressed in pancreatic tumor, including LUM, GSN, TIMP1, transglutaminase 2 (TGM2), and SFN, were evaluated with a multiplexed SRM assay [32]. The receiver operating characteristic (ROC) analysis of the plasma concentration of these proteins indicated that TIMP1, LUM, and GSN had an area–under–curve (AUC) value greater than 0.75 in distinguishing pancreatic cancer from the controls. In a different study, proline-hydroxylated α-fibrinogen was analyzed in plasma using SRM technique [60]. By measuring the concentration of proline-hydroxylated and unmodified α-fibrinogen in the plasma samples from pancreatic cancer patients and healthy controls, the study indicated that the percent hydroxylation of α-fibrinogen and concentration of hydroxylated α-fibrinogen were both significantly greater in the plasma of pancreatic cancer patients, including some of those with a negative test in CA19-9.

ANALYSIS OF PANCREATIC JUICE AND CYST FLUID

Pancreatic Juice

PDAC accounts for more than 90% of all pancreatic neoplasms [61]. Pancreatic juice is rich in proteins secreted from pancreatic duct where PDAC arises, and thus it is a proximate source for investigating tumor-associated proteomics changes. The protein constituents in pancreatic juices have been analyzed using specimens collected from individuals with no apparent pancreatic pathology [62], patients with pancreatic adenocarcinoma [63] and chronic pancreatitis [64]. These nonquantitative studies have identified up to 473 proteins in human pancreatic juice with different pathological states. In addition to the tumor-associated proteins shed into the pancreatic duct, a number of proteins identified in pancreatic juice are digestive enzymes and related proteins. To reveal the proteins that are expressed differentially in PDAC, quantitative proteomics studies were conducted to study the cancer-associated proteome alterations in pancreatic juice. ICAT-based shotgun proteomics was applied to investigate the differential proteins present in cancerous pancreatic juice in comparison with pancreatic juice collected from noncancerous controls [65]. The cancer-related overexpressed proteins (≥twofold) identified included kallikrein 1 (KLK1), IGFBP2, REG1A and REG1B, pancreatic secretory granule membrane major glycoprotein (GP2), SPINK1, pancreatitis-associated protein 1 (PAP1), pancreatic ribonuclease (RNASE1), and T-cell receptor beta chain (TCRB). In addition, a difference gel electrophoresis (DIGE)–based study identified overexpression of matrix metalloproteinase-9 (MMP9), oncogene DJ1 (PARK7), and alpha-1B-glycoprotein (A1BG) in pancreatic juices from pancreatic cancer patients [66]. The comparison of pancreatic juice from patients with PDAC and chronic pancreatitis indicated that some of the over-expressed proteins in cancer were expressed congruently in chronic pancreatitis [67], consistent with the notion that the two diseases share many common clinical and molecular features. An iTRAQ-based quantitative proteomics study further investigated the proteome of pancreatic juices collected from patients with PanIN 3 lesion and healthy controls; and found 20 proteins elevated in PanIN cases [68]. Among them, anterior gradient-2 (AGR2) was further evaluated in a pancreatic juice cohort consisting of patients with PDAC, premalignant lesions (including PanIN 3, PanIN 2, intraductal papillary mucinous neoplasms (IPMNs)), and benign pancreatic disease (including chronic pancreatitis). AGR2 levels in the pancreatic juice were elevated significantly in patients with premalignant conditions (PanINs and IPMNs) as well as pancreatic cancer, compared with the control samples, suggesting its potential value as pancreatic juice biomarker for pancreatic cancer early detection.

It is notable that among the proteins identified in pancreatic juice, there is a low overlap in protein identification among the reported studies. Although this may be in part due to the differences in the methodologies used, it reflects the heterogeneous and dynamic nature of protein profile present in pancreatic juice. A 2-DE study suggested that the level of obstruction of the main pancreatic ducts because of cancer or other diseases was probably the main factor affecting the protein composition, especially the digestive enzymes and related proteins, in pancreatic juice [69]. In addition, bile and blood can be contaminants of pancreatic juice. Identification of large number of blood proteins in pancreatic juice may be an indication of a possible contamination of blood during pancreatic juice collection.

Pancreatic Cyst Fluid

Pancreatic cysts have been increasingly detected with the widespread use of cross-sectional imaging techniques [70]. However, management of increasingly prevalent pancreatic cystic lesions has been a challenging task largely because of the lack of an effective diagnosis method for detecting clinically relevant neoplasm associated with cysts. Pancreatic cyst fluid, which can be obtained via needle aspiration at endoscopic ultrasound, appears to be a suitable source for protein biomarker development. Using 2-DE and mass spectrometry, one study investigated the cyst fluids obtained from a group of patients who were categorized according to their cytology results, including benign (no evidence of benign mucinous epithelium, atypical cells, or carcinoma), benign mucinous epithelium, atypical–suspicious for neoplasm, and malignant cysts [71]. The study suggested that the expression of certain mucins, carcinoembryonic antigen-related cell adhesion molecules (CEACAMs), and S100 proteins in cyst fluid were associated with pancreatic cancer. In a different study, a similar proteomics approach was applied to investigate surgically collected cyst fluids from symptomatic patients who underwent partial pancreatectomy [72]. The study identified up to 727 proteins in the cyst fluids analyzed and showed that different protein patterns were associated with specific cyst types, including serous cystadenomas, mucinous neoplasms (MCN), pancreatic neuroendocrine tumors (NET), malignant IPMN, and pseudo-cyst (PC). The expressions of two proteins, olfactomedin-4 (OLFM4) (identified in MCN and IPMN cyst fluids) and cell surface glycoprotein MUC18 (MUC18) (identified in NET cyst fluid) were confirmed with immunohistochemistry using pancreas tissue.

FUNCTIONAL AND HYPOTHESIS-DRIVEN PROTEOMIC STUDIES

Targeted Interrogation of KRAS Proteins

KRAS is one of the most frequently mutated genes associated with pancreatic cancer, presenting in approximately 90% of PDAC [3]. Mutations in the k-ras gene (e.g., G12D, G13D, G12V) are missense, and such small differences in translated protein structure cannot be measured by Western-blotting or ELISA because no antibody is available to reliably distinguish the wild-type and mutant protein forms. Because of its high specificity in distinguishing molecular mass, mass spectrometry has been applied to detect the wild-type and mutant KRAS proteins in pancreatic tumor tissue, cells, and cyst fluids [73–75]. Stable isotope-labeled synthetic reference peptides representing wild-type and mutant variants of KRAS protein are used as internal standard for absolute quantification. Coupling with immunoprecipitation for protein enrichment, the SRM assays were able to detect mutant KRAS proteins in pancreatic tissue at low femtomole/milligram (fmol/mg) range [74,75]. In a different study, using gel electrophoresis to separate KRAS proteins for SRM analysis, the concentrations of wild-type and mutant KRAS proteins were also measured in pancreatic cyst fluids collected from patients with invasive carcinoma, carcinoma in situ and benign controls [73]. On the basis of the 15 cases tested, wild-type KRAS concentrations in pancreatic cyst fluids varied between 0.08 and 1.1 femtomole/microgram (fmol/µg), whereas mutant KRAS concentrations varied between 0.08 and 0.36 fmol/µg.

Identification of Protein Receptors

Tissue plasminogen activator (tPA) is associated with pancreatic tumor growth and invasion, and its interaction with cell membrane receptors has been related to increased proteolytic activity and transduction of tPA signaling in pancreatic tumor [76]. A proteomics approach utilizing antibody affinity capturing was applied to characterize the tPA receptors in pancreatic cancer cell lines [77]. Using nonpancreatic cancer endothelial cells as a comparison, 31 proteins were identified in the pull-down of tPA; and annexin A2 and galectin 1 were verified to be the functional receptors of tPA in pancreatic cancer [30,76,77].

Determination of Protein Activities

Activity-based proteomics approach enables characterizing enzyme activities in a diseased setting, and was applied to investigate serine hydrolase activity in primary PDAC [78]. Using bifunctional active site-directed probes, which covalently bind the active site of serine hydrolases, to enrich for the proteins for mass spectrometric analysis, the study identified retinoblastoma-binding protein 9 (RBBP9) as a pancreatic tumor associated serine hydrolase with increased activity in pancreatic carcinoma. Although RBBP9 protein abundance was expressed at similar levels in both normal and cancerous tissue, its increased activity associated with pancreatic tumorigenesis may contribute to the suppression of TGF-β signaling [78].

Investigation of Cancer-Associated Cell Invasiveness

Overexpression of palladin (PALLD) in cancer-associated fibroblasts has been related to pancreatic tumor invasion and metastases [79,80]. To discover the mechanism underlying the invasive capability of PALLD-activated stromal fibroblasts in the setting of pancreatic cancer, quantitative proteomics was conducted to examine the invadopodia of activated fibroblasts in comparison with the control quiescent fibroblasts [79]. The podia that invaded through matrix-covered pores of an invasion chamber were isolated and analyzed, leading to the identification of more than 200 differentially expressed proteins in invasive PALLD-activated fibroblasts, including known invadopodia proteins, ras-related proteins, GTP-binding proteins, and proteolytic enzymes. The increased proteolytic enzymes in invadopodia of PALLD-associated fibroblasts enhanced ECM degradation and creation of tunnels through the matrix, thus promoting the invasion of cancer cells through multiple modes of matrix remodeling [81].

POST-TRANSLATIONAL MODIFICATIONS

Protein PTMs occur on many proteins and play important roles in regulating a variety of protein functional activities and cellular physiology. Proteomics investigation of PTMs can reveal unique information uncovering the pathways and molecular events involved in pancreatic tumorigenesis and provide useful clues for clinical application.

Phosphorylation

Protein kinase phosphorylation is central to the regulation and control of cell functions in both normal and disease states. Phosphoproteomics studies were carried out to investigate pancreatic cell lines that have upregulation of tyrosine kinase signaling [82]. Using immunoprecipitation, the enriched tyrosine phosphoproteins were resolved with sodium dodecyl sulfate-polyacrylamide gel electrophoresis (SDS-PAGE), digested, and analyzed by LC MS/MS. The analysis of tyrosine kinase pathways led to the identification of aberrant activation of epidermal growth factor receptor (EGFR) pathway in the PDAC cell line. Mouse xenograft studies demonstrated that the EGFR inhibitor, erlotinib, was effective in reducing the growth of the tumor size, confirming the EGFR pathway to be responsible for the proliferation of these tumors. In a different study, the effect of inhibition of the transketolase activity on signaling pathways in pancreatic cancer cell lines was investigated using 2-DE and MALDI TOF/TOF [83]. Using oxythiamine (OT), a metabolic inhibitor to suppress pancreatic cancer cell proliferation, the study identified 12 phosphor proteins that were suppressed significantly by OT treatment; and further revealed that phosphorylation at serine 78 of heat shock protein 27 (Hsp27) was inhibited dramatically by the treatment. These observations suggested that the inhibition of transketolase pathway may cause a decrease in the phosphorylation of proteins associated with cancer proliferation and survival. Using 2-DE and mass spectrometry, a third study investigated the response of circulating autoantibodies to r-enolase (ENOA) in PDAC patients by examining the expression of ENOA isoforms in pancreatic tissues and cell lines and by quantifying the autoantibody response in sera from PDAC and noncancerous patients [84]. The study found that 62% of PDAC patients produced autoantibodies to two ENOA isoforms (ENOA1, 2) with phosphorylation on serine 419 and found that the presence of autoantibodies against phosphorylated ENOA1, 2 correlated with a significantly better clinical outcomes in advanced patients treated with standard chemotherapy.

Glycosylation

Altered glycosylation has long been recognized as a hallmark in epithelial cancer, including pancreatic cancer. Cancer-associated glycoproteins can be altered in two main ways: (1) protein sites that are normally glycosylated are either hypo- or hyperglycosylated, and (2) the glycan moiety itself is altered. Ultimately, malignant transformation is usually associated with one or both of these types of abnormal glycosylation events, leading to the accumulation of tumor-specific glycoproteins actively involved in the neoplastic progression and metastasis. Glycoproteins that are secreted from pancreatic tumor cells can have abnormal glycosylation compared with normal cells, such as the alterations in sialylation and fucosylation [85]. Tumor-specific glycoproteins, such as mucins (MUC) and CEACAMs [86–91], are involved actively in the neoplastic progression and metastasis of pancreatic cancer. CA19-9, which detects the epitope of sialyl Lewis(a) on mucins and other adhesive molecules, is currently the only clinical blood biomarker for pancreatic cancer [92]. Using lectin affinity chromatography and LC MS/MS, N-glycan profiling studies to compare human sera from pancreatic cancer patients and healthy controls have identified approximately 130 sialylated N-linked glycoproteins [93] and 105 unique carbohydrates, including 44 oligosaccharides that were distinct in the pancreatic cancer serum [94]. Glycomic analysis of pancreatic cyst fluid, including mucinous cystic neoplasms and IPMN, identified 80 N-linked glycans with high mannose or complex structures [95]. The study also observed hyperfucosylation of complex N-linked glycans on several glycoproteins, including triacylglycerol lipase and pancreatic α-amylase. Tissue proteomics studies have demonstrated the enrichment of glycoproteins among the proteins upregulated in PDAC and chronic pancreatitis tissues, implicating their potential roles in malignancy and inflammation [29].

Membrane and secreted proteins are frequently glycoproteins. A study of cell surface glycoproteins from five pancreatic cancer cell lines identified several surface glycoproteins that not only are overexpressed but also play a functional role in tumor cell survival, including integrin β6 (ITGB6), CD46, tissue factor (TF), and chromosome 14 open-reading frame 1 (C14ORF1) [96]. A global-scale glycoproteomics study to systematically profile the N-glycoproteome of pancreatic tumor tissue in comparison with normal pancreas identified a group of glycoproteins with aberrant N-glycosylation occupancy (hyper- or hypoglycosylated) associated with PDAC, including mucin-5AC (MUC5AC), carcinoembryonic antigen-related cell adhesion molecule 5 (CEACAM5), IGFBP3, and galectin-3-binding protein (LGALS3BP) [97]. The study revealed an emerging phenomenon that increased N-glycosylation activity was implicated in several pancreatic cancer pathways, including TGF-β, TNF, NF-kappa-B, and TFEB-related lysosomal changes. The study also found that aberrant glycosylation occupancy corresponding to pancreatic malignancy or inflammation could be not only protein-specific but also glycosylation site-specific, reflecting the complex molecular mechanisms involved in the pathogenesis of pancreatic cancer.

SUMMARY

Pancreatic cancer is a highly lethal disease that is difficult to detect at an early stage when curable treatments are possible. With the advances in mass spectrometry and bioinformatics, proteomics—especially quantitative and functional proteomics—have been increasingly applied to investigate a variety of clinical specimens, ranging from neoplastic tissues to bodily fluids. These translational studies will be pivotal in the efforts toward better diagnosis and therapeutic treatment. Although some of the novel pancreatic cancer–associated proteins discovered in proteomics studies have been under investigation to further define their roles in the pathogenesis of the disease and their potential clinical value, much work remains to be done to follow up the vast information obtained from the discovery studies [98–100]. As an emerging technology, the current challenges in pancreatic cancer proteomics include the limited scope of proteome coverage and the reproducibility issues associated with studies with different methodologies and sample sources. Nonetheless, the reported studies have provided a wealth of knowledge integrating with our existing understanding at genomics level to shed light on the molecular mechanisms underlying pancreatic tumorigenesis and have offered guidance for future experimentation. The integration of proteomics, genomics, systems biology, and other molecular techniques carries a great promise to improve the outcome of pancreatic cancer.

ACKNOWLEDGMENT

This work was supported in part by the National Institutes of Health under grants K25CA137222, R21CA149772, R21CA161575, and R01CA107209, and Canary Foundation.

REFERENCES

[1] Siegel R, Naishadham D, Jemal A. Cancer statistics, 2012. CA Cancer J Clin 2012;62:10–29.

[2] Siegel R, DeSantis C, Virgo K, Stein K, Mariotto A, Smith T, et al. Cancer treatment and survivorship statistics, 2012. CA Cancer J Clin 2012;62:220–41.

[3] Goggins M. Molecular markers of early pancreatic cancer. J Clin Oncol 2005;23:4524–31.

[4] Yeo CJ, Cameron JL, Lillemoe KD, Sitzmann JV, Hruban RH, Goodman SN, et al. Pancreaticoduodenectomy for cancer of the head of the pancreas. 201 patients. Ann Surg 1995;221:721–31.

[5] Van den BG, Arckens L. Recent advances in 2D electrophoresis: an array of possibilities. Expert Rev Proteomics 2005;2:243–52.

[6] Schirmer EC, Yates III JR, Gerace L. MudPIT: a powerful proteomics tool for discovery. Discov Med 2003;3:38–9.

[7] Aebersold R, Mann M. Mass spectrometry-based proteomics. Nature 2003;422:198–207.

[8] Pan S, Aebersold R. Quantitative proteomics by stable isotope labeling and mass spectrometry. Methods Mol Biol 2007;367:209–18.

[9] Gygi SP, Rist B, Gerber SA, Turecek F, Gelb MH, Aebersold R. Quantitative analysis of complex protein mixtures using isotope-coded affinity tags. Nat Biotechnol 1999;17:994–9.

[10] Schmidt A, Kellermann J, Lottspeich F. A novel strategy for quantitative proteomics using isotope-coded protein labels. Proteomics 2005;5:4–15.

[11] Ross PL, Huang YN, Marchese JN, Williamson B, Parker K, Hattan S, et al. Multiplexed protein quantitation in *Saccharomyces cerevisiae* using amine-reactive isobaric tagging reagents. Mol Cell Proteomics 2004;3:1154–69.

[12] Thompson A, Schafer J, Kuhn K, Kienle S, Schwarz J, Schmidt G, et al. Tandem mass tags: a novel quantification strategy for comparative analysis of complex protein mixtures by MS/MS. Anal Chem 2003;75:1895–904.

[13] Ong SE, Blagoev B, Kratchmarova I, Kristensen DB, Steen H, Pandey A, et al. Stable isotope labeling by amino acids in cell culture, SILAC, as a simple and accurate approach to expression proteomics. Mol Cell Proteomics 2002;1:376–86.

[14] Veenstra TD, Martinovic S, Anderson GA, Pasa-Tolic L, Smith RD. Proteome analysis using selective incorporation of isotopically labeled amino acids. J Am Soc Mass Spectrom 2000;11:78–82.

[15] Mirgorodskaya OA, Kozmin YP, Titov MI, Korner R, Sonksen CP, Roepstorff P. Quantitation of peptides and proteins by matrix-assisted laser desorption/ionization mass spectrometry using ^{18}O-labeled internal standards. Rapid Commun Mass Spectrom 2000;14:1226–32.

[16] Choi H, Fermin D, Nesvizhskii AI. Significance analysis of spectral count data in label-free shotgun proteomics. Mol Cell Proteomics 2008;7:2373–85.

[17] Old WM, Meyer-Arendt K, Aveline-Wolf L, Pierce KG, Mendoza A, Sevinsky JR, et al. Comparison of label-free methods for quantifying human proteins by shotgun proteomics. Mol Cell Proteomics 2005;4:1487–502.

[18] Mikesh LM, Ueberheide B, Chi A, Coon JJ, Syka JE, Shabanowitz J, et al. The utility of ETD mass spectrometry in proteomic analysis. Biochim Biophys Acta 2006;1764:1811–22.

[19] Eng J, McCormack AL, Yates JR. An approach to correlate tandem mass spectral data of peptides with amino acid sequences in a protein database. J Am Soc Mass Spectrom 1994;5:976–89.

[20] Perkins DN, Pappin DJ, Creasy DM, Cottrell JS. Probability-based protein identification by searching sequence databases using mass spectrometry data. Electrophoresis 1999;20:3551–67.

[21] Craig R, Beavis RC. TANDEM: matching proteins with tandem mass spectra. Bioinformatics 2004;20:1466–7.

[22] Huttenhain R, Malmstrom J, Picotti P, Aebersold R. Perspectives of targeted mass spectrometry for protein biomarker verification. Curr Opin Chem Biol 2009;13:518–25.

[23] Pan S, Aebersold R, Chen R, Rush J, Goodlett DR, McIntosh MW, et al. Mass spectrometry based targeted protein quantification: methods and applications. J Proteome Res 2009;8:787–97.

[24] Lu Z, Hu L, Evers S, Chen J, Shen Y. Differential expression profiling of human pancreatic adenocarcinoma and healthy pancreatic tissue. Proteomics 2004;4:3975–88.

[25] Shen J, Person MD, Zhu J, Abbruzzese JL, Li D. Protein expression profiles in pancreatic adenocarcinoma compared with normal pancreatic tissue and tissue affected by pancreatitis as detected by two-dimensional gel electrophoresis and mass spectrometry. Cancer Res 2004;64:9018–26.

[26] Chen R, Yi EC, Donohoe D, Pan S, Eng J, Crispin DA, et al. Pancreatic cancer proteome: the proteins that underlie invasion, metastasis, and immunologic escape. Gastroenterology 2005;129:1187–97.

[27] Chen R, Brentnall TA, Pan S, Cooke K, Moyes KW, Lane Z, et al. Quantitative proteomics analysis reveals that proteins differentially expressed in chronic pancreatitis are also frequently involved in pancreatic cancer. Mol Cell Proteomics 2007;6:1331–42.

[28] Pan S, Chen R, Reimel BA, Crispin DA, Mirzaei H, Cooke K, et al. Quantitative proteomics investigation of pancreatic intraepithelial neoplasia. Electrophoresis 2009;30:1132–44.

[29] Pan S, Chen R, Stevens T, Bronner MP, May D, Tamura Y, et al. Proteomics portrait of archival lesions of chronic pancreatitis. PLoS One 2011;6:e27574.

[30] Roda O, Ortiz-Zapater E, Martinez-Bosch N, Gutierrez-Gallego R, Vila-Perello M, Ampurdanes C, et al. Galectin-1 is a novel functional receptor for tissue plasminogen activator in pancreatic cancer. Gastroenterology 2009;136:1379–90.

[31] Chen R, Pan S, Ottenhof NA, de Wilde RF, Wolfgang CL, Lane Z, et al. Stromal galectin-1 expression is associated with long-term survival in resectable pancreatic ductal adenocarcinoma. Cancer Biol Ther 2012;13:899–907.

[32] Pan S, Chen R, Brand RE, Hawley S, Tamura Y, Gafken PR, et al. Multiplex targeted proteomic assay for biomarker detection in plasma: a pancreatic cancer biomarker case study. J Proteome Res 2012;11:1937–48.

[33] Bausch D, Thomas S, Mino-Kenudson M, Fernández-del CC, Bauer TW, Williams M, et al. Plectin-1 as a novel biomarker for pancreatic cancer. Clin Cancer Res 2011;17:302–9.

[34] Kelly KA, Bardeesy N, Anbazhagan R, Gurumurthy S, Berger J, Alencar H, et al. Targeted nanoparticles for imaging incipient pancreatic ductal adenocarcinoma. PLoS Med 2008;5:e85.

[35] Kagawa S, Takano S, Yoshitomi H, Kimura F, Satoh M, Shimizu H, et al. Akt/mTOR signaling pathway is crucial for gemcitabine resistance induced by Annexin II in pancreatic cancer cells. J Surg Res 2012;178:758–67.

[36] Sato T, Kita K, Sugaya S, Suzuki T, Suzuki N. Extracellular release of annexin II from pancreatic cancer cells and resistance to anticancer drug-induced apoptosis by supplementation of recombinant annexin II. Pancreas 2012;41:1247–54.

[37] Wang Y, Kuramitsu Y, Ueno T, Suzuki N, Yoshino S, Iizuka N, et al. Differential expression of up-regulated cofilin-1 and down-regulated cofilin-2 characteristic of pancreatic cancer tissues. Oncol Rep 2011;26:1595–9.

[38] Naidoo K, Jones R, Dmitrovic B, Wijesuriya N, Kocher H, Hart IR, et al. Proteome of formalin-fixed paraffin-embedded pancreatic ductal adenocarcinoma and lymph node metastases. J Pathol 2012;226:756–63.

[39] Neupane D, Korc M. 14-3-3sigma Modulates pancreatic cancer cell survival and invasiveness. Clin Cancer Res 2008;14:7614–23.

[40] Cui Y, Wu J, Zong M, Song G, Jia Q, Jiang J, et al. Proteomic profiling in pancreatic cancer with and without lymph node metastasis. Int J Cancer 2009;124:1614–21.

[41] Brown LF, Guidi AJ, Schnitt SJ, Van De WL, Iruela-Arispe ML, Yeo TK, et al. Vascular stroma formation in carcinoma in situ, invasive carcinoma, and metastatic carcinoma of the breast. Clin Cancer Res 1999;5:1041–56.

[42] Liotta LA, Kohn EC. The microenvironment of the tumour-host interface. Nature 2001;411:375–9.

[43] Rhim AD, Mirek ET, Aiello NM, Maitra A, Bailey JM, McAllister F, et al. EMT and dissemination precede pancreatic tumor formation. Cell 2012;148:349–61.

[44] Lowenfels AB, Maisonneuve P, Cavallini G, Ammann RW, Lankisch PG, Andersen JR, et al. Pancreatitis and the risk of pancreatic cancer. International Pancreatitis Study Group. N Engl J Med 1993;328:1433–7.

[45] Malka D, Hammel P, Maire F, Rufat P, Madeira I, Pessione F, et al. Risk of pancreatic adenocarcinoma in chronic pancreatitis. Gut 2002;51:849–52.

[46] Rosty C, Geradts J, Sato N, Wilentz RE, Roberts H, Sohn T, et al. p16 Inactivation in pancreatic intraepithelial neoplasias (PanINs) arising in patients with chronic pancreatitis. Am J Surg Pathol 2003;27:1495–501.

[47] Shekouh AR, Thompson CC, Prime W, Campbell F, Hamlett J, Herrington CS, et al. Application of laser capture microdissection combined with two-dimensional electrophoresis for the discovery of differentially regulated proteins in pancreatic ductal adenocarcinoma. Proteomics 2003;3:1988–2001.

[48] Sheikh AA, Vimalachandran D, Thompson CC, Jenkins RE, Nedjadi T, Shekouh A, et al. The expression of S100A8 in pancreatic cancer-associated monocytes is associated with the Smad4 status of pancreatic cancer cells. Proteomics 2007;7:1929–40.

[49] Li C, Heidt DG, Dalerba P, Burant CF, Zhang L, Adsay V, et al. Identification of pancreatic cancer stem cells. Cancer Res 2007;67:1030–7.

[50] Dai L, Li C, Shedden KA, Lee CJ, Li C, Quoc H, et al. Quantitative proteomic profiling studies of pancreatic cancer stem cells. J Proteome Res 2010;9:3394–402.

[51] Liumbruno G, D'Alessandro A, Grazzini G, Zolla L. Blood-related proteomics. J Proteomics 2010;73:483–507.

[52] Omenn GS, States DJ, Adamski M, Blackwell TW, Menon R, Hermjakob H, et al. Overview of the HUPO Plasma Proteome Project: results from the pilot phase with 35 collaborating laboratories and multiple analytical groups, generating a core dataset of 3020 proteins and a publicly-available database. Proteomics 2005;5:3226–45.

[53] Deng R, Lu Z, Chen Y, Zhou L, Lu X. Plasma proteomic analysis of pancreatic cancer by 2-dimensional gel electrophoresis. Pancreas 2007;34:310–7.

[54] Faca VM, Song KS, Wang H, Zhang Q, Krasnoselsky AL, Newcomb LF, et al. A mouse to human search for plasma proteome changes associated with pancreatic tumor development. PLoS Med 2008;5:e123.

[55] Kakisaka T, Kondo T, Okano T, Fujii K, Honda K, Endo M, et al. Plasma proteomics of pancreatic cancer patients by multi-dimensional liquid chromatography and two-dimensional difference gel electrophoresis (2D-DIGE): up-regulation of leucine-rich alpha-2-glycoprotein in pancreatic cancer. J Chromatogr B Analyt Technol Biomed Life Sci 2007;852:257–67.

[56] Pan S, Chen R, Crispin DA, May D, Stevens T, McIntosh MW, et al. Protein alterations associated with pancreatic cancer and chronic pancreatitis found in human plasma using global quantitative proteomics profiling. J Proteome Res 2011;10:2359–76.

[57] Sinclair J, Timms JF. Quantitative profiling of serum samples using TMT protein labelling, fractionation and LC-MS/MS. Methods 2011;54:361–9.

[58] Tonack S, Aspinall-O'Dea M, Jenkins RE, Elliot V, Murray S, Lane CS, et al. A technically detailed and pragmatic protocol for quantitative serum proteomics using iTRAQ. J Proteomics 2009;73:352–6.

[59] Yan L, Tonack S, Smith R, Dodd S, Jenkins RE, Kitteringham N, et al. Confounding effect of obstructive jaundice in the interpretation of proteomic plasma profiling data for pancreatic cancer. J Proteome Res 2009;8:142–8.

[60] Yoneyama T, Ohtsuki S, Ono M, Ohmine K, Uchida Y, Yamada T, et al. Quantitative targeted absolute proteomics-based large-scale quantification of proline-hydroxylated alpha-fibrinogen in plasma for pancreatic cancer diagnosis. J Proteome Res 2013;12:753–62.

[61] Mergo PJ, Helmberger TK, Buetow PC, Helmberger RC, Ros PR. Pancreatic neoplasms: MR imaging and pathologic correlation. Radiographics 1997;17:281–301.

[62] Doyle CJ, Yancey K, Pitt HA, Wang M, Bemis K, Yip-Schneider MT, et al. The proteome of normal pancreatic juice. Pancreas 2012;41:186–94.

[63] Gronborg M, Bunkenborg J, Kristiansen TZ, Jensen ON, Yeo CJ, Hruban RH, et al. Comprehensive proteomic analysis of human pancreatic juice. J Proteome Res 2004;3:1042–55.

[64] Paulo JA, Kadiyala V, Banks PA, Steen H, Conwell DL. Mass spectrometry-based (GeLC-MS/MS) comparative proteomic analysis of endoscopically (ePFT) collected pancreatic and gastroduodenal fluids. Clin Transl Gastroenterol 2012;3:e14.

[65] Chen R, Pan S, Yi EC, Donohoe S, Bronner MP, Potter JD, et al. Quantitative proteomic profiling of pancreatic cancer juice. Proteomics 2006;6:3871–9.

[66] Tian M, Cui YZ, Song GH, Zong MJ, Zhou XY, Chen Y, et al. Proteomic analysis identifies MMP-9, DJ-1 and A1BG as overexpressed proteins in pancreatic juice from pancreatic ductal adenocarcinoma patients. BMC Cancer 2008;8:241.

[67] Chen R, Pan S, Cooke K, Moyes KW, Bronner MP, Goodlett DR, et al. Comparison of pancreas juice proteins from cancer versus pancreatitis using quantitative proteomic analysis. Pancreas 2007;34:70–9.

[68] Chen R, Pan S, Duan X, Nelson BH, Sahota RA, de Rham S, et al. Elevated level of anterior gradient-2 in pancreatic juice from patients with pre-malignant pancreatic neoplasia. Mol Cancer 2010;9:149.

[69] Zhou L, Lu Z, Yang A, Deng R, Mai C, Sang X, et al. Comparative proteomic analysis of human pancreatic juice: methodological study. Proteomics 2007;7:1345–55.

[70] Kwon RS, Simeone DM. The use of protein-based biomarkers for the diagnosis of cystic tumors of the pancreas. Int J Proteomics 2011;2011:413646.

[71] Ke E, Patel BB, Liu T, Li XM, Haluszka O, Hoffman JP, et al. Proteomic analyses of pancreatic cyst fluids. Pancreas 2009;38:e33–42.

[72] Cuoghi A, Farina A, Z'graggen K, Dumonceau JM, Tomasi A, Hochstrasser DF, et al. Role of proteomics to differentiate between benign and potentially malignant pancreatic cysts. J Proteome Res 2011;10:2664–70.

[73] Halvey PJ, Ferrone CR, Liebler DC. GeLC-MRM quantitation of mutant KRAS oncoprotein in complex biological samples. J Proteome Res 2012;11:3908–13.

[74] Ruppen-Canas I, Lopez-Casas PP, Garcia F, Ximenez-Embun P, Munoz M, Morelli MP, et al. An improved quantitative mass spectrometry analysis of tumor specific mutant proteins at high sensitivity. Proteomics 2012;12:1319–27.

[75] Wang Q, Chaerkady R, Wu J, Hwang HJ, Papadopoulos N, Kopelovich L, et al. Mutant proteins as cancer-specific biomarkers. Proc Natl Acad Sci USA 2011;108:2444–9.

[76] Ortiz-Zapater E, Peiro S, Roda O, Corominas JM, Aguilar S, Ampurdanes C, et al. Tissue plasminogen activator induces pancreatic cancer cell proliferation by a non-catalytic mechanism that requires extracellular signal-regulated kinase 1/2 activation through epidermal growth factor receptor and annexin A2. Am J Pathol 2007;170:1573–84.

[77] Roda O, Chiva C, Espuna G, Gabius HJ, Real FX, Navarro P, et al. A proteomic approach to the identification of new tPA receptors in pancreatic cancer cells. Proteomics 2006;6(Suppl. 1):S36–41.

[78] Shields DJ, Niessen S, Murphy EA, Mielgo A, Desgrosellier JS, Lau SK, et al. RBBP9: a tumor-associated serine hydrolase activity required for pancreatic neoplasia. Proc Natl Acad Sci USA 2010;107:2189–94.

[79] Brentnall TA, Lai LA, Coleman J, Bronner MP, Pan S, Chen R. Arousal of cancer-associated stroma: overexpression of palladin activates fibroblasts to promote tumor invasion. PLoS One 2012;7:e30219.

[80] Salaria SN, Illei P, Sharma R, Walter KM, Klein AP, Eshleman JR, et al. Palladin is overexpressed in the non-neoplastic stroma of infiltrating ductal adenocarcinomas of the pancreas, but is only rarely overexpressed in neoplastic cells. Cancer Biol Ther 2007;6:324–8.

[81] Goicoechea SM, Garcia-Mata R, Staub J, Valdivia A, Sharek L, McCulloch CG, et al. Palladin promotes invasion of pancreatic cancer cells by enhancing invadopodia formation in cancer-associated fibroblasts. Oncogene 2013 Mar 25. doi: 10.1038/onc.2013.68. [Epub ahead of print].

[82] Harsha HC, Jimeno A, Molina H, Mihalas AB, Goggins MG, Hruban RH, et al. Activated epidermal growth factor receptor as a novel target in pancreatic cancer therapy. J Proteome Res 2008;7:4651–8.

[83] Zhang H, Cao R, Lee WN, Deng C, Zhao Y, Lappe J, et al. Inhibition of protein phosphorylation in MIA pancreatic cancer cells: confluence of metabolic and signaling pathways. J Proteome Res 2010;9:980–9.

[84] Tomaino B, Cappello P, Capello M, Fredolini C, Sperduti I, Migliorini P, et al. Circulating autoantibodies to phosphorylated alpha-enolase are a hallmark of pancreatic cancer. J Proteome Res 2011;10:105–12.

[85] Zhao J, Patwa TH, Qiu W, Shedden K, Hinderer R, Misek DE, et al. Glycoprotein microarrays with multi-lectin detection: unique lectin binding patterns as a tool for classifying normal, chronic pancreatitis and pancreatic cancer sera. J Proteome Res 2007;6:1864–74.

[86] Chaturvedi P, Singh AP, Chakraborty S, Chauhan SC, Bafna S, Meza JL, et al. MUC4 mucin interacts with and stabilizes the HER2 oncoprotein in human pancreatic cancer cells. Cancer Res 2008;68:2065–70.

[87] Remmers N, Bailey JM, Mohr AM, Hollingsworth MA. Molecular pathology of early pancreatic cancer. Cancer Biomark 2010;9:421–40.

[88] Simeone DM, Ji B, Banerjee M, Arumugam T, Li D, Anderson MA, et al. CEACAM1, a novel serum biomarker for pancreatic cancer. Pancreas 2007;34:436–43.

[89] Singh AP, Chaturvedi P, Batra SK. Emerging roles of MUC4 in cancer: a novel target for diagnosis and therapy. Cancer Res 2007;67:433–6.

[90] Swanson BJ, McDermott KM, Singh PK, Eggers JP, Crocker PR, Hollingsworth MA. MUC1 is a counter-receptor for myelin-associated glycoprotein (Siglec-4a) and their interaction contributes to adhesion in pancreatic cancer perineural invasion. Cancer Res 2007;67:10222–9.

[91] Yue T, Goldstein IJ, Hollingsworth MA, Kaul K, Brand RE, Haab BB. The prevalence and nature of glycan alterations on specific proteins in pancreatic cancer patients revealed using antibody-lectin sandwich arrays. Mol Cell Proteomics 2009;8:1697–707.

[92] Goonetilleke KS, Siriwardena AK. Systematic review of carbohydrate antigen (CA 19-9) as a biochemical marker in the diagnosis of pancreatic cancer. Eur J Surg Oncol 2007;33:266–70.

[93] Zhao J, Simeone DM, Heidt D, Anderson MA, Lubman DM. Comparative serum glycoproteomics using lectin selected sialic acid glycoproteins with mass spectrometric analysis: application to pancreatic cancer serum. J Proteome Res 2006;5:1792–802.

[94] Zhao J, Qiu W, Simeone DM, Lubman DM. N-linked glycosylation profiling of pancreatic cancer serum using capillary liquid phase separation coupled with mass spectrometric analysis. J Proteome Res 2007;6:1126–38.

[95] Mann BF, Goetz JA, House MG, Schmidt CM, Novotny MV. Glycomic and proteomic profiling of pancreatic cyst fluids identifies hyperfucosylated lactosamines on the N-linked glycans of overexpressed glycoproteins. Mol Cell Proteomics 2012;11:M111.

[96] Lee CN, Heidbrink JL, McKinnon K, Bushman V, Olsen H, FitzHugh W, et al. RNA interference characterization of proteins discovered by proteomic analysis of pancreatic cancer reveals function in cell growth and survival. Pancreas 2012;41:84–94.

[97] Pan S, Chen R, Tamura Y, Crispin DA, Lai LA, May DH, et al. Quantitative glycoproteomics analysis reveals changes in N-glycosylation level associated with pancreatic ductal adenocarcinoma. J Proteome Res 2014;Jan 28. [Epub ahead of print].

[98] Grote T, Logsdon CD. Progress on molecular markers of pancreatic cancer. Curr Opin Gastroenterol 2007;23:508–14.

[99] Harsha HC, Kandasamy K, Ranganathan P, Rani S, Ramabadran S, Gollapudi S, et al. A compendium of potential biomarkers of pancreatic cancer. PLoS Med 2009;6:e1000046.

[100] Pan S, Brentnall TA, Kelly K, Chen R. Tissue proteomics in pancreatic cancer study: discovery, emerging technologies, and challenges. Proteomics 2013;13:710–21.

CHAPTER 10

Proteomic Differences and Linkages between Chemoresistance and Metastasis of Pancreatic Cancer Using Knowledge-Based Pathway Analysis

Jin-Gyun Lee, Kimberly Q. McKinney, Sun-Il Hwang

Proteomics and Mass Spectrometry Research Laboratory, Carolinas HealthCare System, Charlotte, NC, USA

Contents

Introduction	221
Proteomic Analysis at Subcellular Level	222
Protein Identification and Data Compiling	224
Comparative Analysis of Differentially Expressed Proteins	225
Biological Network Analysis	230
Canonical Pathway Analysis Using MetaCore™	233
Vimentin Expression and Chemoresistance	238
Vimentin Knockdown in Panc-1 Cells	239
Sensitivity on GEM Treatment of Vimentin Knockdown Panc-1	241
Conclusion	241
References	242

INTRODUCTION

Pancreatic cancer (PC) has been recognized as one of the most life-threatening diseases because of the lack of diagnostic methods in the early stage as well as its rapid progression [1,2]. Among the well-known key barriers for the effective cure of PC are chemoresistance and metastasis [3–5], which complicate therapeutic strategies. A thorough understanding of the specific cellular and molecular mechanisms of PC development and progression is required for early detection strategies and effective therapy [5].

Aggressive growth behavior makes PC resistant to chemotherapy, radiotherapy, and immunotherapy [6–8]. Gemcitabine (GEM) has been recognized as a primary chemotherapeutic agent, which may increase relative survival rates [9,10], although it showed limited improvement. The poor prognosis of PC is derived from the unpredictable and uncontrollable metastatic pattern, which comes along with the development of chemoresistance. Recently, some transcription factors have been shown to play a key role in epithelial-to-mesenchymal transition (EMT). One of these transcription factors, Snail, has been reported to be one of the markers related to resistance against chemotherapy [11]. Metastasis is a multistep process including the loss of cell-to-cell adhesion, which promotes cell motility and migration–invasion into surrounding tissues, as well as transport through the blood stream. Chemoresistance has been considered to be an integrated process with metastatic progression, although the identified markers are not sufficient so far to hypothesize the interconnection between the two biological networks.

This chapter introduces knowledgebase pathway analysis. This analysis has been performed using comparative data sets generated by the subcellular proteomics of matched pairs of PC cell lines by phenotypic and genotypic grouping. Specifically, Su8686 and BXPC-3 were utilized as representatives for GEM-sensitive cell lines, MiaPaCa-2 and Panc-1 for GEM-resistant cell lines, BXPC-3 and Capan-2 for primary cell lines, and Su8686 and Capan-1 for metastatic cell lines. Identified proteins with upregulation from the GEM-resistant and metastasis group compared with the baseline (GEM sensitive or primary) were processed using MetaCore™ (Thomson Reuters, NY, USA) analysis, which provided biological information through the generation of pathway maps with high data relevancy. During the course of analysis, lists of proteins with signal-to-noise (STN) were uploaded into the web-based application, which clustered relevant proteins into specific biological networks. MetaCore™ analysis provided the most relevant biological processes, from which plausible linkages between development of chemoresistance and metastatic progression were identified. This data was further supported using gene knockdown and GEM treatment experiments. The knowledgebase pathway analysis has demonstrated that it may provide useful systemic information regarding correlation of protein data sets in a high-throughput data mining approach that generates disease marker candidates for therapeutic targeting with a minimal time investment.

PROTEOMIC ANALYSIS AT SUBCELLULAR LEVEL

A brief work flow for the proteomic analysis followed by pathway analysis is introduced in Figure 10.1A. Proteomic analysis was performed using six cell lines—namely, Panc-1, BXPC-3, MiaPaCa-2, Su8686, Capan-1, and

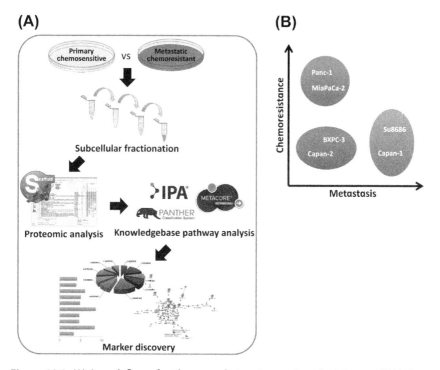

Figure 10.1 (A) A work flow of pathway analysis using proteomic data sets. (B) Various phenotype and genotype of pancreatic adenocarcinoma cells. (For color version of this figure, the reader is referred to the online version of this book.)

Capan-2, for which phenotypic and genotypic characteristics are depicted in Figure 10.1B.

Capan-1, Su8686, and MiaPaCa-2 cells are classified as metastatic cell lines generated from PC metastatic lesions of the patients while BXPC-3, Capan-2, Panc-1, and MiaPaCa-2 as primary cell lines, derived from primary pancreatic tumor tissue [1,5]. The cell lines have been well known to show different sensitivity to chemotherapeutics, such as GEM [4]. The six cell lines were classified as either drug sensitive or resistant by their sensitivity to GEM treatment as demonstrated by viability assays. Capan-1, Capan-2, Su8686, and BXPC-3 cells are classified as chemosensitive, while Panc-1 and MiaPaCa-2 cell lines are considered chemoresistant.

Cells were obtained from the American Type Culture Collection (ATCC; Manassas, VA, USA), and cultured in ATCC-recommended media with 10% fetal bovine serum. Cells were maintained at 37 °C under humidified 5% CO_2 and grown to 80% confluence in culture dishes and used for the experiments. Trypsinized cells were washed with phosphate-buffered saline (PBS) three times, and then subcellular fractionation was performed using the Proteo

Extract Subcellular Proteome Extraction Kit (Calbiochem, CA, USA) according to the manufacturer's protocol. Four fractions were generated: fraction 1 for cytosolic proteins, fraction 2 for membrane proteins, fraction 3 for nuclear proteins, and fraction 4 for cytoskeletal proteins. Then, 30 µg of denatured protein from the subcellular fractions from each cell line were separated on sodium dodecyl sulfate polyacrylamide gel electrophoresis (SDS-PAGE) followed by in-gel digestion by the method reported previously. Peptides were extracted from the gel matrix by adding 100 µL 50% (v/v) acetonitrile (ACN) containing 5% (v/v) formic acid and incubated at room temperature for 30 min three times. The extracts were dried under vacuum and then were suspended in 10% (v/v) ACN containing 3% (v/v) formic acid to be subjected to liquid chromatography with tandem mass spectrometry (LC MS/MS).

Peptide samples were separated on a Nano-Acquity ultra performance liquid chromatography system with a Nano-Acquity C_{18} trap column (5 µm, 180 µm × 20 mm) and a Nano-Acquity BEH130 C_{18} analytical column (1.7 µm, 75 µm × 150 mm) (Waters Corporation, Milford, MA, USA) and then analyzed by a high-resolution linear ion trap mass spectrometer (Linear Trap Quadrupole/Orbitrap-XL, Thermo Finnigan, San Jose, CA, USA) equipped with a nano-scale electrospray source (Thermo Finnigan, San Jose, CA, USA). A linear gradient system that consisted of binary mobile phases (A, water with 0.1% formic acid; B, ACN with 0.1% formic acid) flowing from 5% mobile phase B to 45% mobile phase B for 75 min at the flow rate of 0.35 µL/min was employed for separation of peptides. Tandem MS scan was conducted by a data dependent scan for the top-10 intense ions acquired from each full MS scan using the dynamic exclusion option.

PROTEIN IDENTIFICATION AND DATA COMPILING

MS spectra were searched in the human International Protein Index (IPI) database v3.72 FASTA database (86,392 entries) using the SEQUEST search algorithm (SRF v.5) of the Bioworks software v3.3.1sp1 (Thermo Fisher Scientific, San Jose, CA, USA) with the following parameters: parent mass tolerance of 10 ppm, fragment tolerance of 0.5 Da (monoisotopic), variable modification on methionine of 16 Da (oxidation), and maximum missed cleavage of two sites assuming the digestion enzyme trypsin. Data were compiled with Scaffold software (v3_06_03, Proteome Software, Portland, OR, USA) for comparison of spectral counts with filtering criteria of two peptides minimum; XCorr scores of greater than 1.9, 2.3, and 3.4 for singly, doubly, and triply charged peptides; and deltaCn scores of greater than 0.10.

COMPARATIVE ANALYSIS OF DIFFERENTIALLY EXPRESSED PROTEINS

Raw spectral counts from duplicate analysis of each fraction were compared within the cell line group of GEM-sensitive versus resistant and primary versus metastatic individually. For the identification of proteins involved in GEM resistance, Su8686 and BXPC-3 versus MiaPaCa-2 and Panc-1 were compared. For the identification of proteins involved in metastasis, BXPC-3 and Capan-2 versus Su8686 and Capan-1 were compared. Comparative analysis was performed by the method based on the power law global error model (PLGEM) [12,13] to identify statistically significant protein changes by STN and p-value according to previous method [14]. PLGEM software was downloaded from http://www.bioconductor.org and imported into our web-based interface working on a Firefox platform. Although PLGEM was developed using a normalized spectral abundance factor (NSAF) as input, its performance with a limited number of replicates has been shown to improve when raw spectral count rather than NSAF is used. Therefore, raw spectral count was used as the input in our PLGEM analysis. Estimated false-discovery rates for PLGEM-generated significance lists were estimated using the Benjamini–Hochberg estimator [15]. The list of proteins given by PLGEM analysis with STN and p-value was filtered by the degree of change and the significance. Proteins that showed high significance ($p < 0.01$) were chosen from among those showing increased expression in each comparison group (sensitive versus resistant and primary versus metastatic). The most upregulated proteins identified from the subcellular fractions are shown in Tables 10.1 and 10.2.

As shown in Table 10.1, vimentin, a member of cytoskeletal protein was found mostly within fraction 4, and is highly overexpressed in both Mia-PaCa-2 and Panc-1 compared with Su8686 and BXPC-3. Also prominent is the upregulation of proteins in the cytokeratin family, especially keratin type 1, which showed higher cellular levels overall. Peripherin is another one of the most upregulated proteins in fraction 4. The marked changes in cytoskeletal proteins implies that the development of chemoresistance may involve enhanced cell adhesion through cytoskeletal modifications or that cytoskeleton remodeling is a protective cellular response to drug influx or drug-receptor binding. Table 10.2 presents a number of proteins upregulated that are related to cytoskeletal remodeling, cell-to-cell junction, and EMT. Interestingly, vimentin was increased in Su8686, one of the metastatic cell lines. Anterior gradient protein 2 (AGR2) was increased in metastatic cell lines. AGR2 is well known to be present in various cancer cell types and is regulated by hypoxia inducing factor-1 (HIF-1) [16,17]. Because the EMT

Table 10.1 List of Proteins with Significant Up-regulation in GEM Resistant Cell Lines

				Raw Spectral Counts							
				Drug Sensitive				Drug Resistant			
				Su8686		BXPC-3		MiaPaCa-2		Panc-1	
Protein ID	Description	STN	p-Value	1st	2nd	1st	2nd	1st	2nd	1st	2nd
Fraction 1											
IPI00418471	Vimentin	5.71	0.0001	6	5	0	0	88	84	28	26
IPI00009865	Keratin, type I cytoskeletal 10	5.18	0.0001	168	170	163	136	334	321	284	244
IPI00021812	Neuroblast differentiation-associated protein AHNAK (Fragment)	3.98	0.0004	17	15	8	3	99	71	19	17
IPI00218914	Retinal dehydrogenase 1	3.78	0.0005	0	0	0	0	49	57	0	0
IPI00220327	Keratin, type II cytoskeletal 1	3.37	0.0008	173	174	155	128	266	262	235	204
Fraction 2											
IPI00418471	Vimentin	14.56	0.0000	38	36	5	5	371	395	106	117
IPI00440493	ATP synthase alpha chain, mitochondrial precursor	8.54	0.0001	54	51	47	69	286	290	102	108
IPI00303476	ATP synthase beta chain, mitochondrial precursor	7.81	0.0001	85	99	121	127	359	346	168	174
IPI00007765	Stress-70 protein, mitochondrial precursor	5.45	0.0003	105	120	68	65	231	234	142	135
IPI00328753	Isoform 1 of Kinectin	5.33	0.0003	46	42	33	33	94	87	132	131

Fraction	IPI	Protein	Ratio	p-value								
Fraction 3	IPI00220327	Keratin, type II cytoskeletal 1	3.53	0.0004	221	219	232	197	349	370	315	342
	IPI00009865	Keratin, type I cytoskeletal 10	3.40	0.0004	253	231	231	182	367	360	323	340
	IPI00021304	Keratin, type II cytoskeletal 2 epidermal	2.65	0.0010	101	104	117	88	183	181	162	157
	IPI00030363	Acetyl-CoA acetyltransferase, mitochondrial precursor	2.43	0.0012	26	24	8	4	63	63	30	30
	IPI00150057	Isoform 2 of SWI/SNF-related matrix-associated actin-dependent regulator of chromatin subfamily C member 2	2.29	0.0015	2	3	6	3	8	9	32	39
Fraction 4	IPI00418471	Vimentin	26.29	0.0000	302	319	13	15	1852	1741	1296	1298
	IPI00013164	Peripherin	7.77	0.0004	27	25	5	3	179	175	137	123
	IPI00239405	Isoform 1 of Nesprin-2	7.19	0.0005	18	16	5	5	139	132	118	114
	IPI00217963	Keratin, type I cytoskeletal 16	5.76	0.0009	4	4	20	17	176	139	36	28
	IPI00554788	Keratin, type I cytoskeletal 18	5.34	0.0011	764	804	348	369	698	670	1051	1025

Table 10.2 List of Proteins with Significant Up-regulation in Metastatic Cell Lines

					Raw Spectral Counts							
					Primary				Metastatic			
					BXPC-3		Capan-2		Su8686		Capan-1	
	Protein ID	Description	STN	p-Value	1st	2nd	1st	2nd	1st	2nd	1st	2nd
Fraction 1	IPI00334627	Similar to annexin A2 isoform 1	3.90	0.0005	122	112	63	58	98	86	286	323
	IPI00002459	annexin VI isoform 2	3.41	0.0008	4	3	3	2	44	47	19	25
	IPI00014424	Elongation factor 1-alpha 2	3.32	0.0008	116	112	175	171	281	247	247	241
	IPI00418169	annexin A2 isoform 1	2.93	0.0012	41	30	15	16	30	24	124	114
	IPI00246975	Glutathione S-transferase Mu 3	2.71	0.0016	6	8	0	0	6	5	57	47
Fraction 2	IPI00472102	Heat shock protein 60	9.77	0.0000	77	90	261	239	476	508	557	527
	IPI00386854	HNRPA2B1 protein	4.27	0.0001	9	8	7	9	9	15	103	100
	IPI00296337	Isoform 1 of DNA-dependent protein kinase catalytic subunit	4.24	0.0001	33	43	46	50	30	40	214	203
	IPI00413728	Isoform 1 of Spectrin alpha chain, brain	4.06	0.0002	23	37	49	45	49	59	166	168
	IPI00005614	Isoform Long of Spectrin beta chain, brain 1	3.97	0.0002	18	22	30	28	41	47	128	123

	IPI	Protein										
Fraction 3	IPI00021812	Neuroblast differentiation-associated protein AHNAK (Fragment)	3.25	0.0004	88	48	70	94	296	274	138	161
	IPI00004671	Golgin subfamily B member 1	2.08	0.0023	5	3	17	24	0	0	100	99
	IPI00007427	AGR2	1.86	0.0032	45	33	130	138	136	140	180	194
	IPI00009865	Keratin, type I cytoskeletal 10	1.79	0.0035	143	125	163	153	177	153	301	325
	IPI00019359	Keratin, type I cytoskeletal 9	1.38	0.0073	47	39	38	41	36	29	118	134
Fraction 4	IPI00167941	Midasin	2.99	0.0013	5	5	2	0	79	85	21	11
	IPI00418471	Vimentin	2.60	0.0017	10	12	53	47	202	216	0	0
	IPI00334775	Hypothetical protein DKFZp761K0511	2.36	0.0022	32	29	7	10	58	63	94	81
	IPI00007289	Alkaline phosphatase, placental type precursor	1.89	0.0038	0	0	10	10	0	0	67	54
	IPI00007752	Tubulin beta-2C chain	1.88	0.0038	4	7	10	14	34	37	43	37

process can be induced by tumor growth factor-β (TGF-β) dependent EMT induction pathways as well as by hypoxic conditions[18,19], it may be assumed that the metastasis of PC is related to hypoxia–induced EMT [20–22]. From Tables 10.1 and 10.2, it may be hypothesized that development of both chemoresistance and metastasis possibly share common cellular pathways in which cytoskeletal proteins such as vimentin play pivotal roles.

BIOLOGICAL NETWORK ANALYSIS

Three biological pathway analysis programs were utilized for further analysis of PLGEM data. The input data was generated by filtration of the PLGEM upregulated protein data set using a p-value cutoff of 0.01. Because of the majority of upregulated proteins residing in cytoskeletal fraction, only cytoskeletal proteins (fraction 4) were chosen for the downstream pathway analysis.

Figure 10.2 shows the top-10 biological networks from the three pathway analysis tools used—namely, MetaCore™, Thomson Reuters, MN, USA;

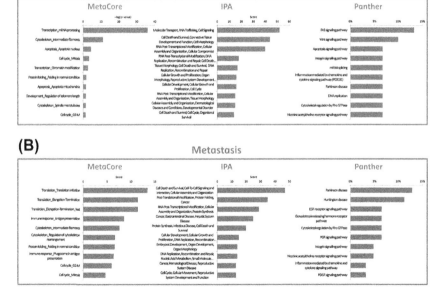

Figure 10.2 *Top-10 Biological Networks Provided by the Analysis Using MetaCore™, IPA®, and Panther Classification System.* Proteomic data sets from (A) GEM-sensitive versus GEM-resistant cell lines and (B) primary versus metastatic cell lines were used for the comparative analysis. (For color version of this figure, the reader is referred to the online version of this book.)

IPA®, Ingenuity Systems, CA, USA; and Panther Classification System v8.1 (http://www.pantherdb.org/). Each pathway tool uses a different data enrichment algorithm and may provide different results. The Panther Classification System is a public source for classification of proteins and genes according to family and subfamily, molecular function, associated biological processes, and pathways. The input data for MetaCore™ and IPA® were prepared as a Microsoft Excel spreadsheets containing protein identification, fold change (e.g., STN), and *p*-value; however, the Panther Classification System only required a list of IPI protein accession numbers.

Figure 10.2A and B exhibits the top significant networks calculated from the drug-resistance group and metastasis group, respectively. The significance of the respective pathway maps were expressed as −log(*p*-value), score, and percent for MetaCore™, IPA®, and Panther analysis. The top-10 biological networks generated by MetaCore™ and IPA® are representative of the same or similar pathways, although the pathway nomenclature differs. The top-10 networks from MetaCore™ were found to be correlated with those of IPA® when comparing a list of genes involved in each pathway. In Figure 10.2(A), most of the top-10 networks from MetaCore™ indicate that the upregulated proteins in GEM-resistant cell lines are related to cytoskeleton remodeling, mRNA processing for transcription, cell cycle, and cell death, which also are shown in the top networks from IPA®. For example, the network titled by MetaCore™ as transcription_mRNA processing corresponds to the networks from IPA® entitled molecular transport/RNA trafficking and RNA post-transcriptional modification/DNA replication, recombination and repair. The network from MetaCore™ cytoskeleton_intermediate filaments network describes cellular networks similar with connective tissue development and function, cellular assembly and organization, and tissue morphology within IPA®. Likewise, Metacore's Apoptosis_apoptotic nucleus networks also correspond to cell death and survival, cellular growth, and proliferation networks from IPA®. The scores of the networks were slightly different, which is thought to come from the difference in algorithms for enrichment processing. Because Panther analysis was conducted with the list of proteins without fold change or *p*-value, the significance of the top-10 networks was expressed as the percentage of identified proteins that participated in corresponding canonical pathways. These pathways still include similar networks, such as cytoskeletal regulation, apoptosis signaling pathways, and DNA replication.

From the biological network analysis of the two data sets shown in Figure 10.2A and B, one of the common biological networks with high relevance is the cytoskeleton_intermediate filaments network, which includes keratin 1, keratin 14, lamin B, keratin 16, keratin 8, peripherin, SYNE2, keratin 8/18, vimentin, nestin, keratin 18, lamin B1, desmuslin, and lamin A/C. Because vimentin is one of the most overexpressed proteins in both data sets, it is expected that vimentin could be a key protein in the development of chemoresistance and metastasis of PC.

Classification analysis was performed with the data sets from GEM resistant and metastatic cell lines individually using MetaCore™ enrichment analysis, which consists of matching gene IDs of possible targets for the "common", "similar", and "unique" sets with gene IDs in functional ontologies in MetaCore™. The probability of a random intersection between a set of IDs and a set of ontology entities is expressed by the p-value of hypergeometric intersection. The lower p-value indicates higher relevance of the entity to the data set and thus shows a higher rating for the entity. Figure 10.3 summarizes the classification by functional ontologies using enrichment analysis from the data set of GEM-sensitive versus -resistant cell lines, and also showing vimentin involvement in top-ranked pathways and diseases.

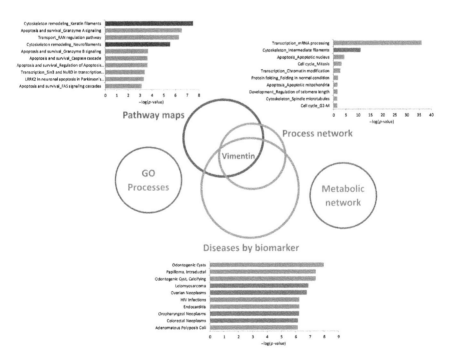

Figure 10.3 *Classification by Functional Ontologies Given by the Enrichment Analysis Using MetaCore™.* Proteomic data set from GEM-sensitive versus -resistant cell lines was used for the analysis. (For color version of this figure, the reader is referred to the online version of this book.)

Interestingly, in both drug resistance and metastasis, the cytoskeleton remodeling pathway by keratin filaments and neurofilaments was revealed to be the most relevant pathway with the lowest p-values (Figure 10.4).

CANONICAL PATHWAY ANALYSIS USING METACORE™

Canonical pathway maps represent a comprehensive set of human cellular signaling and metabolic pathways. All maps are created based on published peer reviewed literature. Experimental data are visualized on the maps as red (upregulation) histograms, in which case height corresponds to the degree of increased expression for particular genes or proteins. Enrichment analysis with the lists of proteins from the data sets of drug-resistant cell lines and metastatic cell lines has provided two highly relevant pathways: cytoskeleton remodeling by keratin filaments and cytoskeleton remodeling by neurofilaments (Figure 10.5A and B).

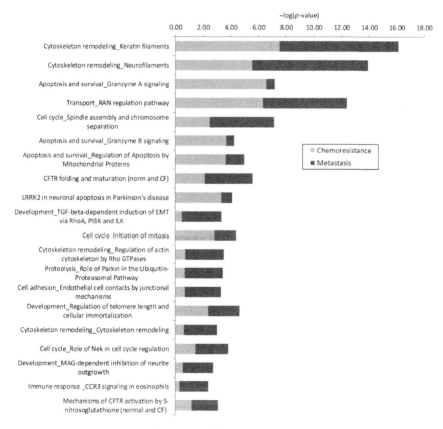

Figure 10.4 *Comparative Pathway Maps from GEM Resistance and Metastasis Data Sets.*

(A)

(B)

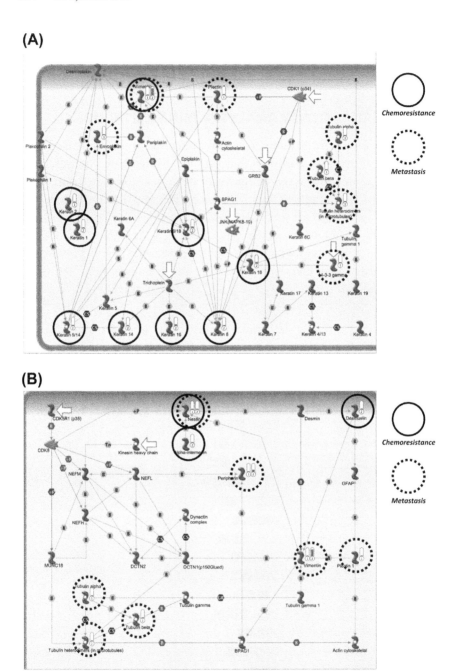

Figure 10.5 (A) Canonical pathway presenting the cytoskeletal remodeling by keratin filaments. (B) Canonical pathway presenting the cytoskeletal remodeling by neurofilaments. (For color version of this figure, the reader is referred to the online version of this book.)

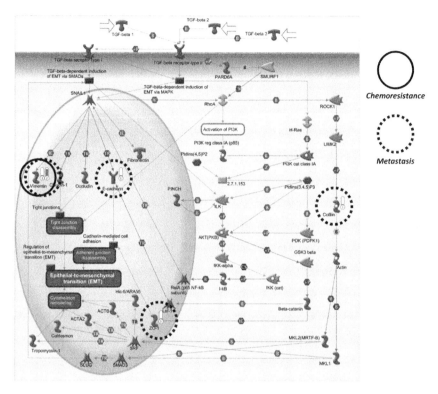

Figure 10.6 *Canonical Pathway Presenting the Development TGF-β-Dependent Induction of EMT via RhoA, PI3K, and ILK.* (For color version of this figure, the reader is referred to the online version of this book.)

Two additional pathways with high relevance were identified by grouping the network objects related with cytoskeleton remodeling: (1) TGF-β-dependent induction of EMT via RhoA, PI3K, and ILK; and (2) cell adhesion by endothelial cell contacts by junctional mechanisms (Figures 10.6 and 10.7).

It has been well known that chemoresistance of the cancer cell is deeply related to the regulation of keratin and integrin gene expression. These proteins are recognized biomarkers in the metastasis of cancer [23,24]. This regulatory process includes a signaling reaction involving the extracellular matrix (ECM) and integrins, which are members of a transmembrane receptor family that play essential roles in cell attachment and signal transduction from the extracellular environment [25,26]. Usually, integrins mediate the linkage between the ECM system and the intracellular actin filament system, which promotes cell-to-cell adhesion [27]. At the same time, the ligation of integrin with ECM ligands triggers a variety of intracellular signaling, which regulates cell migration, differentiation, and proliferation [28–30].

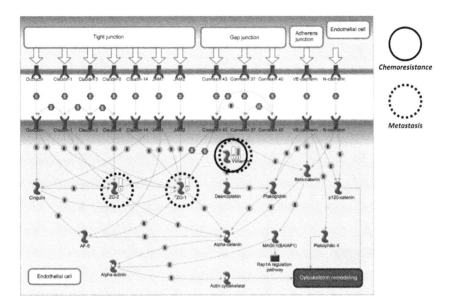

Figure 10.7 *Canonical Pathway Presenting Cell Adhesion and Endothelial Cell Contacts by Junctional Mechanisms.* (For color version of this figure, the reader is referred to the online version of this book.)

The integrin-signaling system is an important pathway for cancer cell signaling and development of chemoresistance.

Figure 10.5A demonstrates how marker proteins upregulated in GEM resistant cell lines are correlated with each other with high significance in the pathway of cytoskeleton remodeling by the alteration of keratin filaments. Keratin family proteins, which are major components of the pathway, were found to be upregulated in the GEM-resistant cell lines overall. In general, integrins mostly interact with ECM ligands to trigger intracellular signal transduction with one exception, that is, integrin α6β4 links to the keratin filament system in epithelial cells [31], which may explain the suggested relationship in our data between the keratin filament system and integrin-mediated signaling within the setting of chemoresistance. Actually, the observed spectral counts of integrin α protein in the GEM-resistant Panc-1 cell line was found to be larger than that of GEM sensitive cell lines (data not shown). This finding supports the position that the development of chemoresistance may accompany increased cell-to-cell interconnection via integrin-mediated keratin filament rearrangement.

Recently, integrin mediated intracellular signal transduction has been reported to also regulate various cytoplasmic proteins, such as phosphatidylinositol-3 kinase (PI3K) [32,33], the serine–threonine kinase AKT, and the mitogen-activated protein kinase/extracellular regulated kinase (MAPK/ERK) [34,35]. Additionally, integrin ligand binding has been reported to activate focal adhesion kinase (FAK), integrin-linked kinase (ILK), and Src kinases that are related to EMT [36–38]. Figure 10.6 shows the canonical pathway of the development of EMT via PI3K and ILK, in which some of the proteins, such as vimentin, upregulated in GEM-resistant cell lines are involved.

Although Figure 10.6 is suggestive that the PI3K- and ILK-mediated EMT pathway has a partial role in chemoresistance of PC as evidenced by the upregulation of common proteins like vimentin, most of the involved protein identifications are from the data generated by the metastatic cell lines. As shown in Figure 10.6, EMT is regulated by tight junction disassembly, adherent junction disassembly, and cytoskeleton remodeling. Metastasis of cancer cells via mesenchymal transition is known to be initiated by the disassembly of the cell-to-cell junction (tight junction or adherent junction), which results in cell movement and motility [39,40]. Meanwhile, development of chemoresistance is triggered by the integrin–keratin filament system, which results in increased cellular adhesion and produces a tight protective barrier. From Figure 10.5, it may be assumed that the development of chemoresistance and metastasis undergo cytoskeleton remodeling in the opposing ways. It is interesting, however, that vimentin is overexpressed in GEM-resistant cell lines and metastatic cell lines, being involved in both the cytokeratin and EMT pathways.

As shown in Figure 10.7, vimentin overexpression was correlated to the mechanism of cell adhesion by endothelial cell contacts.

On the other hand, one of the common mechanisms of cancer cell movement is mesenchymal-type movement, inducing EMT [41]. Metastatic cancer progression by EMT consists of two phases. The first phase includes desmosomal disruption, cell spreading, and partial separation at cell-to-cell borders, and the second phase involves the induction of cell motility, repression of cytokeratin expression, and activation of vimentin expression [42,43]. Cytokeratin expression also is regulated by the p63 factor in epithelial cancer [44]. Figure 10.5B shows the canonical pathway of cytoskeleton remodeling by neurofilaments with upregulated cytoplasmic intermediate filament proteins in metastatic cell lines. The cytoskeleton consists of three major structural categories, that is, actin filaments, microtubules, and intermediate filaments (IFs), which are interconnected with one another [45]. Cells usually are connected or assembled by the IFs or interactions with various types of ECM ligands, such as fibronectin, vitronectin, collagen, and laminin [46]. Figure 10.5B shows the changes in cytoplasmic IF proteins, like vimentin, peripherin, nestin, and desmuslin, without keratin overexpression. Plectin-1, which was overexpressed in our metastatic cell line data, is responsible for the maintenance of cellular and tissue integrity by the coordinated interconnection of three distinct cytoskeletal filament systems [47]. Additionally, this figure demonstrates how tubulins, upregulated in metastatic cell lines, form microtubules, which are components of the cytoskeleton that maintain cell structure in conjunction with microfilaments and IFs [48]. On the basis of our proteomic data showing the repression of keratin and overexpression of vimentin, it may be assumed that metastasis of PC is developed mostly via the EMT pathway.

Enrichment analysis by MetaCore™ provided important information about the relationship between chemoresistance and metastasis. Namely, that two common pathways involved in cytoskeleton remodeling were identified from the data sets of GEM-resistant cell lines and metastatic cell lines. The development of chemoresistance in PC has been proven to include cytoskeleton remodeling via the alteration of keratin filaments. Upregulated proteins from metastatic cell lines have been shown to be involved in cytoskeleton remodeling by the change of neurofilaments and the EMT pathway. The pathway analysis results were suggestive that cytoskeleton-remodeling processes contribute to the development of not only chemoresistance but also metastasis of PC, although specifically through different mechanisms of action. Furthermore, regulation of vimentin expression has been revealed as a common denominator at the intersection of these pathways.

VIMENTIN EXPRESSION AND CHEMORESISTANCE

Vimentin is expressed by cells undergoing cell-to-cell adhesion, EMT, and cytoskeleton remodeling, cellular processes observed during metastatic progression of epithelial cancers [49]. Vimentin recently has been reported as one of the most increased proteins in multiple metastatic PC cell lines [50]. Figure 10.8 shows various pathway in which vimentin has been known to be involved.

From the enrichment analysis using MetaCore™, vimentin was revealed to be one of the potential markers linked to both chemoresistance and metastasis. Vimentin overexpression and its role in the metastasis of cancer cells has been well documented by a number of previous studies; however, the specific effect of vimentin expression on chemoresistance is still unclear. In this chapter, chemosensitization of Panc-1 cells by abrogation of vimentin expression and subsequent GEM treatment was introduced to test the hypothesis generated by the knowledgebase pathway analysis.

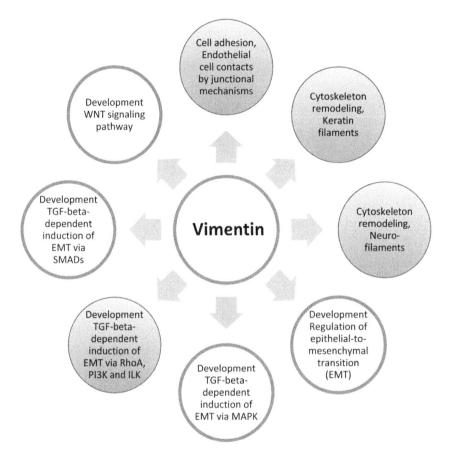

Figure 10.8 *Vimentin has been Known to Participate Various Biological Networks, Mostly Related to the Maintenance of Cellular Structure (e.g., Cytoskeleton Remodeling, EMT).* (For color version of this figure, the reader is referred to the online version of this book.)

Vimentin Knockdown in Panc-1 Cells

Panc-1 cells were plated and incubated overnight in complete media in six well plates. The following morning, media was removed and replaced with Optimem media and transfected with 50 pmol vimentin oligonucleotides complexed with 6 µL RNAiMax transfection reagent in a final volume of 2.5 mL. Control samples included transfection reagent alone or no treatment at all. Cells were incubated for 4 h, then 2.5 mL of complete media were added and samples were incubated at the representative time points. At the time of harvest, wells were washed two times with 5 mL PBS, and then were aspirated completely. Then, 100 µL of 1X-RIPA with 2X-protease inhibitor cocktail solutions were added

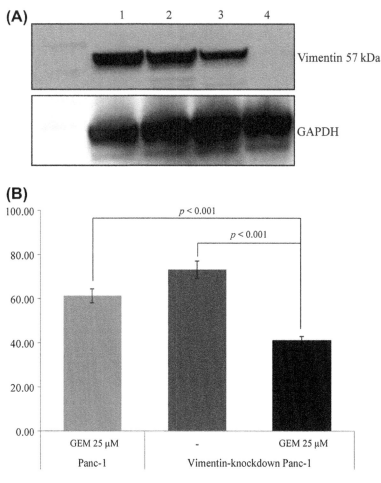

Figure 10.9 (A) Vimentin expression was inhibited completely with small interfering ribonucleic acid transfection at 144 h: (1) 24 h, (2) 48 h, (3) 72 h, (4) 144 h. (B) Panc-1 vimentin knockdown cells showed significantly ($p < 0.001$) decreased viability with 25 µM GEM 72 h treatment.

to the well. Cells were scraped from the monolayer and transferred to a 1.5 mL centrifuge tube. Cell lysates then were centrifuged and transferred to clean tubes where total protein concentrations were determined via bicinchoninic acid assay. Then, 30 µg of each sample were separated by SDS-PAGE and immunoblotting for detection of vimentin expression was carried out using standard Western blotting procedures. Results indicate complete knockdown of vimentin expression at 144 h (Figure 10.9A). This indicates a good condition for knockdown of vimentin expression and subsequent GEM treatment.

Sensitivity on GEM Treatment of Vimentin Knockdown Panc-1

Sensitivity of vimentin-deficient Panc-1 cells to GEM treatment was evaluated by 3-(4,5-dimethylthiazol-2-yl)-2,5-diphenyltetrazolium bromide (MTT cytotoxicity assay). Monolayer Panc-1 cells were trypsinized and suspended in the culture medium and $200\,\mu L$ of a single-cell suspension containing 3.5×10^4 cells/mL were seeded into each well of a 96-well culture plate. After 3 h incubation at 37 °C in a humidified 95% air/5% CO_2 incubator, small interfering ribonucleic acid complexes for vimentin knockdown were added at 3 pmol per well in 12 wells. After incubation for 72 h, GEM was added to final concentration of $25\,\mu M$ into each transfected well. GEM treatment also was carried out in untransfected wells and negative control wells (lipid transfection reagent with no oligonucleotide present). After further incubation for 72 h, cytotoxicity was measured by a cell viability assay based on the colorimetric method using MTT assay. Cell viability of GEM-treated cells was compared with untreated cells where viability was determined by dividing the OD_{570} of the treated cells by the OD_{570} of the untreated, untransfected cells. Ratios were multiplied by 100 to generate percent viability. The means and standard errors of means were calculated for all experiments. The data were subjected to one-way analysis of variance followed by Duncan's multiple-range test to determine whether means were significantly different from the control. As shown in Figure 10.9B, Panc-1 cell viability with $25\,\mu M$ GEM treatment was identified to be decreased significantly by gene knockdown, which support the theory that vimentin overexpression may contribute to the development of chemoresistance of PC. This result is suggestive that decreased or absent vimentin expression may sensitize chemoresistant PC to respond chemotherapy and therefore vimentin could be a promising molecular target against chemoresistance.

CONCLUSION

This chapter introduced differences and linkages between chemoresistance and metastasis identified by knowledgebase pathway analysis. Proteomic data sets from the matched pairs of cell lines representing chemosensitive versus chemoresistant and primary versus metastatic PC cells. From MetaCore™ analysis, two common pathways related to cytoskeletal remodeling were identified with high relevance. On the basis of this data, we support the theory that development of chemoresistance in PC accompanies cytokeratin overexpression, which mediates increased cellular protection against drugs, whereas metastastatic progress of PC involves the repression of keratin and vimentin overexpression. Common proteins with upregulation in both pathways were identified, with vimentin being chief among these and highly involved in both biological processes. Vimentin is a well-known biomarker in terms of the metastatic progress of cancer. Interestingly, the level of vimentin expression was higher in chemoresistant cell lines than in sensitive cell lines as well. The putative role of vimentin in chemoresistance was demonstrated by a gene knockdown experiment in which vimentin knockdown decreased chemoresistance and thus viability with GEM treatment. These results imply that chemoresistance of PC is developed along with metastasis, and both of the biological processes share specific proteins, such as vimentin, which drive these phenotypic changes. On the basis of the clear evidence revealing the contribution of vimentin to GEM resistance in our experimental system, we believe that global proteomics combined with knowledgebase pathway analysis may provide opportunities to develop systems-based biological understanding of disease markers and associated pathways.

REFERENCES

[1] Dunphy EP. Pancreatic cancer: a review and update. Clin J Oncol Nurs 2008;12: 735–41.
[2] Eckel F, Schneider G, Schmid RM. Pancreatic cancer: a review of recent advances. Expert Opin Investig Drugs 2006;15:1395–410.
[3] Li M, Jiang M, Yan X, Wang F, Luo F. Metastatic pancreatic cancer response to treatment with cetuximab and gemcitabine plus capecitabine: a case report and review of the literature. Tumori 2010;96:764–7.
[4] Di Marco M, Di Cicilia R, Macchini M, Nobili E, Vecchiarelli S, Brandi G, et al. Metastatic pancreatic cancer: is gemcitabine still the best standard treatment? (Review). Oncol Rep 2010;23:1183–92.
[5] Deer EL, Gonzalez-Hernandez J, Coursen JD, Shea JE, Ngatia J, Scaife CL, et al. Phenotype and genotype of pancreatic cancer cell lines. Pancreas 2010;39:425–35.
[6] Murtaza I, Saleem M, Adhami VM, Hafeez BB, Mukhtar H. Suppression of cFLIP by lupeol, a dietary triterpene, is sufficient to overcome resistance to TRAIL-mediated apoptosis in chemoresistant human pancreatic cancer cells. Cancer Res 2009;69:1156–65.
[7] Mimeault M, Hauke R, Batra SK. Recent advances on the molecular mechanisms involved in the drug resistance of cancer cells and novel targeting therapies. Clin Pharmacol Ther 2008;83:673–91.
[8] Egberts JH, Cloosters V, Noack A, Schniewind B, Thon L, Klose S, et al. Anti-tumor necrosis factor therapy inhibits pancreatic tumor growth and metastasis. Cancer Res 2008;68:1443–50.
[9] Plunkett W, Huang P, Gandhi V. Preclinical characteristics of gemcitabine. Anticancer Drugs 1995;6(Suppl. 6):7–13.
[10] Burris 3rd HA, Moore MJ, Andersen J, Green MR, Rothenberg ML, Modiano MR, et al. Improvements in survival and clinical benefit with gemcitabine as first-line therapy for patients with advanced pancreas cancer: a randomized trial. J Clin Oncol 1997;15:2403–13.

[11] Yin T, Wang C, Liu T, Zhao G, Zha Y, Yang M. Expression of snail in pancreatic cancer promotes metastasis and chemoresistance. J Surg Res 2007;141:196–203.

[12] Pavelka N, Fournier ML, Swanson SK, Pelizzola M, Ricciardi-Castagnoli P, Florens L, et al. Statistical similarities between transcriptomics and quantitative shotgun proteomics data. Mol Cell Proteomics 2008;7:631–44.

[13] Pavelka N, Pelizzola M, Vizzardelli C, Capozzoli M, Splendiani A, Granucci F, et al. A power law global error model for the identification of differentially expressed genes in microarray data. BMC Bioinformatics 2004;5:203.

[14] Lee YY, McKinney KQ, Ghosh S, Iannitti DA, Martinie JB, Caballes FR, et al. Subcellular tissue proteomics of hepatocellular carcinoma for molecular signature discovery. J Proteome Res 2011;10:5070–83.

[15] Benjamini Y, Drai D, Elmer G, Kafkafi N, Golani I. Controlling the false discovery rate in behavior genetics research. Behav Brain Res 2001;125:279–84.

[16] Dumartin L, Whiteman HJ, Weeks ME, Hariharan D, Dmitrovic B, Iacobuzio-Donahue CA, et al. AGR2 is a novel surface antigen that promotes the dissemination of pancreatic cancer cells through regulation of cathepsins B and D. Cancer Res 2011;71: 7091–102.

[17] Hong XY, Wang J, Li Z. AGR2 expression is regulated by HIF-1 and contributes to growth and angiogenesis of glioblastoma. Cell Biochem Biophys 2013.

[18] Zavadil J, Bottinger EP. TGF-beta and epithelial-to-mesenchymal transitions. Oncogene 2005;24:5764–74.

[19] Ai Z, Fischer A, Spray DC, Brown AM, Fishman GI. Wnt-1 regulation of connexin43 in cardiac myocytes. J Clin Investig 2000;105:161–71.

[20] Cheng ZX, Sun B, Wang SJ, Gao Y, Zhang YM, Zhou HX, et al. Nuclear factor-kappaB-dependent epithelial to mesenchymal transition induced by HIF-1alpha activation in pancreatic cancer cells under hypoxic conditions. PloS One 2011;6:e23752.

[21] Bao B, Ali S, Ahmad A, Azmi AS, Li Y, Banerjee S, et al. Hypoxia-induced aggressiveness of pancreatic cancer cells is due to increased expression of VEGF, IL-6 and miR-21, which can be attenuated by CDF treatment. PloS One 2012;7:e50165.

[22] Salnikov AV, Liu L, Platen M, Gladkich J, Salnikova O, Ryschich E, et al. Hypoxia induces EMT in low and highly aggressive pancreatic tumor cells but only cells with cancer stem cell characteristics acquire pronounced migratory potential. PloS One 2012;7:e46391.

[23] Zutter MM. Integrin-mediated adhesion: tipping the balance between chemosensitivity and chemoresistance. Adv Exp Med Biol 2007;608:87–100.

[24] Aoudjit F, Vuori K. Integrin signaling in cancer cell survival and chemoresistance. Chemother Res Pract 2012:283181.

[25] Wegener KL, Campbell ID. Transmembrane and cytoplasmic domains in integrin activation and protein-protein interactions (review). Mol Membr Biol 2008;25:376–87.

[26] Haas TA, Plow EF. Integrin-ligand interactions: a year in review. Curr Opin Cell Biol 1994;6:656–62.

[27] Grzesiak JJ, Ho JC, Moossa AR, Bouvet M. The integrin-extracellular matrix axis in pancreatic cancer. Pancreas 2007;35:293–301.

[28] Hutchings H, Ortega N, Plouet J. Extracellular matrix-bound vascular endothelial growth factor promotes endothelial cell adhesion, migration, and survival through integrin ligation. FASEB J 2003;17:1520–2.

[29] Conti JA, Kendall TJ, Bateman A, Armstrong TA, Papa-Adams A, Xu Q, et al. The desmoplastic reaction surrounding hepatic colorectal adenocarcinoma metastases aids tumor growth and survival via alphav integrin ligation. Clin Cancer Res 2008;14:6405–13.

[30] Wang D, Sun L, Zborowska E, Willson JK, Gong J, Verraraghavan J, et al. Control of type II transforming growth factor-beta receptor expression by integrin ligation. J Biol Chem 1999;274:12840–7.

[31] Sansing HA, Sarkeshik A, Yates JR, Patel V, Gutkind JS, Yamada KM, et al. Integrin alphabeta1, alphavbeta, alpha6beta effectors p130Cas, Src and talin regulate carcinoma invasion and chemoresistance. Biochem Biophys Res Commun 2011;406:171–6.

[32] Krishnamurthy M, Li J, Fellows GF, Rosenberg L, Goodyer CG, Wang R. Integrin {alpha}3, but not {beta}1, regulates islet cell survival and function via PI3K/Akt signaling pathways. Endocrinology 2011;152:424–35.

[33] Murillo CA, Rychahou PG, Evers BM. Inhibition of alpha5 integrin decreases PI3K activation and cell adhesion of human colon cancers. Surgery 2004;136:143–9.

[34] McDonald PC, Oloumi A, Mills J, Dobreva I, Maidan M, Gray V, et al. Rictor and integrin-linked kinase interact and regulate Akt phosphorylation and cancer cell survival. Cancer Res 2008;68:1618–24.

[35] Wang J, Zhang Z, Xu K, Sun X, Yang G, Niu W, et al. Suppression of integrin alphaupsilonbeta6 by RNA interference in colon cancer cells inhibits extracellular matrix degradation through the MAPK pathway. International journal of cancer. J Int Cancer 2008;123:1311–7.

[36] Michael KE, Dumbauld DW, Burns KL, Hanks SK, Garcia AJ. Focal adhesion kinase modulates cell adhesion strengthening via integrin activation. Mol Biol Cell 2009;20: 2508–19.

[37] Zhu XY, Liu N, Liu W, Song SW, Guo KJ. Silencing of the integrin-linked kinase gene suppresses the proliferation, migration and invasion of pancreatic cancer cells (Panc-1). Genet Mol Biol 2012;35:538–44.

[38] Gil D, Ciolczyk-Wierzbicka D, Dulinska-Litewka J, Zwawa K, McCubrey JA, Laidler P. The mechanism of contribution of integrin linked kinase (ILK) to epithelial-mesenchymal transition (EMT). Adv Enzyme Regul 2011;51:195–207.

[39] Elsum IA, Martin C, Humbert PO. Scribble regulates an EMT-polarity pathway through modulation of MAPK-ERK signaling to mediate junction formation. J Cell Sci 2013.

[40] Liu Y, Dean DC. Tumor initiation via loss of cell contact inhibition versus Ras mutation: do all roads lead to EMT? Cell Cycle 2010;9:897–900.

[41] Jiang P, Enomoto A, Takahashi M. Cell biology of the movement of breast cancer cells: intracellular signalling and the actin cytoskeleton. Cancer Lett 2009;284:122–30.

[42] Chaw SY, Majeed AA, Dalley AJ, Chan A, Stein S, Farah CS. Epithelial to mesenchymal transition (EMT) biomarkers–E-cadherin, beta-catenin, APC and Vimentin–in oral squamous cell carcinogenesis and transformation. Oral Oncol 2012;48:997–1006.

[43] Boyer B, Tucker GC, Valles AM, Franke WW, Thiery JP. Rearrangements of desmosomal and cytoskeletal proteins during the transition from epithelial to fibroblastoid organization in cultured rat bladder carcinoma cells. J Cell Biol 1989;109:1495–509.

[44] Lindsay J, McDade SS, Pickard A, McCloskey KD, McCance DJ. Role of DeltaNp-63gamma in epithelial to mesenchymal transition. J Biol Chem 2011;286:3915–24.

[45] Semenov AV. Elements of cytoskeleton and pathogenesis of allergic reactions. 1. Elements of cytoskeleton and their functions (a literature review). Klin Lab Diagn 2002:3–11.

[46] Inoue S. Cell biological effects of fibronectin and collagen on the organization of keratin intermediate filaments and microtubules in cultured human keratinocytes. Nihon Hifuka Gakkai Zasshi 1988;98:709–20.

[47] Bausch D, Thomas S, Mino-Kenudson M, Fernandez-del CC, Bauer TW, Williams M, et al. Plectin-1 as a novel biomarker for pancreatic cancer. Clin Cancer Res 2011;17:302–9.

[48] Drukman S, Kavallaris M. Microtubule alterations and resistance to tubulin-binding agents (review). Int J Oncol 2002;21:621–8.

[49] Satelli A, Li S. Vimentin in cancer and its potential as a molecular target for cancer therapy. Cell Mol Life Sci 2011;68:3033–46.

[50] McKinney KQ, Lee JG, Sindram D, Russo MW, Han DK, Bonkovsky HL, et al. Identification of differentially expressed proteins from primary versus metastatic pancreatic cancer cells using subcellular proteomics. Cancer Genomics Proteomics 2012;9:257–63.

CHAPTER 11

RNAi Validation of Pancreatic Cancer Antigens Identified by Cell Surface Proteomics

Candy N. Lee[1,2], Tao He[1,4], Ian McCaffrey[1,6], Charles E. Birse[1,3], Katherine McKinnon[1,7], Bruno Domon[1,8], Steven M. Ruben[1], Paul A. Moore[1,5]

[1]Department of Protein Therapeutics, Celera, Rockville, MD, USA, [2]Pfizer, South San Francisco, CA, USA, [3]Celera, Alameda, CA, USA, [4]Pfizer, Cambridge, MA, USA, [5]MacroGenics Inc., Rockville, MD, USA, [6]Genentech, South San Francisco, CA, USA, [7]NCI, Bethesda, MD, USA, [8]Luxembourg Clinical Proteomics Center, CRP-Sante, Luxembourg

Contents

Introduction	245
Proteomics Platform for the Identification of Novel Plasma Membrane Proteins	247
Biological Samples for Analysis	247
Enrichment for Cell Surface Glycoproteins	253
Quantitative Proteomics Using ICAT Technology	255
Expression Validation Methods	260
Validation of Expression in Tumor Cells by IHC	261
Validation of Expression in Tumor Cells and Membrane Localization by FACS	263
Functional Validation by RNA Interference	266
Summary	272
References	273

INTRODUCTION

Unlike most other cancers, incidences of pancreatic cancer have been on the rise [1,2]. It is the fourth leading cause of cancer death in the United States; in 2013, an estimated 45,220 men and women will be diagnosed with pancreatic cancer, and 38,460 will die from this disease [3]. Pancreatic cancer is a challenging disease as symptoms experienced by patients are often nonspecific. Since there are no early detection tools available, patients are often diagnosed at a late stage. As such, even with today's best treatment efforts, only 5% of pancreatic cancer patients will survive 5 years beyond their initial diagnosis [4,5].

With only 15–20% of cases deemed to be operable, the standard of care for nonresectable patients remains to be treatment with the chemotherapeutic gemcitabine [6]. It is discouraging to note that gemcitabine provides a median survival rate of only 6 months. Though a number of alternative treatment options have been in clinical testing, the majority of these have failed to demonstrate improvements. The most promising so far is FOL-FIRINOX, a chemotherapeutic combination (oxaliplatin, irinotecan, fluorouracil, and leucovorin) that has been proven under phase III clinical trial setting to extend overall survival rate to 11.1 months [4]. Whilst this result is encouraging, it is clear that there is an urgent need for the identification of new diagnostic and therapeutic strategies for this disease.

In recent years, there has been increasing interest in targeted approaches for cancer. For certain types of cancers, such as breast cancer [7], chronic myeloid leukemia [8], lymphomas [9], and non-small cell lung cancer [10], this approach has been proven to be very effective. For pancreatic cancer, development of targeted therapy has been more challenging [11]. Genetically, pancreatic ductal adenocarcinoma (PDA, the most common form of pancreatic cancer), universally carry one of four defects: activating KRAS2 oncogene (70–90% of tumors), inactivation of p16/CDKN2A gene (75–80% of tumors), TP53 abnormality (50–75% of tumors), and deletion in SMAD4 gene (50–60% of tumors) [12,13]. Unfortunately, none of these mutations is targetable by the two approaches that have proven to be successful for cancer treatment: targeted small molecules and antibody-based therapies. Whilst strategies that target druggable enzymes downstream of these modifications are being pursued, they have so far been ineffective in the clinical setting. For example, inhibitors for farnesyltransferase, an enzyme that is important for Ras activation, demonstrated no survival benefit for pancreatic cancer patients when compared to standard therapy [13].

Cell surface proteins account for more than two-thirds of known drug targets [14]. These proteins are easily accessible and play significant, functional roles in tumorigenesis and are involved in processes such as cell proliferation, cell adhesion, and cell invasion. The identification of cell surface proteins that specifically target pancreatic cancer may therefore yield novel treatment targets for this disease. However, due to their hydrophobic nature and low abundance, it has been difficult to identify new candidates for drug therapy.

Proteomics is a technique that offers the opportunity to identify hundreds of differentially expressed proteins. This often leaves the researcher with the daunting task of having too many potential targets to validate [15,16]. One of the goals in our laboratory is to reduce sample complexity so the proteomic can be performed at greater depth. This enabled us to obtain a focused list of differentials, each of which can then be thoroughly validated using an array of well-defined expression and functional validation methods [16]. To this end, we isolated cell surface membrane proteins from cell lines and performed LC-MS/MS on this specific subcellular compartment [17,18]. The expression validation platform and the RNAi target validation platform that was utilized to assign roles these proteins play in pancreatic tumorigenesis will be described. Example proteins that were identified and validated using this platform, namely Tissue Factor, Integrin Beta 6, and Na^+/K^+ ATPase Beta 3, will be presented. We provide here a first report of identification and validation of Na^+/K^+ ATPase Beta 3 subunit as a pancreatic cancer target. We believe this strategy, as outlined in Figure 11.1, has allowed us to identify potentially valuable therapeutic and diagnostic targets.

Proteomics Platform for the Identification of Novel Plasma Membrane Proteins
Biological Samples for Analysis
Proteomics is a tool that offers the opportunity to identify thousands of new targets for biomarkers and therapeutics development. Given the numbers of proteins that could potentially be discovered, it is vital that a focused identification and validation platform be employed.

The process must first begin with samples that appropriately represent the disease in question. The samples may include blood/serum, urine, or pancreatic juice from patients, tissues from surgically obtained samples, or disease-relevant cell lines. Given the clinical ease of obtaining blood and urine samples, they represent excellent potential sources of biomarkers. To this end, numerous proteomic-based profiling studies utilizing serum or urine have been published [19–22]. For example in the Xue study [21], potential diagnostic panels with apolipoprotein C-II (ApoC-II) and apolipoprotein A-II (ApoA-II) as biomarkers were identified from profiling of 20 resectable and 18 stage IV pancreatic cancer patient serum samples following comparisons with control serum samples from healthy volunteers. Similarly, in a study by Weeks et al. [19], urine samples from pancreatic cancer patients were compared to urine samples from healthy volunteers and chronic pancreatitis patients, and this study permitted the identification of a number of proteins associated with pancreatic cancer, including annexin A2, gelsolin, and CD59 [19].

Due to proximity to the pancreas, pancreatic juice can also represent a rich source of biomarkers for pancreatic cancer [23–25]. However, since endoscopic retrograde cholangiopancreatography, the process from which pancreatic juice is obtained, is a complex process that carries a risk of development of

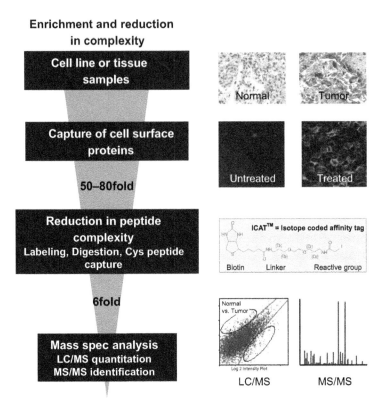

Figure 11.1 *Schematic Diagram of the Proteomics Process Developed for Identification of Overexpressed Tumor Antigens.* In this process, either cell lines or tissue samples can be utilized. Cell surface glycoproteins are first captured by sodium periodate treatment of live cells. Capture of these glycoproteins led to a 50 to 80-fold reduction in sample complexity. The samples were then labeled with ICAT™, digested with trypsin, and the collection of cysteine-containing peptide fraction further led to another six-fold reduction in sample complexity. Relative quantitation is then performed using LC/MS, followed by MS/MS identification. (For color version of this figure, the reader is referred to the online version of this book.)

pancreatitis, proteomic analysis of pancreatic juice from nondiseased humans for use as comparisons to pancreatic cancer patient samples has been limited [26]. These limited studies include the work by Doyle et al. [24], who completed profiling experiments with pancreatic fluid from three patients with no significant pancreatic pathology. They then compared their results with the published results from Goggins's group [27], who performed proteomics on samples from three pancreatic cancer patients. One hundred twenty proteins were subsequently identified as only expressed in the tumor samples, including putative tumor markers azurocidin, carcinoembryonic antigen (CEA), insulin-like growth factor (ILGF) binding protein 2, lipocalin 2, mucin 1 (MUC1), pancreatitis-associated protein/hepatocarcinoma-intestinepancreas (PAP/HIP), and tumor rejection antigen. Another study was performed by Tian et al. [25], who performed comparisons of pancreatic juice from nine pancreatic ductal adenocarcinoma patients with nine cancer-free controls. In this study, 14 proteins were found to be upregulated in the cancerous samples, including MMP-9, DJ-1, and A1BG. A third study was published by Parks et al. [23], who used 2-D gel electrophoresis combined with MALDI-TOF-MS, and identified 35 proteins, including BIG2, PRDX6, and REG1a, that were upregulated by at least two-fold in pancreatic cancer patients compared to normal control and chronic pancreatitis controls.

These studies clearly demonstrate the feasibility of using serum, urine, and pancreatic juice to identify biomarkers and potential proteins for a diagnostic panel. Secreted proteins from the serum or pancreatic juice may also serve as potential therapeutic targets. Of course, a more direct means of identifying therapeutic and diagnostic targets is from the analysis of neoplastic cells from tissues, or cell lines that represent the relevant disease.

Unlike some forms of cancers, pancreatic tissue is not readily available, and the acquisitions of quality tissue from pancreatic cancer patients represent a significant challenge. Firstly, biopsies are not often indicated given the remote location of the organ within the body, and the serious safety risks the procedure itself carries for the patient that includes tumor seeding, and development of complications such as pancreatic leak and pancreatitis [28]. Secondly, it may not be possible to obtain tissues that represent all stages of disease. Pancreatic cancer is often diagnosed at a later stage, so tissues that represent early stages of cancer development may be impossible to obtain [6,29]. It may also not be possible to obtain tissues that present the most advanced stages of the disease, since patients with advanced disease are not candidates for surgery [6] Furthermore, since the pancreatic organ is full of proteases, the task of obtaining enough quality protein for proteomic analysis from these precious sources can be challenging [30].

In the literature, a restricted number of proteomic studies performed with resected, whole tissue patient specimens have been reported. These studies mainly focused on the use of gel-based fractionation, usually by two-dimensional gel electrophoresis (2-DE) followed by mass spectrometry identification [31–34]. For example, Chen et al. [32] analyzed tissues from three pairs of pancreatic cancer samples and compared the samples to adjacent noncancerous tissues resected from the same patient, and found that S100A11 and galectin-3 were overexpressed in pancreatic cancer.

Chung et al. [33] performed 2-DE proteomic analysis on 10 pairs of PDAC specimens and matched adjacent normals, and identified galectin-1 as a potential biomarker. Similarly, Qi et al. [31] utilized tissues from eight matched PDAC and noncancerous tissues and identified TBX4 to be expressed on PDAC samples. Another example is the study by Shen et al. [34], who utilized frozen tissue from the National Cancer Institute Human Tissue Network and completed proteomic analysis on whole tissue homogenates from pancreatic adenocarcinoma tissues compared to normal adjacent, normal, and chronic pancreatitis tissues. In this study, galectin-1 was validated by IHC and western blot to be elevated in pancreatic cancer.

It should be remembered though that since tissue is made up of a heterogeneous population of cells, proteomic analysis of whole tissues may lead to the identification of proteins that are upregulated in the cancer specimens due to the differences in proportion of cell types rather than due to true elevation following dysregulation of a biological process. In a normal mature pancreas, ductal epithelial cells make up 14% of normal pancreatic tissue [35]. In contrast, pancreas from a pancreatic cancer patient may consist of 30–90% of tumor ductal epithelial cells.

As such, proteins identified directly through a comparison of the epithelial cells isolated from tumor versus normal samples may serve as better therapeutic candidates. One technique that has been utilized to capture a pure population of ductal epithelial cells is laser capture microdissection (LCM) [36,37]. However, as only several hundred to a few thousand cells can be isolated by using this technique, only a limited number of proteomic studies on pancreatic cancer have been performed with LCM-resected cells. As the study by Shekouh et al. [38] outlined, sample size from LCM is so low that even quantification of protein yield was not possible with conventional techniques. Instead, following the isolation of pancreatic epithelial cells, Shekouh et al. [38] had to utilize silver staining and densitometry to ensure that equal amounts of proteins from the normal and disease controls were loaded onto 2-D gels. In this limited study, five proteins, including S100A6, were found to be upregulated in pancreatic tumor epithelial cells but not in normal cells. What is apparent from this study is that protein yield can severely limit the types of proteomic analysis that can be accomplished. For us, protein yield is especially important since we wanted to focus our efforts on the proteomics of cell surface membrane proteins for the identification of potential therapeutic targets. As this class of proteins is predicted to be of low abundance, an approach that will allow protein to be isolated at a higher yield is clearly required [39].

Preparation of single cell suspension from the heterogeneous tissue may offer the opportunity for a greater number of epithelial cells to be isolated, and therefore an increase in protein yield can be obtained. Mechanical and enzymatic dissociation of pancreatic tissue has been previously described [40,41]. By using chelating agent EDTA in combination with trypsin, Li et al. [41] demonstrated that it was feasible to dissociate murine pancreas into a single suspension with >90% viability. Using snap frozen tissue, Boyd et al. [40] isolated keratin 7, and keratin 8 positive pancreatic adenocarcinoma cells by combining mechanical cell dissociation with flow cytometry. In our laboratory, we developed a similar process that permitted the isolation of single cell suspensions of epithelial cells prepared from surgically resected human neoplastic lesions and normal tissue specimens. This process has so far been adopted successfully for colon, lung, and kidney cancers (Figure 11.2). By using a series of mechanical disaggregation and enzymatic

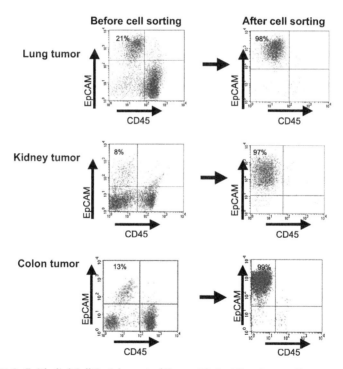

Figure 11.2 *Epithelial Cell Enrichment of Tumor Clinical Specimens.* Tumor specimens are first dissociated into single cell suspensions and red cells are lysed (left panel). Suspension cells are then enriched by flow cytometry or bead capture for EpCAM+ epithelial cells. (For color version of this figure, the reader is referred to the online version of this book.)

digestion steps, we first prepared a single cell suspension from resected tissue samples. Red blood cells were then removed through addition of ACK lysis buffer. This was followed by a depletion of CD45+ hematopoietic cells by flow cytometry, and selection of epithelial cell surface antigen (ECSA/ EpCam) positive cells by a bead-based enrichment process (Dynal CELLection Epithelial Enrich kit, Invitrogen, Carlsbad, CA). Greater than 80% enrichment of epithelial cells was achieved by using this isolation method. Since EpCAM positive cells from the pancreas also contain tumor-initiating cells, a mechanical/enzymatic tissue dissociation process followed by an antibody-based selection similar to the process described herein may allow a highly enriched population of pancreatic epithelial cells to be isolated [42,43].

In the absence of available tissue, cell line models can serve as a valid alternative for the proteomic identification process. Cell line models are not only readily available but are well defined and represent difference stages of

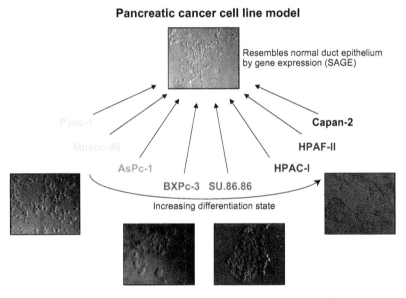

Pancreatic cancer cell line model

Resembles normal duct epithelium by gene expression (SAGE)

Panc-1

Mpanc-96

AsPc-1

BXPc-3   SU.86.86

Increasing differentiation state

Capan-2

HPAF-II

HPAC-I

Figure 11.3 *Pancreatic Cell Line Models Represent Different Stages of Pancreatic Cancer Differentiation.* Hs766t cell line was chosen as the normal comparator since this cell line has been shown by SAGE to have a genetic signature that is similar to normal ductile epithelial cells. From left (least differentiated) to right (most differentiated): PANC-1 and MPANC-96 (poorly differentiated cell lines), ASPC-1 (poorly to moderately differentiated cell line), BXPC-3 and HPAC (moderately differentiated cell lines), Su86.86 and HPAF (moderately to well-differentiated cell lines), and Capan-2 (well-differentiated cell line). (For color version of this figure, the reader is referred to the online version of this book.)

pancreatic cancer differentiation (see Figure 11.3). A number of groups, including ours, have used these models for proteomic identification [18,30]. For example, McKinney et al. [30] used cell lines to identify differences in protein expression between metastatic site–derived cell lines verses primary tumor cell lines. In this study, they identified vimentin to be expressed only on Su.86.86 (a cell line of metastatic origin) but not in BXPC-3 and Capan-2 (cell lines derived from primary tumors). In our own study using pancreatic cancer cell line models [18], we looked at differences between the "normoid" cell line Hs766T and PANC-1 (poorly differentiated), BXPC-3 (moderately differentiated), HPAC (moderately to well differentiated), and Capan-2 (well differentiated) cell lines. By using a decoupled ICAT process described in the following section, we not only looked at global differences between tumor and normal cells but also identified proteins that are upregulated at difference stages of tumor development. It should be highlighted that we also utilized an activity-based process to isolate a specific subcellular compartment, namely the cell surface membrane compartment, to increase our ability to find therapeutically relevant targets.

Enrichment for Cell Surface Glycoproteins

As has already been demonstrated in the numerous studies published to date, many proteins can potentially be identified by differential proteomic analysis [15,16]. Proteomics can therefore provide complicated results if not utilized effectively. We chose to focus our proteomics work on plasma membrane proteins, since we were interested in identifying potential therapeutic targets. Out of 120 known protein targets of marketed drugs, two-thirds are represented by plasma membrane proteins [14,44]. Their functional significance highlights their importance in drug discovery and development; they not only play a vital role in the regulation of cell signaling but are also important for cell–cell interactions as well as metabolite and ion transport. The ability to target cell surface proteins using antibody-based approaches, irrespective of the existence of a druggable domain, further contributes to their amenability as therapeutic targets.

Though it is estimated that approximately 20–30% of genes within the human genome are represented by membrane proteins, detailed analysis of this protein class has traditionally been difficult to accomplish [45–47]. As membrane proteins are hydrophobic, they are almost impossible to solubilize. Furthermore, most membrane proteins are of low abundance. A number of subcellular fractionation methods have been described, but most of these methods allow all membrane proteins, not just cell surface membrane proteins, to be identified [48–50]. For example, the ProteoExtract kit (Calbiochem, Billerica, MA) used by Paulo et al. [49] led to the identification of 47–48% membrane proteins, in addition to 34–36% cytoplasmic proteins and 8–12% nuclear proteins.

As such, a novel method that specifically enriched for cell surface proteins for LC-MS/MS analysis was developed [17,18,51]. Most transmembrane proteins are glycosylated. As previously described, we utilized sodium periodate to oxidize glycoproteins on the cell surface (see Figure 11.4(A)) [18,52,53].

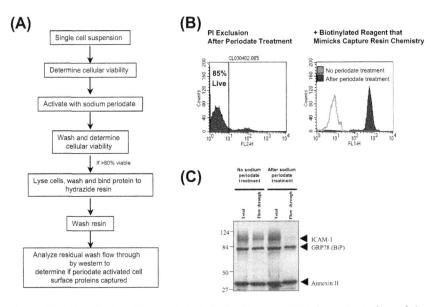

Figure 11.4 *Cell Surface Glycoprotein Isolation Process.* (A) Schematic outline of the glycoprotein isolation process. Cell surface glycoproteins are first activated by sodium periodate treatment. Since the cells remain >95% viable, only cell surface glycoproteins were activated. The oxidized glycoproteins can then be captured on a hydrazide resin. (B) Flow cytometry confirmation of cell viability (left panel) and glycoprotein oxidation (right panel). >95% cell viability was confirmed by PI exclusion. Flow cytometry binding assay using a fluorescently labeled hydrazide probe confirms oxidation of cell surface glycoproteins. (C) Western blot of protein samples before sodium periodate treatment and after treatment. In the absence of periodate activation, no oxidized glycoproteins are captured on the hydrazide resin. Both intracellular protein GRP78 and cell surface protein ICAM-1 are eluted following resin washing. After sodium periodate activation, cell surface proteins such as ICAM-1 are captured on the hydrazide resin and are therefore not eluted following washing of the resin. Intracellular protein GRP78 is not oxidized and therefore is not captured on the resin. (For color version of this figure, the reader is referred to the online version of this book.)

Cellular viability played a key role in ensuring that only cell surface glycoproteins were oxidized. To this end, we utilized a concentration of sodium periodate, i.e., 1 mM for pancreatic cells, that permitted oxidation of glycoproteins. As the cells remained intact, only cell surface glycoproteins were oxidized. In our experiments, cells typically remained >85% viable following sodium periodate treatment (see Figure 11.4(B)). Following sodium periodate treatment and confirming viability, the cells are washed and lysed, and periodate-treated proteins are captured on a hydrazide resin. A visualization of the resin capture process was possible by staining cells with a biotinylated agent that mimics the resin capture process and analyzing the samples by flow cytometry (Figure 11.4(B)). As shown in Figure 11.4(C), capture of these oxidized glycoproteins on the hydrazide resin allowed us to specifically enrich for cell surface proteins such as ICAM-1, but endoplasmic reticulum proteins such as GRP-78 are eluted from the column and can be detected in the residual wash flow through.

Quantitative Proteomics Using ICAT Technology

As demonstrated in the published studies mentioned previously, numerous proteomic studies have already been performed on pancreatic cancer serum, urine, pancreatic juice, tissue, and cell lines. Many of these studies relied on using gel-based fractionation methods (usually two-dimensional gel electrophoresis, or 2-DE) followed by identification by mass spectrometry. That is, protein samples from the normal controls and tumor comparisons are run (usually separately) on different gels, and any protein spots that appear to have a difference in intensity between the two samples are extracted and identified by mass spectrometry. This technique has been popular since it permits the comparison of intact proteins, thereby making it possible to identify posttranslation modifications, proteolytic cleavage, and polypeptide variations [54]. However, not only is it difficult to compare gel spots from experiment to experiment, but the spots may contain multiple proteins, and very acidic and basic proteins are not usually well presented on a standard gel [54]. This method is also biased against membrane proteins due their hydrophobic nature, and against low abundant proteins due to limits in dynamic range. Since the technique has a dynamic range of 10^4, the excessive presence of actin at 10^8 molecules per cell will mask any proteins that are expressed at levels less than 10^5 molecules per cell [50]. This method will therefore exclude membrane proteins such as cell surface receptors, which are expressed at 100 to 1000 molecules per cell.

This, plus the fact that 2-DE is a low throughput method that has been difficult to automate, led us to use alternative methods for quantitating differences in protein expression in our tumor versus "normoid" pancreatic cell lines. Given these limitations, we chose to use the uncoupled ICAT approach for proteomics analysis [17].

Isotope coded affinity tag (ICAT) is a probe that is made up of a biotin tag, a linker, and iodoaceramide handle. The linker maybe a light version (8 hydrogen atoms) or a heavy version (8 deuterium atoms). In this method, ICAT reagent is first added to the protein mixture to label cysteine residues on peptides. Digestion with trypsin followed by purification of cysteine-containing peptides by liquid chromatography allowed further reduction in the complexity of the protein mixture for LC/MS quantitation. In our laboratory, we went further and developed a decoupled ICAT process that has a distinct advantage over a coupled ICAT process. As outlined in the paper published by Kim et al. [17], and as illustrated in Figure 11.5, the coupled process of using a light version of ICAT on one sample versus the usage of the heavy version of ICAT on a second sample limits the analysis to a pair-wise comparison. In our proteomic analysis of cell lines from different stages of differentiation, we wanted to use a technique that will not only allow us to identify proteins that are upregulated in tumor cells but also to complete multiplex analysis that will allow us to look at expression of proteins across different stages of disease development. In the decoupled approach, as shown in Figure 11.5, both the tumor and normal samples are labeled separately using the same version of the ICAT reagent. Peptide ion peaks of LC/MS maps from normal and tumor samples are aligned based on mass-to-charge ratio (m/z), corrected retention time (RT), and charge state (z). Peptide ion peaks were detected from the LC/MS maps by using RESPECT™ software. The intensities of ions in each map were then compared to the mean intensities of those ions across all maps in the alignment. Using ions with mean intensities in the 10th–90th percentiles, and unconstrained nonlinear optimization, it was possible for a normalization factor to be generated for each map. This minimizes the sum of the differences between intensities of each ion and the mean intensity for that ion across all maps. Scatter plot of the aligned peptide ions can be produced by using Spotfire™ (TIBCO Spotfire, Somerville, MA), and from there differential ratios could be calculated. Peptide ions, in our case those with a differential expression of greater than three-fold between tumor and normal samples, were then selected for LC-MS/MS–based peptide sequencing, and peptide/protein identification can be accomplished by using MASCOT (Matrix Science, London, UK).

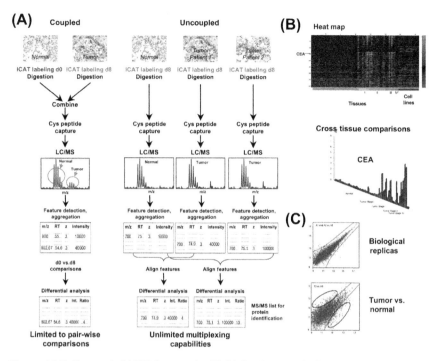

Figure 11.5 *Decoupled ICAT Process for Multiplex Proteomic Comparisons.* (A) Traditional proteomic analysis using ICAT is limited to pair-wise comparisons. In the decoupled process, each sample is labeled separately with the same ICAT reagent. Peptide ion peaks are detected and aligned based on mass-to-charge ratio (*m/z*), corrected retention time (RT), and charge state (*z*). Scatter plots of the aligned peptide ions are produced, and differential ratios can be calculated. (B) Example heat map of peptides that can be generated using the decoupled approach. Expression of any protein, e.g., CEA shown, can be compared across numerous tissues and cell lines. (C) Scatter plot of peptide alignment between biological replicas, 99.4% of the common features' intensities are within three-fold for BXPC3 replicates compared to 80.0% for that of BXPC3 versus Hs766T. (For color version of this figure, the reader is referred to the online version of this book.)

As illustrated in Figure 11.5(B), this method permits multiplex analysis and the generation of heat map comparisons across disease states, and even across disease areas. As shown in Figure 11.5(C), for each cell line, the reproducibility of intensities of common features between process replicates is greater than that of a tumor versus normal comparison, indicating that the differences observed between tumor and normal samples are significant. In our example, 99.4% of the common features' intensities are within three-fold for BXPC3 replicates compared to 80.0% for that of BXPC3 versus Hs766T.

Figure 11.6 shows the peptide intensity plot of tissue factor Na^+/K^+ ATPase Beta 3 (also known as CD298) and Integrin Beta 6 (β6) from decoupled proteomics analysis. Tissue factor is a 47-kDa membrane-bound glycoprotein that is expressed by many cancer cells, including pancreatic cancer cells [55]. The expression of tissue factor has been demonstrated to correlate with tumor progression, with the highest levels observed in poorly differentiated tumors [56]. In xenograph models, pancreatic cancer cells that produce tissue factor consistently produced tumors that are larger in size than pancreatic cancer cells that don't produce tissue factor [57]. The family of integrin heterodimeric receptors plays key roles in cell adhesion, invasion, migration, and proliferation differentiation [58]. The subunit Integrin β6 is unique since it can only partner with the alpha v (αv) subunit. Its expression has been shown to be exclusive to developing and cancerous epithelial cells, and to epithelial cells undergoing wound healing. A number of studies, including studies performed on ovarian, colon, and pancreatic cancer, have correlated Integrin αvβ6 expression with progression into advance stages of disease [59–61]. Na^+/K^+ ATPase is a family of isoenzymes that are found on the plasma membrane that catalyzes the efflux of cytoplasmic Na^+ and uptake of extracellular K^+ [62]. The isoenzyme consists of alpha subunits, beta subunits, and FXYD proteins. Diversity of this isoenzyme comes from the association of different molecular forms of the alpha (alpha1, alpha2, alpha3, and alpha4) and beta (beta1, beta2, and beta3) subunits. The catalytic alpha subunit hydrolyzes ATP and transports the cations. The beta subunits, including beta3-type subunit, and FXYD proteins may contribute the function of Na^+/K^+ ATPase in different tissues [63,64]. Steroidal cardiac Na^+/K^+ ATPase inhibitors have been demonstrated to have antitumor activity in prostate and lung xenografts [65].

As shown in Figure 11.6, tissue factor, Integrin β6, and Na^+/K^+ ATPase Beta 3 were identified to be overexpressed in pancreatic cancer cell lines. The decoupled process allowed us to perform comparative analysis across different pancreatic cell lines and tissues, even with tissues from other organs. As such, tissue factor was found to be overexpressed in not only pancreatic cancer cell lines but also in lung and breast cancer cell lines, as well as in conditioned media from colon and breast cancer cell lines. Similarly, Integrin β6 was shown to be overexpressed in breast cell lines, lung cell lines, gastric tissues, and colon stem cells; whilst Na^+/K^+ ATPase Beta 3 was found to be overexpressed in pancreatic, liver, lung, ovarian, kidney, and colon tumor cell lines, as well as in colon cancer stem cells and lung tumor tissues.

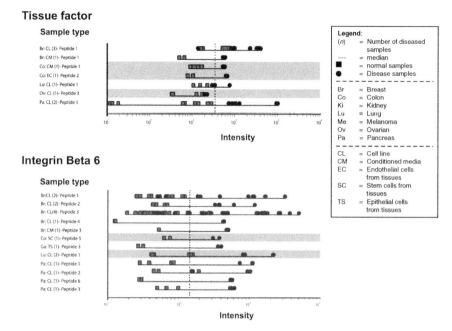

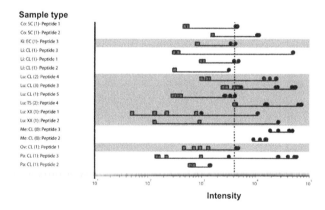

Figure 11.6 *Peptide Intensity Plots for Tissue Factor, Integrin Beta 6, and Na⁺/K⁺ ATPase Beta 3.* Black squares: intensity of peptides from normal samples; black circles: intensity of peptides from tumor samples; dotted line: median intensity of all peptides for each protein. Differential expression of each peptide sequence in breast (Br), colon (Co), kidney (Ki), lung (Lu), melanoma (Me), ovarian (Ov), and pancreatic (Pa) cancer samples versus normal comparators are shown. Samples analyzed include samples from cell lines (CL), conditioned media (CM), endothelial cells from tissues (EC), stem cells from tissues (SC), and epithelial cells from tissue (TS).

It should be noted that the proteomics identification platform should really only serve as a beginning; it is only following validation with other expression methods, and functional validation with methods such as RNAi, that any given target we identified becomes important. These platforms, using tissue factor, Integrin Beta 6, and Na^+/K^+ ATPase Beta 3 as examples, will be described next.

Expression Validation Methods

Given the complexity of performing proteomics on tissues from pancreatic cancer patients, we chose to complete our proteomics identification by using cell lines. Whilst cell lines provide a valuable source of homologous cells to work with, they have well-documented, distinct disadvantages [66,67]. For example, since they have been in culture for numerous passages, it is recognized that most cell lines have acquired a molecular phenotype that differs from the phenotype of primary cells. Furthermore, since the origins of a number of cell lines have been in dispute, whether cell lines truly represent the intended disease has been called into question.

Thus, to verify what we discover from our cell line proteomics discovery platform, a robust validation platform must be put into place. Figure 11.7 shows an example schematic of the validation process that we had employed. In the outlined schematic, the expression validation process depended on the availability of antibodies against the intended target. In our validation scheme, if antibodies were available, immunohistochemistry (IHC) was utilized to confirm expression on tumor pancreatic tissues versus normal tumor tissues. Validation of expression on vital organs was also completed. To validate cell surface membrane localization, FACS and immunofluorescence were utilized. Western blotting was used to validate expression in cell lines if other methods were not readily available. If antibodies against the target of interest were not available, quantitative PCR was used as a first step expression validation tool, and production of antibodies directed against the intended target were initiated once validated by mRNA. Details of two of these methods we most often utilized for expression validation, namely IHC and quantitative flow cytometry, will be described in more detail following. Once candidates are validated to be expressed in pancreatic cancer, they may serve as potential candidates for biomarker development. It is also possible to further functionally validate these candidates by RNAi, neutralizing antibody, and/or small molecule tool compounds. Validation of function is essentially for determining value of any candidate for therapeutic development. Further details of RNAi for functional validation will be described below.

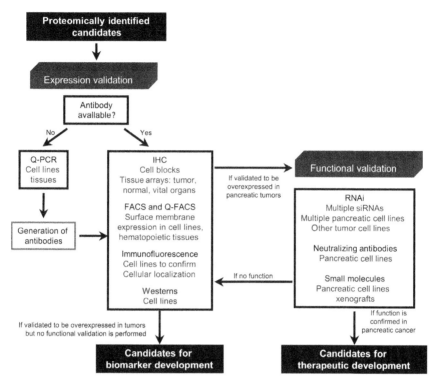

Figure 11.7 *Schematic of the Validation Process for Proteomically Identified Candidates.* Each candidate identified from proteomic analysis first undergoes expression validation. Validation of protein expression is dependent on antibody availability. If appropriate antibodies are available, expression is validated by IHC, FACS/Q-FACs, immunofluorescence, and/or western blotting. If no antibodies are initially available, candidates are first validated by Q-PCR before generation of antibodies is triggered. Once antibodies are generated, the protein candidates are further validated. If expression is confirmed, the candidates may serve as candidates for biomarker development. All candidates validated to be overexpressed in pancreatic tumors are functionally validated by RNAi. If neutralizing antibodies or tool compounds for targets of interest are available, further functional validation is completed. Candidates for therapeutics development are selected from those candidates identified to play a functional role in pancreatic cancer. (For color version of this figure, the reader is referred to the online version of this book.)

Validation of Expression in Tumor Cells by IHC

IHC could be one of the most powerful expression validation techniques if an experienced pathologist is involved with the interpretation of the results. Not only is it possible to determine differences in staining intensity, and therefore expression levels, but it also provides a means of visualization of the subcellular location of any given protein. What makes this technique particularly useful is the fact that tissue arrays are now readily available [68].

Tissue arrays typically contain cylindrical tissue samples from thousands of different archival tissue blocks, thereby allowing a pathologist to rapidly analyze hundreds of patient samples simultaneously. For example, LifeSpan Biosciences have an internal collection of over 2 million tissue specimens, including tissue arrays for pancreatic tissues from primary and metastatic cells. Using tissue arrays, it was possible for us to validate our proteomic findings from a number of patients and determine if the targets that were identified were truly upregulated in pancreatic cancer [18]. Since tissue arrays are available for normal and tumor tissues, including tissues from other organs, it was possible to determine if the targets we identified were of therapeutic value. That is, by using IHC, expression of target protein in vital organs such as the heart, lungs, brain, liver, etc. can be determined early on, and any target with intense staining in the vital organs can be quickly de-prioritized [69]. This is especially important since a similar level of staining within vital organs and tumor tissues suggests that it may not be possible to obtain an adequate therapeutic window from which patients could be treated without affecting a vital organ. Furthermore, since it is possible to perform IHC on other cancer tissues, added value can be provided by IHC validation since a target's application across different tumor types can also be determined.

Figure 11.8 shows the expression validation of tissue factor, an example target that was identified through our proteomics platform. As shown in Figure 11.8(A), tissue factor expression was found to be expressed on all 10 pancreatic carcinoma samples from different subjects tested. When examined closely, the positive staining was identified to be membranous, and nuclear staining was not encountered. Expression was also found in the majority of lung carcinomas and occasional samples of ovary, prostate, colon, and breast carcinomas (see Figure 11.8(B) for staining in NSCLC and prostate cancer). Figure 11.8(C) shows staining of tissue factor on normal tissues. Either no, or very weak, staining was detected in all normal tissues tested to date. Prominent positivity was present in the reserve cell layer of respiratory epithelium, basal epithelial cells in the prostate, pneumocytes, and renal glomerular visceral epithelial cells. Focal positivity was present in neuroendocrine cells in the intestine, testicular fibroblasts, ovarian follicles, adrenal medulla, and in developing follicles in the ovary. Only rare staining was present in cardiac myocytes. The majority of positive staining in normal tissues was found to be cytoplasmic. This data therefore suggests that it might be possible to target tissue factor therapeutically; the difference in expression levels of tissue factor in pancreatic cancer compared to normal

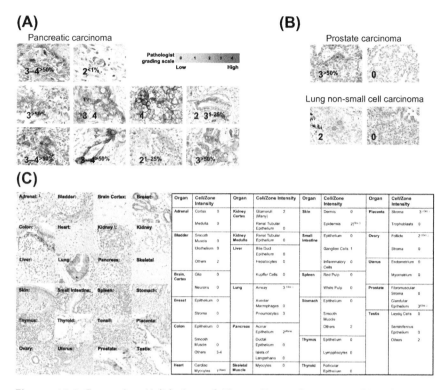

Figure 11.8 *Expression Validation of Tissue Factor by Immunohistochemistry (IHC).* Numbers on each image (40×) indicate pathologist grading scale and percentage of section showing staining. (A) Tissue factor staining in pancreatic carcinomas. (B) Tissue factor staining in prostate and non-small cell lung cancer. (C) Left: Tissue factor staining in representative normal tissue sections; Right: pathologist score of cell types within each normal organ. Occ = occasional staining. (For color version of this figure, the reader is referred to the online version of this book.)

vital organs would provide a therapeutic index from which on target adverse events could be minimized. A differential response to therapeutics may also be possible with tissue factor, since expression was identified to be within the cytoplasm of normal cells, but membranous in pancreatic cancer cells.

Validation of Expression in Tumor Cells and Membrane Localization by FACS

A second technique that we employed for expression validation is quantitative flow cytometry (Q-FACS) [70,71]. As a highly specific technique, flow cytometry makes it possible to quickly, and simultaneously, measure numerous cellular physical parameters on a large number of suspension cells. The usage of flow cytometry also makes it feasible to confirm cell surface localization of the protein target in question. The measurement of these physical parameters, such as receptors on a cell, can be quantified and compared between laboratories by using commercially available fluorescent calibration beads [70,72]. By using bead standards combined with a known fluorochrome-to-antibody ratio, the fluorescence axis can be calibrated to calculate the number of fluorochrome molecules attached to the cell. Using this technique, also known as quantitative flow cytometry, it is possible to quantify the number of membrane proteins per cell. A number of methods are available, based on the types of standards employed. We chose to use the Quantum Simply Cellular System (Bangs Laboratories, Fishers, IN), which utilizes Type IIIC calibration standards. This particular type of standard is reported to produce the best spectra matching since the beads bind the same conjugated antibody as the cell sample [71].

Quantum Simply Cellular System kits consist of five polystyrene microbead sets, where each set is labeled with a predetermined number of ligands on each bead. As shown in Figure 11.9(A), following staining with a specific fluorochrome-conjugated antibody, each population of beads will produce a distinct fluorescent signal on the flow cytometer. A calibration curve for the antibody can then be established by using linear regression analysis and plotting the mean fluorescent intensity against its assigned antibody binding capacity (ABC). By labeling the cells with the same antibody as the beads, and by using the same instrument settings on the flow cytometer, the ABC for the cells can be calculated from the calibration cure. The calculated antibody binding capacity ultimately correlates to the number of antigenic sites present on the cell surface.

As an example, Figure 11.9(B) shows the relative copy number of tissue factor on seven pancreatic cell lines. Compared to the normoid cell line HS766t, tissue factor was found to be greater than 12-fold overexpressed in the more differentiated cell lines—namely, the moderately differentiated cell lines (BXPC-3, SU.86.86), moderately to well-differentiated cell lines (HPAC1, HPAF-II), and well-differentiated cell lines (Capan-2). However, no difference was reported in the least, poorly differentiated cell line (PANC-1). As shown in Figure 11.9(C), there is good correlation between the QFACS data and the proteomics data. By both QFACS and quantitative proteomics, tissue factor was found to be overexpressed in the moderately differentiated cell line BXPC-3, moderately to well-differentiated cell line HPAC, and well-differentiated Capan-2, as compared to "normoid" cell line Hs766t. At the same time, it was determined by both techniques that

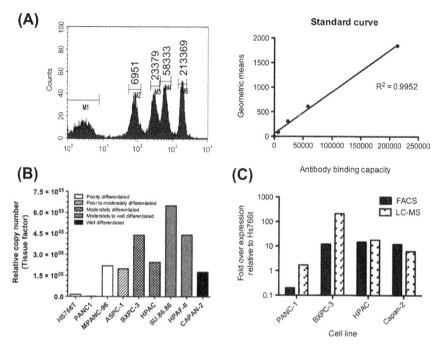

Figure 11.9 *Expression Validation of Tissue Factor by Quantitative Flow Cytometry (Q-FACS).* (A) Left: QSC Beads coated with goat anti-mouse antibody with known antibody binding capacity values are incubated with a PE-conjugated tissue factor antibody, and geometric mean fluorescence for each bead population is recorded by flow cytometry. Right: standard curve for tissue factor antibody. (B) Left: copy number of tissue factor in pancreatic cancer cell lines; (C) Right: fold overexpression of tissue factor in pancreatic cancer cell lines PANC-1, BXPC-3, HPAC, and CAPAN-2 compared to reference cell line HS766t. Black bars=fold overexpression calculated by QFACS; White line bars=fold overexpression calculated by LC-MS. (For color version of this figure, the reader is referred to the online version of this book.)

tissue factor was not overexpressed in the poorly differentiated cell line MPANC96 cells. Therefore, for tissue factor, we were able to verify our proteomics findings by quantitative flow cytometry.

A second application of Q-FACS is the ability to quantitate any given target on specific populations of hematopoietic cells. Hematoxicity, especially myelosuppression, is a major dose-limited factor in drug development [73]. Disruption to the different specific lineages of the hematopoietic development process may have different clinical consequences. Disruption to erythrocyte development may lead to anemia, disruptions to the development of granulocytes may lead to neutropenia, disruptions to the development of monocytes may lead to immunosuppression, and disruptions to the development of platelets may lead to thrombocytopenia. Cytopenia is often an indicator for tolerable dose and frequency of administration. By using QFACS, it is possible to quantitate the expression of a particular cell surface protein in different hematopoietic cell populations and compare these values to the tumor cells in question. It is therefore possible to utilize this information as part of a package to predict if a therapeutic index exists that will allow the targeting of tumor cells and not hematopoietic cells.

Functional Validation by RNA Interference

Large-scale genomics and proteomic studies have ushered in a new era of discovery for cancer research [15]. The challenge now is not only to verify the variations in expression of proteins in the tumor cell but to map out the specific roles the dysregulated proteins play in the context of disease. Whilst it is recognized that protein function is not essential for therapeutic antibody development, knowledge of the underlying mechanism will still provide key information necessary for developing a strategic path. Not only will functionality provide vital information regarding how best to disrupt protein function but this information may also be used to predict potential adverse reactions and reveal mechanisms of resistance [74,75]. The generation and optimization of small molecule inhibitors for a given protein target involves a lengthy and costly process—a lead scaffold must first be identified from screening compound libraries, followed by substantial medicinal chemistry efforts in enhancing specificity and sensitivity [76]. As such, mechanistic information will help decipher if a small molecule screening campaign is worth pursuing. Similarly, tool grade antibodies are expensive and time consuming to produce and validate, and naked antibodies with robust antitumor activities are rarely available [69,77]. Thus, the underlying mechanism of an antigen will determine if it is even feasible to target the protein antigen by using a naked antibody, or if the antibody requires drug or radiolabeling, or if other modifications such as glycoengineering will be required. Therefore, a functional validation method that can quickly and cheaply decipher a protein's role in tumor development should first be employed before embarking on a journey toward small molecule or antibody development.

Since its inception in 1998, RNA interference (RNAi) has quickly developed into a vital tool for high-throughput target validation [78]. Its importance is highlighted by the fact that a mere eight years following its discovery, its founders, Craig Mellow and Andrew Fire, were awarded the Nobel Prize in Physiology or Medicine (2006). Compared to antisense and ribozyme technology, RNAi is more robust, enabling more efficient down-regulation of a target gene with a lower dose, and is also more specific [79,80]. Unlike antisense, RNAi takes advantage of a naturally occurring cellular process that is thought to be a defense mechanism against viruses. Numerous comprehensive reviews of the RNAi mechanism have been published, including review articles by Cejka et al. [79], Hannon et al. [81], Meister et al. [82], and Kim et al. [83]. A simplification of the RNAi mechanism is as follows: during the first RNAi initiating step, an RNase III endo-nuclease called Dicer acts to cleave foreign long double-stranded RNA entered into the cellular cytoplasm. The cleavage products are shorter, 21 to 23 nucleotide strands known as small interfering RNA (siRNA). The siRNA is then passed onto the RNA-induced silencing complex (RISC), through RNA-binding proteins, the TAR-RNA–binding protein (TRBP), PACT, and Argonaute-2 (Ago-2) enzyme that are complexed with Dicer. Once the double-stranded siRNA is bound to RISC, the "passenger" (or less thermodynamically stable) strand is cleaved and released by Ago-2, thereby activating RISC. The complex then utilizes the "guide" (or more thermodynamically stable) strand to target its exact complementary mes-senger RNA sequence. Subsequent cleavage of the target messenger RNA by Ago-2 prevents transcription of the target sequence.

This natural mechanism can be adapted to validate cancer targets, since RNAi mediated gene knockdown is a universal mechanism, and the RNAi machinery remains intact in the cancer cell [84]. Experimentally, the RNAi process in the pancreatic cancer cell could either be mediated by using syn-thetic siRNA that is transiently transfected into a cell or by using short hairpin (sh) RNA plasmid constructs where siRNAs are produced from Dicer processing of transcribed shRNA [85]. For target validation purposes, the synthetic siRNA method is the method of choice; they are cheap to manufacture, readily available, and can easily be introduced into a cell via transient transfections. Since the effect is transient, they are more likely to mimic a therapeutic response. For example, siRNA against BCR-ABL imi-tated the apoptotic response induced by imatinib in K562 CML cells [86]. Whilst we will focus our attention in this chapter on the siRNA method, it should be pointed out that the shRNA method does possess several distinct advantages. For example, for difficult-to-transfect cells, RNAi experiments are still possible through the use of an infection method for shRNA delivery [85]. Secondly, since the plasmids can be stability integrated into the DNA, long-term evaluations of nonlethal genes are possible. Thus, if the phenotype is not detectable within the transient transfection time frame, i.e., within five days, shRNA can provide an effective, alternative way of RNAi screening. However, there are a number of disadvantages to the shRNA method, including the need for cloning and stable transfection of the plasmid constructs. Furthermore, since genomic integration into the DNA may induce unexpected changes, we chose to validate our short list of proteomic targets by using synthetic siRNA.

There were a number of other considerations that needed to be addressed before we embarked on an RNAi validation program. Firstly, siRNA target sequences must be optimized in order to ensure specificity and reduce the potential for off-target effects. Secondly, cellular assays that appropriately address the biological functionality in question must be optimized. Thirdly, depending on the cellular assay, the RNAi screening format must be chosen, and RNAi transfection conditions must be optimized for each cell type in question.

For a thorough RNAi validation program, siRNAs against the target of interest must be specific, and the effects must be reproducible by siRNAs that target different portions of the mRNA sequence. Any off-target effects must be minimized, whilst specific mRNA knockdown activity must be optimized. A set of initial rules governing siRNA design was published by Elbashir et al., in 2001 [87], and these design rules continues to evolve [88]. To date, there have been a number of publications in this area, and quite sophisticated algorithms have been developed [89]. Essentially, considerations into siRNA design can be thought of as those parameters that influence activity or potency, and those parameters that influence specificity. Potency is known to be influenced by parameters that determine the accessibility of the target sequence, which include parameters such as overall siRNA G/C content, structure of mRNA target region, strand selection, and positional preferences of specific bases [90–92]. siRNA specificity is critical in reducing the likelihood of nonspecific effects; though rules are not fully defined, parameters that govern specificity include homology to other target sequences and presence of immunogenic sequences within the siRNA duplex [89,93,94].

For our initial screens, we utilized a pool of four siRNAs that target the same mRNA, but within different regions. Not only did this allow us to increase our throughput and decrease reagent consumption, but screening with siRNA pools has also been demonstrated to increase the likelihood of finding putative hits, and generate a more severe penetrant phenotype [95]. To confirm hits from our initial screens, follow-up experiments were performed with individual duplexes, and any effective duplexes were titrated down to 1 nM. The same phenotype produced by at least two siRNAs targeting different regions within the same mRNA is far less likely to be due to sequence dependent off-target effect, such as miRNA effects [96]. Furthermore, since the RNAi machinery is saturable, phenotypic and knockdown verification with a low concentration of siRNA can reduce chances of the phenotype being the result of an off-target effect [97].

Another consideration is the high-throughput layout of the experiment. There are a number of different RNAi experimental formats, and the format chosen largely depends on throughput requirements and the types of cell assays available. siRNA transfections can be performed by traditional forward transfections, whereby cells are first plated, and followed by addition of siRNA-transfection reagent complex to cells. Alternatively, siRNA can be performed by reverse transfection, whereby cells are plated onto wells already containing siRNA-transfection reagent complex. One advantage to forward transfections is that master plates with siRNA/transfection reagents can be made, and multiple plates for different cell assays can be transfected by using aliquots from the same master plates [98]. Automation using forward transfections are feasible; for example, Chung et al. [98] automated their platform by utilizing robotic liquid handling systems, separating the RNA procedure into making the master or intermediate plates first, followed by transfection, and completed a genome-scale siRNA screen in HeLa cells. Many laboratories, though, prefer reverse transfection for automation and genome-wide screens; not only does this method reduce experimental time by one day, as cells do not need to be plated the day before transfection, but since microtiter plates or siRNA chips are now readily available (much akin to microarray technology), this method is highly suitable for HTS [99].

In our laboratory, we utilized a forward transfection platform and took advantage of commercially available siRNA libraries. This platform allowed us to functionally validate our proteomically identified targets in a number of pancreatic cancer cell lines, including cell lines from the more differentiated stages that do not form confluent monolayers. For cell lines that are more fragile, the seeding of cells a day prior to transfections allowed the cells to "settle down" before they were transfected, which in our hands helped us to decrease transfection-induced cellular toxicity (results not published). For initial screening, we wanted to focus our biological assessments on two fundamental processes in cancer: apoptosis and proliferation. Unless proper controls are in place and cells are growing confidently, it is easy to mistake transfection toxicity with proper biological function. It was also important for us to access knockdown simultaneously with every experiment, so that biological differences are always confirmed by target knockdown. The forward transfection platform we adopted allowed us to assess mRNA knockdown and assess multiple biological functions simultaneously from the same transfection.

A robust RNAi validation platform is only possible if a transfection agent that allows high transfectivity whilst maintaining cellular viability can be identified. Traditionally, siRNA transfections can be carried out by using lipid-based transfection reagents or by using electroporation. For our purposes, since our aim is to perform RNAi in a high-throughput manner, lipid-based transfection became the method of choice. Our functional validation process began with the optimization of cell numbers for each assay. During this process the assay limits are identified, including initial cell seeding numbers, since cells should still be in log phase growth within the time frame of the biological assay, usually within four days of a siRNA transient transfection. If too many cells are plated at the beginning of the experiment and are in lag phase by the time of the biological assay (that is, cells have already stopped proliferating), a wrong assessment of function could be made. Subculturing of adherent pancreatic cancer cells before assay readout is not advisable for high-throughput format, since this will simply induce assay errors due to inadequate dissociation of cells from plates, and errors due to inadequate mixing before cell dilutions are re-plated.

Once assay limits and proper cell seeding numbers are identified for each assay, a panel of transfection reagents were typically tested in various dose-ranging conditions, where the initial doses are normally tested in $0.5\,\mu l$ increments, up to $2.5\,\mu l$ per $100\,\mu l$ volume. In our forward transfection platform, the optimization experiments were always carried out by simultaneous mRNA knockdown and alamar blue toxicity assessment. As shown in Figure 11.10(A), the transfection reagent and volume is always chosen where the cells transfected with negative control siRNA are at least 90% live, including scrambled negative, and nontargeting firefly luciferase siRNA, and mRNA knockdown assessed the day after transfection is maximum with housekeeper control cyclophilin siRNA (>90% efficient).

Figure 11.10(B) shows RNAi knockdown results of tissue factor, Integrin β6, and Na^+/K^+ ATPase Beta 3 subunit. As shown, 24 h following tissue factor, Integrin β6, and Na^+/K^+ ATPase Beta 3 siRNA transfection, over 75% knockdown was observed. Three days following tissue factor or Integrin Beta 6 siRNA transfection, a dose-dependent inhibition of cell growth, as measured by cellular metabolic activity, was observed in MPANC96 and

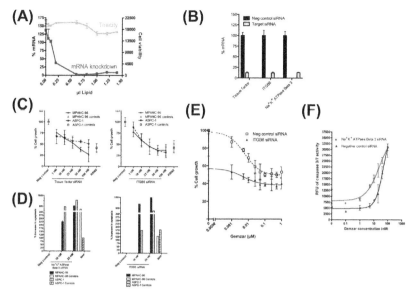

Figure 11.10 *RNAi Functional Validation of Tissue Factor, Integrin Beta 6 and Na⁺/K⁺ ATPase Beta 3 in Pancreatic Cancer Cell Lines.* (A) Optimization of transfection conditions. Amount of transfection reagent chosen for RNAi experiments typically provides >90% knockdown with housekeeper control siRNA one day following transfection, and exhibits minimal toxicity. (B) Knockdown of tissue factor, Integrin Beta 6 and Na⁺/K⁺ ATPase Beta 3 mRNA. (C) Alamar blue cell proliferation following titration of tissue factor, and Integrin Beta 6 siRNA in ASPC-1 and MPANC-96 cell lines. Data is plotted as a percentage of the scrambled negative control. The positive control, ribonucleotide reductase M2 polypeptide (RRM2) siRNA, is also shown. (D) Apoptotic cell death, as measured by caspase 3/7 activity, following transfection of ITGB6 or Na⁺/K⁺ ATPase Beta 3 siRNA into MPANC96 or ASPC-1 cell lines. Results shown are relative to scrambled negative control. Positive control, XIAP, is also indicated. (E) Alamar blue proliferation following transfection with 1 nM Integrin Beta 6 siRNA (black triangles) or negative control siRNA (white squares) plus 0–1 µM Gemzar in MPANC-96 cells (F) Caspase 3/7 apoptosis of BXPC-3 cells following transfection with 25 nM Na⁺/K⁺ ATPase Beta 3 siRNA or negative control siRNA plus 0–100 nM Gemzar. (For color version of this figure, the reader is referred to the online version of this book.)

ASPC-1 cell lines (Figure 11.10(C)). Similar inhibitory effects were observed for our positive control X-linked Inhibitor of Apoptosis Protein (XIAP) which is known to inhibit proliferation of cancer cells in vitro and in vivo [100]. As anticipated, no inhibitory effects were observed for the negative control siRNA. Knockdown of Integrin β6 and Na⁺/K⁺ ATPase Beta 3 mRNA also induced apoptosis in both MPANC96 and ASPC-1 cell lines. As shown in Figure 11.10(D), the level of caspase 3/7 induction was comparable or higher than the positive control XIAP.

As discussed in earlier sections, the standard of care for the nonresectable pancreatic cancer patients is treatment with gemcitabine. Therefore, any efficacy assessment during a clinical trial must be referenced to this standard treatment. For our in vitro functional validation platform, either an additive or synergistic apoptotic or antiproliferative effect when gemcitabine treatment is combined with target knockdown will add significant value and increase a protein's priority for further development.

MPANC96 cells were either transfected with 25 nM of negative control siRNA or Integrin β6 siRNA (Figure 11.10(E)). The cells were treated with no gemcitabine or increasing concentrations of gemcitabine, from 1 nM up to 0.1 µM. As shown in Figure 11.10(D), gemcitabine treatment alone induced a dose-dependent inhibition of MPANC96 proliferation, with maximum inhibition of ~50% observed with treatment with >50 nM gemcitabine treatment. Meanwhile, with only 1 nM of integrin β6 siRNA, 57% decrease in proliferation was observed in MPANC96 cells. The decrease in proliferation was greater than 50% when 1 nM of integrin β6 siRNA was combined with 5 nM of gemcitabine, with greater than 60% growth inhibition reached when siRNA treatment was combined with 50 nM or greater of gemcitabine. An additive effect on apoptosis was also observed when Na$^+$/K$^+$ ATPase Beta 3 siRNA was combined with Gemzar (Figure 11.10(F)). When the cells were treated with either 0.1, 1, or 10 nM Gemzar, the level of caspase 3/7 activity increases by approximately two-fold when treatment with Gemzar was combined with Na$^+$/K$^+$ ATPase Beta 3 siRNA. This additive effect was not observed at the highest levels of Gemzar tested (100 nM), suggesting that the highest level of apoptosis was reached.

SUMMARY

In this chapter, we described the high-throughput LC-MS–based proteomics platform that was developed in our laboratory. Since access to quality pancreatic tissues at a high yield was not possible, and considering the goal of our platform is to discover novel cell surface glycoproteins, we completed our proteomics analysis using pancreatic cell line models. By putting a robust expression validation platform in place that included IHC and quantitative flow cytometry methods, not only was it possible to verify expression in pancreatic tumor tissues but it was also possible to determine if any given proteins were upregulated in other tumor types. As we also extended expression validation to vital organs within a healthy volunteer, our platform enabled us to formulate initial insights regarding possible therapeutic windows and therefore develop a strategic plan forward for diagnostic and therapeutic development. We further added value to our proteomics discovery by developing a functional validation platform using RNAi. Thus, it was possible to decipher if our expression-based discovery played any role in the functional dysregulation of a pancreatic tumor cell. Certainly, it is our hope that the work from this novel platform will ultimately lead to the discovery of new targets for the diagnosis and treatment of pancreatic cancer.

ACKNOWLEDGMENTS

The authors wish to thank Jenny L. Heidbrink, Victoria Bushman, Erin Brand, Jim Norton, Jun Kim, Brian Feild, Roxanne Armstrong, Henrik Olsen, Will Fitzhugh, Jim Duff, Ping Zhang and Katherine Paweletz, for their technical assistance. We also wish to thank Samuel Broder, Robert Booth and Scott Patterson for their advise on this project.

REFERENCES

[1] Yeo TP, Lowenfels AB. Demographics and epidemiology of pancreatic cancer. Cancer J 2012;18:477–84.

[2] Michaud DS. Epidemiology of pancreatic cancer. Minerva Chir 2004;59:99–111.

[3] Siegel R, Naishadham D, Jemal A. Cancer statistics, 2013. CA Cancer J Clin 2013;63:11–30.

[4] Chiu J, Yau T. Metastatic pancreatic cancer: are we making progress in treatment? Gastroenterol Res Pract 2012;2012:898–931.

[5] Saif MW. Is there a standard of care for the management of advanced pancreatic cancer? Highlights from the Gastrointestinal Cancers Symposium. Orlando, FL, USA. January 25–27, 2008. JOP 2008;9:91–8.

[6] Paulson AS, Tran Cao HS, Tempero MA, Lowy AM. Therapeutic advances in pancreatic cancer. Gastroenterology 2013;144:1316–26.

[7] Ahn ER, Vogel CL. Dual HER2-targeted approaches in HER2-positive breast cancer. Breast Cancer Res Treat 2012;131:371–83.

[8] Jain P, Kantarjian H, Cortes J. Chronic myeloid leukemia: overview of new agents and comparative analysis. Curr Treat Options Oncol 2013;14:127–43.

[9] Dotan E, Aggarwal C, Smith MR. Impact of rituximab (Rituxan) on the treatment of B-cell non-Hodgkin's lymphoma. P T 2010;35:148–57.

[10] Kaneda H, Yoshida T, Okamoto I. Molecularly targeted approaches herald a new era of non-small-cell lung cancer treatment. Cancer Manag Res 2013;5:91–101.

[11] Bayraktar S, Rocha-Lima CM. Advanced or metastatic pancreatic cancer: molecular targeted therapies. Mt Sinai J Med 2010;77:606–19.

[12] Wong HH, Lemoine NR. Pancreatic cancer: molecular pathogenesis and new therapeutic targets. Nat Rev Gastroenterol Hepatol 2009;6:412–22.

[13] Hidalgo M, Von Hoff DD. Translational therapeutic opportunities in ductal adenocarcinoma of the pancreas. Clin Cancer Res 2012;18:4249–56.

[14] Hopkins AL, Groom CR. The druggable genome. Nat Rev Drug Discov 2002;1:727–30.

[15] Ryan TE, Patterson SD. Proteomics: drug target discovery on an industrial scale. Trends Biotechnol 2002;20:S45–51.

[16] Patterson S. Selecting targets for therapeutic validation through differential protein expression using chromatography-mass spectrometry. Bioinformatics 2002;18(Suppl. 2):S181.

[17] Kim YJ, Zhan P, Feild B, Ruben SM, He T. Reproducibility assessment of relative quantitation strategies for LC-MS based proteomics. Anal Chem 2007;79:5651–8.

[18] Lee CN, Heidbrink JL, McKinnon K, Bushman V, Olsen H, FitzHugh W, et al. RNA interference characterization of proteins discovered by proteomic analysis of pancreatic cancer reveals function in cell growth and survival. Pancreas 2012;41:84–94.

[19] Weeks ME, Hariharan D, Petronijevic L, Radon TP, Whiteman HJ, Kocher HM, et al. Analysis of the urine proteome in patients with pancreatic ductal adenocarcinoma. Proteomics Clin Appl 2008;2:1047–57.

[20] Bhattacharyya S, Siegel ER, Petersen GM, Chari ST, Suva LJ, Haun RS. Diagnosis of pancreatic cancer using serum proteomic profiling. Neoplasia 2004;6:674–86.

[21] Xue A, Gandy RC, Chung L, Baxter RC, Smith RC. Discovery of diagnostic biomarkers for pancreatic cancer in immunodepleted serum by SELDI-TOF MS. Pancreatology 2012;12:124–9.

[22] Koopmann J, Zhang Z, White N, Rosenzweig J, Fedarko N, Jagannath S, et al. Serum diagnosis of pancreatic adenocarcinoma using surface-enhanced laser desorption and ionization mass spectrometry. Clin Cancer Res 2004;10:860–8.

[23] Park JY, Kim SA, Chung JW, Bang S, Park SW, Paik YK, et al. Proteomic analysis of pancreatic juice for the identification of biomarkers of pancreatic cancer. J Cancer Res Clin Oncol 2011;137:1229–38.

[24] Doyle CJ, Yancey K, Pitt HA, Wang M, Bemis K, Yip-Schneider MT, et al. The proteome of normal pancreatic juice. Pancreas 2012;41:186–94.

[25] Tian R, Wei LM, Qin RY, Li Y, Du ZY, Xia W, et al. Proteome analysis of human pancreatic ductal adenocarcinoma tissue using two-dimensional gel electrophoresis and tandem mass spectrometry for identification of disease-related proteins. Dig Dis Sci 2007;53(1):65–72.

[26] Lail LM, Cotton PB. Risks of endoscopic retrograde cholangiopancreatography and therapeutic applications. Gastroenterol Nurs 1990;12:239–45.

[27] Goggins M. Identifying molecular markers for the early detection of pancreatic neoplasia. Semin Oncol 2007;34:303–10.

[28] Goldin SB, Bradner MW, Zervos EE, Rosemurgy 2nd AS. Assessment of pancreatic neoplasms: review of biopsy techniques. J Gastrointest Surg 2007;11:783–90.

[29] Kaur S, Baine MJ, Jain M, Sasson AR, Batra SK. Early diagnosis of pancreatic cancer: challenges and new developments. Biomark Med 2012;6:597–612.

[30] McKinney KQ, Lee JG, Sindram D, Russo MW, Han DK, Bonkovsky HL, et al. Identification of differentially expressed proteins from primary versus metastatic pancreatic cancer cells using subcellular proteomics. Cancer Genomics Proteomics 2012;9:257–63.

[31] Qi T, Han J, Cui Y, Zong M, Liu X, Zhu B. Comparative proteomic analysis for the detection of biomarkers in pancreatic ductal adenocarcinomas. J Clin Pathol 2008;61:49–58.

[32] Chen JH, Ni RZ, Xiao MB, Guo JG, Zhou JW. Comparative proteomic analysis of differentially expressed proteins in human pancreatic cancer tissue. Hepatobiliary Pancreat Dis Int 2009;8:193–200.

[33] Chung JC, Oh MJ, Choi SH, Bae CD. Proteomic analysis to identify biomarker proteins in pancreatic ductal adenocarcinoma. ANZ J Surg 2008;78:245–51.

[34] Shen J, Person MD, Zhu J, Abbruzzese JL, Li D. Protein expression profiles in pancreatic adenocarcinoma compared with normal pancreatic tissue and tissue affected by pancreatitis as detected by two-dimensional gel electrophoresis and mass spectrometry. Cancer Res 2004;64:9018–26.

[35] Githens S. The pancreatic duct cell: proliferative capabilities, specific characteristics, metaplasia, isolation, and culture. J Pediatr Gastroenterol Nutr 1988;7:486–506.

[36] Espina V, Wulfkuhle JD, Calvert VS, VanMeter A, Zhou W, Coukos G, et al. Laser-capture microdissection. Nat Protoc 2006;1:586–603.

[37] Waanders LF, Chwalek K, Monetti M, Kumar C, Lammert E, Mann M. Quantitative proteomic analysis of single pancreatic islets. Proc Natl Acad Sci USA 2009;106:18902–7.

[38] Shekouh AR, Thompson CC, Prime W, Campbell F, Hamlett J, Herrington CS, et al. Application of laser capture microdissection combined with two-dimensional electrophoresis for the discovery of differentially regulated proteins in pancreatic ductal adenocarcinoma. Proteomics 2003;3:1988–2001.

[39] Prinz T, Muller J, Kuhn K, Schafer J, Thompson A, Schwarz J, et al. Characterization of low abundant membrane proteins using the protein sequence tag technology. J Proteome Res 2004;3:1073–81.

[40] Boyd ZS, Raja R, Johnson S, Eberhard DA, Lackner MR. A tumor sorting protocol that enables enrichment of pancreatic adenocarcinoma cells and facilitation of genetic analyses. J Mol Diagn 2009;11:290–7.

[41] Li D, Peng SY, Zhang ZW, Feng RC, Li L, Liang J, et al. Complete disassociation of adult pancreas into viable single cells through cold trypsin-EDTA digestion. J Zhejiang Univ Sci B 2013;14:596–603.

[42] Palagani V, El Khatib M, Kossatz U, Bozko P, Muller MR, Manns MP, et al. Epithelial mesenchymal transition and pancreatic tumor initiating CD44+/EpCAM+ cells are inhibited by gamma-secretase inhibitor IX. PLoS One 2012;7:e46514.

[43] van der Gun BT, Melchers LJ, Ruiters MH, de Leij LF, McLaughlin PM, Rots MG. EpCAM in carcinogenesis: the good, the bad or the ugly. Carcinogenesis 2010;31:1913–21.

[44] Bledi Y, Inberg A, Linial M. PROCEED: a proteomic method for analysing plasma membrane proteins in living mammalian cells. Brief Funct Genomic Proteomic 2003;2:254–65.

[45] Lander ES, Linton LM, Birren B, Nusbaum C, Zody MC, Baldwin J, et al. Initial sequencing and analysis of the human genome. Nature 2001;409:860–921.

[46] Venter JC, Adams MD, Myers EW, Li PW, Mural RJ, Sutton GG, et al. The sequence of the human genome. Science 2001;291:1304–51.

[47] Fagerberg L, Jonasson K, von Heijne G, Uhlen M, Berglund L. Prediction of the human membrane proteome. Proteomics 2010;10:1141–9.

[48] Arachea BT, Sun Z, Potente N, Malik R, Isailovic D, Viola RE. Detergent selection for enhanced extraction of membrane proteins. Protein Expr Purif 2012;86:12–20.

[49] Paulo JA, Gaun A, Kadiyala V, Ghoulidi A, Banks PA, Conwell DL, et al. Subcellular fractionation enhances proteome coverage of pancreatic duct cells. Biochim Biophys Acta 2013;1834:791–7.

[50] Rabilloud T. Membrane proteins and proteomics: love is possible, but so difficult. Electrophoresis 2009;30(Suppl. 1):S174–180.

[51] Domon B, McCaffery I, Ryan TE, Applera Corporation, United States assignee. Selective capture and enrichment of proteins expressed on the cell surface United States Patents US 7348416. March 28, 2008.

[52] Aggarwal S, He T, Fitzhugh W, Rosenthal K, Feild B, Heidbrink J, et al. Immune modulator CD70 as a potential cisplatin resistance predictive marker in ovarian cancer. Gynecol Oncol 2009;115:430–7.

[53] Fang DD, Kim YJ, Lee CN, Aggarwal S, McKinnon K, Mesmer D, et al. Expansion of CD133(+) colon cancer cultures retaining stem cell properties to enable cancer stem cell target discovery. Br J Cancer 2010;102:1265–75.

[54] Tannu NS, Hemby SE. Two-dimensional fluorescence difference gel electrophoresis for comparative proteomics profiling. Nat Protoc 2006;1:1732–42.

[55] Kasthuri RS, Taubman MB, Mackman N. Role of tissue factor in cancer. J Clin Oncol 2009;27:4834–8.

[56] Khorana AA, Ahrendt SA, Ryan CK, Francis CW, Hruban RH, Hu YC, et al. Tissue factor expression, angiogenesis, and thrombosis in pancreatic cancer. Clin Cancer Res 2007;13:2870–5.

[57] Hobbs JE, Zakarija A, Cundiff DL, Doll JA, Hymen E, Cornwell M, et al. Alternatively spliced human tissue factor promotes tumor growth and angiogenesis in a pancreatic cancer tumor model. Thromb Res 2007;120(Suppl. 2):S13–21.

[58] Bandyopadhyay A, Raghavan S. Defining the role of integrin alpha v beta 6 in cancer. Curr Drug Targets 2009;10:645–52.

[59] Ahmed N, Riley C, Rice GE, Quinn MA, Baker MS. Alpha v beta 6 integrin-A marker for the malignant potential of epithelial ovarian cancer. J Histochem Cytochem 2002;50:1371–80.

[60] Yang GY, Xu KS, Pan ZQ, Zhang ZY, Mi YT, Wang JS, et al. Integrin alpha v beta 6 mediates the potential for colon cancer cells to colonize in and metastasize to the liver. Cancer Sci 2008;99:879–87.

[61] Hezel AF, Deshpande V, Zimmerman SM, Contino G, Alagesan B, O'Dell MR, et al. TGF-beta and alpha v beta 6 integrin act in a common pathway to suppress pancreatic cancer progression. Cancer Res 2012;72:4840–5.

[62] Suhail M. Na, K-ATPase: ubiquitous multifunctional transmembrane protein and its relevance to various pathophysiological conditions. J Clin Med Res 2010;2: 1–17.

[63] Yamanaka Y, Onda M, Uchida E, Yokomuro S, Hayashi T, Kobayashi T, et al. Immunohistochemical localization of Na^+, K^+-ATPase in human normal and malignant pancreatic tissues. Nihon Ika Daigaku Zasshi 1989;56:579–83.

[64] Ueno S, Takeda K, Noguchi S, Kawamura M. Significance of the beta-subunit in the biogenesis of $Na^+/K(+)$-ATPase. Biosci Rep 1997;17:173–88.

[65] Dimas K, Papadopoulou N, Baskakis C, Prousis KC, Tsakos M, Alkahtani S, et al. Steroidal cardiac Na^+/K^+ ATPase inhibitors exhibit strong anti-cancer potential in vitro and in prostate and lung cancer xenografts in vivo. Anticancer Agents Med Chem 2013, [Epub ahead of print].

[66] Kaur G, Dufour JM. Cell lines: valuable tools or useless artifacts. Spermatogenesis 2013;2:1–5.

[67] Yoshino K, Iimura E, Saijo K, Iwase S, Fukami K, Ohno T, et al. Essential role for gene profiling analysis in the authentication of human cell lines. Hum Cell 2006;19:43–8.

[68] Voduc D, Kenney C, Nielsen TO. Tissue microarrays in clinical oncology. Semin Radiat Oncol 2008;18:89–97.

[69] Carter P, Smith L, Ryan M. Identification and validation of cell surface antigens for antibody targeting in oncology. Endocr Relat Cancer 2004;11:659–87.

[70] Mittal R, Bruchez MP. Calibration of flow cytometry for quantitative quantum dot measurements. Curr Protoc Cytom 2009. [Chapter 6], Unit 6, 26.

[71] Schwartz A, Marti GE, Poon R, Gratama JW, Fernandez-Repollet E. Standardizing flow cytometry: a classification system of fluorescence standards used for flow cytometry. Cytometry 1998;33:106–14.

[72] Wu Y, Campos SK, Lopez GP, Ozbun MA, Sklar LA, Buranda T. The development of quantum dot calibration beads and quantitative multicolor bioassays in flow cytometry and microscopy. Anal Biochem 2007;364:180–92.

[73] Rich IN. In vitro hematotoxicity testing in drug development: a review of past, present and future applications. Curr Opin Drug Discov Devel 2003;6:100–9.

[74] Deftereos SN, Andronis C, Friedla EJ, Persidis A, Persidis A. Drug repurposing and adverse event prediction using high-throughput literature analysis. Wiley Interdiscip Rev Syst Biol Med 2011;3:323–34.

[75] Berlow N, Davis LE, Cantor EL, Seguin B, Keller C, Pal R. A new approach for prediction of tumor sensitivity to targeted drugs based on functional data. BMC Bioinformatics 2013;14:239.

[76] Hughes JP, Rees S, Kalindjian SB, Philpott KL. Principles of early drug discovery. Br J Pharmacol 2010;162:1239–49.

[77] Bordeaux J, Welsh A, Agarwal S, Killiam E, Baquero M, Hanna J, et al. Antibody validation. Biotechniques 2010;48:197–209.

[78] Mohr S, Bakal C, Perrimon N. Genomic screening with RNAi: results and challenges. Annu Rev Biochem 2010;79:37–64.

[79] Cejka D, Losert D, Wacheck V. Short interfering RNA (siRNA): tool or therapeutic? Clin Sci (Lond) 2006;110:47–58.

[80] Rayburn ER, Zhang R. Antisense, RNAi, and gene silencing strategies for therapy: mission possible or impossible? Drug Discov Today 2008;13:513–21.

[81] Hannon GJ. RNA interference. Nature 2002;418:244–51.

[82] Meister G, Landthaler M, Dorsett Y, Tuschl T. Sequence-specific inhibition of microRNA- and siRNA-induced RNA silencing. RNA 2004;10:544–50.

[83] Kim D, Rossi J. RNAi mechanisms and applications. Biotechniques 2008;44:613–6.

[84] Billy E, Brondani V, Zhang H, Muller U, Filipowicz W. Specific interference with gene expression induced by long, double-stranded RNA in mouse embryonal teratocarcinoma cell lines. Proc Natl Acad Sci USA 2001;98:14428–33.

[85] Moore CB, Guthrie EH, Huang MT, Taxman DJ. Short hairpin RNA (shRNA): design, delivery, and assessment of gene knockdown. Methods Mol Biol 2010;629:141–58.

[86] Wilda M, Fuchs U, Wossmann W, Borkhardt A. Killing of leukemic cells with a BCR/ABL fusion gene by RNA interference (RNAi). Oncogene 2002;21:5716–24.

[87] Elbashir SM, Martinez J, Patkaniowska A, Lendeckel W, Tuschl T. Functional anatomy of siRNAs for mediating efficient RNAi in *Drosophila melanogaster* embryo lysate. Embo J 2001;20:6877–88.

[88] Reynolds A, Leake D, Boese Q, Scaringe S, Marshall WS, Khvorova A. Rational siRNA design for RNA interference. Nat Biotechnol 2004;22:326–30.

[89] Bramsen JB, Kjems J. Development of therapeutic-grade small interfering RNAs by chemical engineering. Front Genet 2012;3:154.

[90] Chan CY, Carmack CS, Long DD, Maliyekkel A, Shao Y, Roninson IB, et al. A structural interpretation of the effect of GC-content on efficiency of RNA interference. BMC Bioinformatics 2009;10(Suppl. 1):S33.

[91] Gredell JA, Berger AK, Walton SP. Impact of target mRNA structure on siRNA silencing efficiency: a large-scale study. Biotechnol Bioeng 2008;100:744–55.

[92] Snead NM, Wu X, Li A, Cui Q, Sakurai K, Burnett JC, et al. Molecular basis for improved gene silencing by Dicer substrate interfering RNA compared with other siRNA variants. Nucleic Acids Res 2013;41:6209–21.

[93] Semizarov D, Kroeger P, Fesik S. siRNA-mediated gene silencing: a global genome view. Nucleic Acids Res 2004;32:3836–45.

[94] Schwarz DS, Ding H, Kennington L, Moore JT, Schelter J, Burchard J, et al. Designing siRNA that distinguish between genes that differ by a single nucleotide. PLoS Genet 2006;2:e140.

[95] Parsons BD, Schindler A, Evans DH, Foley E. A direct phenotypic comparison of siRNA pools and multiple individual duplexes in a functional assay. PLoS One 2009;4:e8471.

[96] Echeverri CJ, Perrimon N. High-throughput RNAi screening in cultured cells: a user's guide. Nat Rev Genet 2006;7:373–84.

[97] Hutvagner G. Small RNA asymmetry in RNAi: function in RISC assembly and gene regulation. FEBS Lett 2005;579:5850–7.

[98] Chung N, Locco L, Huff KW, Bartz S, Linsley PS, Ferrer M, et al. An efficient and fully automated high-throughput transfection method for genome-scale siRNA screens. J Biomol Screen 2008;13:142–8.

[99] Rantala JK, Makela R, Aaltola AR, Laasola P, Mpindi JP, Nees M, et al. A cell spot microarray method for production of high density siRNA transfection microarrays. BMC Genomics 2011;12:162.

[100] Vogler M, Walczak H, Stadel D, Haas TL, Genze F, Jovanovic M, et al. Small molecule XIAP inhibitors enhance TRAIL-induced apoptosis and antitumor activity in preclinical models of pancreatic carcinoma. Cancer Res 2009;69:2425–34.

Systems and Network Understanding of Pancreatic Cancer Signaling

The Significance of the Feedback Loops between Kras and Ink4a in Pancreatic Cancer

Baltazar D. Aguda
DiseasePathways LLC, Bethesda, MD, USA

Contents

Introduction 281
Threshold of Kras Activation 282
Kras Effector Pathways in PDAC Development 285
Negative versus Positive Feedback Loops between Kras and Ink4a 288
Ink4a against microRNAs in the Control of Kras 289
Concluding Remarks 291
References 293

INTRODUCTION

Molecular feedback mechanisms lend robustness and the ability of living cells to respond and adapt to their environment. As a means to ward off cancer, for example, the expression of proto-oncogenes in response to growth factors is normally followed by the expression of tumor suppressor genes. Myc and p53—a proto-oncogene and a tumor suppressor gene, respectively—are good examples of genes with concomitant expressions; and, in fact, several molecular pathways (direct and indirect) by which Myc upregulates p53, as well as pathways by which p53 downregulates Myc, have been identified (see [1] for a review). Thus, negative feedback loops (nFBLs) between Myc and p53 exist (and we have analyzed and modeled how these nFBLs coordinate cell proliferation and differentiation [1]). In this chapter, we investigate the nFBL between two genes, Kras and Ink4a, that are implicated in the early stages of pancreatic ductal adenocarcinoma (PDAC) development. Oncogenic mutations in Kras and loss or deficiency of Ink4a are exhibited by an overwhelming majority of PDAC patients [2–5] and in various other human cancers [6].

Molecular Diagnostics and Treatment of Pancreatic Cancer

The significance of the Kras–Ink4a nFBL may be related to its role in determining thresholds of Kras activation. Note that individuals with oncogenic Kras mutations can remain normal and healthy, perhaps because a certain threshold of Kras activity has not been reached. To explore this idea, we discuss the possible factors determining this threshold in the section Threshold of Kras Activation. At the single molecule level, Kras switches between inactive and active protein conformations; but, at the level of protein population (in a single cell), Kras activity behaves more like a rheostat rather than a switch [7]. We shall discuss how positive feedback from Kras effector signaling pathways to Kras itself can influence the value of Kras activation threshold. A few of these effector pathways are considered in the section Kras Effector Pathways in PDAC Development, with discussion of their potential control points and the effects of their perturbations on the cell cycle and apoptosis—processes that ultimately determine the rate of tumor growth.

In our review of Myc-p53 interactions [1], we indicated pathways by which Myc downregulates p53 in abnormal conditions (as in various cancers). The mutual downregulation between Myc and p53 constitutes a positive feedback loop (pFBL) that weakens the normal nFBL between them. A similar pFBL can occur between Kras and Ink4a. In the section Negative versus Positive Feedback Loops between Kras and Ink4a, we discuss a case where Kras indirectly downregulates Ink4a, thus forming a pFBL between Kras and Ink4a. This pFBL creates a potentially unstable situation where Ink4a is suppressed and a runaway Kras activation may ensue.

In the section Ink4a against microRNAs in the Control of Kras, we give examples of Kras-mediated pathways that affect the expressions of microRNAs (miRs) whose targets feed back to Kras. Although these feedbacks are all pFBLs, they are different in details: one set is characterized by mutual upregulation between Kras and a miR, while the other set involves mutual antagonism between Kras and a miR. This section illustrates how the nFBL between Kras and Ink4a may play a role in suppressing the deregulatory effects of the miR-mediated pFBLs that can amplify Kras activity.

In the last section, Concluding Remarks, we give a summary of the complexity and confounding features of these Kras pathways, and the role that mathematical and computational modeling can play to increase our understanding of the system.

THRESHOLD OF KRAS ACTIVATION

Activating mutations in the KRAS gene (e.g., KrasG12D) may also be found in normal healthy individuals and are therefore not reliable markers for PDAC [8,9]. It is believed that Kras proteins must be activated beyond a certain threshold before initiating cell transformation. We define a "threshold" to mean a particular level of an input signal below which there is no (or insignificant) response and above which there is a significant response (a binary switch would have a zero or full response below or above the threshold, respectively). As we shall see in this section, there can be different thresholds of Kras activation—one viewed at the single-protein level where switching between structural conformations occurs, and another at the protein population level where Kras effector pathways are involved, particularly those that positively feed back to Kras.

A property of a Ras (Kras, Hras, Nras) protein that makes it an appropriate decision element for signal transmission is the ability to act as a binary switch between different structural conformations depending on whether it is bound to GDP (guanosine diphosphate) or GTP (guanosine triphosphate) (see Figure 12.1 and Refs [10–12]). GTP-bound Ras is said to be active because it can interact with proteins involved at the head of Ras effector pathways. GDP-bound Ras has significantly reduced ability for such interactions and is therefore referred to as inactive. Guanine nucleotide exchange factors (GEFs) catalyze Ras activation by stimulating the exchange between the GDP bound to Ras and cytosolic GTP. On the other hand, GTPase-activating proteins (GAPs) inactivate Ras by catalyzing the hydrolysis of bound GTP to GDP. Ras itself has an intrinsic GAP activity. The detailed mechanism and kinetics of these processes have been and are being investigated (for example, see Refs [12–15]).

In a population of Ras proteins (in a single cell), because of the variable ratios between active and inactive Ras proteins, the activity of the ensemble of Ras proteins is expected to behave more like a rheostat [7]—one in which the overall Kras population activity is monotonously regulated and without noticeable switching features. Activating mutations in the Kras gene have been found to drastically change the ratio of GDP-bound to GTP-bound Ras. Under basal resting conditions, it is estimated that the percentage of GTP-bound Ras is less than 5% for wild-type Ras, compared to over 50% for Ras with oncogenic mutations [16]. Among the possible reasons for the increased levels of GTP-bound Ras mutants, insensitivity to GAPs and significant reduction of the intrinsic GTPase activity of Kras have been shown to be the primary reasons [8,17–19].

As depicted in Figure 12.1, Kras effector pathways can induce cells to produce cytokines, growth factors, and inflammatory mediators that drive Kras activation in autocrine or paracrine manner in a cell population [7,8]. For example, it has been shown by various groups [8,20] that the NF-κB

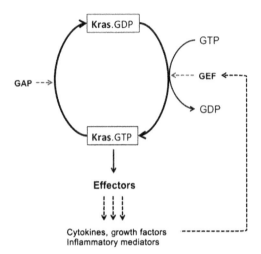

Figure 12.1 *The Kras GTPase Cycle Showing Cycling between GDP-Bound and GTP-Bound Kras, Catalyzed by a GAP (GTPase activating proteins) and a GEF (Guanine nucleotide exchange factor).* The long dashed curve represents positive feedback loops from molecules induced by Kras effector pathways. *Figure is modified from Ref. [7].*

pathway is involved in the pFBL that drives Kras activity to prolonged and sustained levels (this loop involves an NF-κB target, Cox-2, which is an enzyme that induces several mediators of inflammation such as PGE2).

The positive feedback to the KRas GTPase cycle (see Figure 12.1) generates an interesting threshold on Kras activity. We have shown earlier [21] that a positive feedback to a cyclic reaction can create a threshold that depends on the total level of the proteins involved in the cycle (in the present case, the total of inactive and active Kras proteins). Our previous results are summarized in Figure 12.2. In Figure 12.2(B), the steady state level of active Ras ($R_{a,ss}$) is plotted against total Ras protein (R_{total}). It was shown that below a certain level of R_{total} (this level is indicated by $R\star$ in Figure 12.2(B)), active Ras always goes to zero at steady state (the "s" above the zero horizontal line for R_{total} less than $R\star$ in the figure indicates that the zero steady state is stable—in the sense that any perturbation out of the zero state always returns to zero eventually; in other words, there could be transient Ras activities, but these transients eventually go to zero). This zero steady state still exists beyond $R\star$ but is now unstable (shown by the dashed line in Figure 12.2(B) and labeled "u") in the sense that a small perturbation will always increase until a positive value of the steady state is reached; this locus of positive steady states is shown by the solid diagonal line to the right

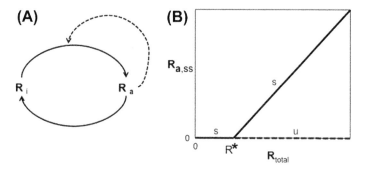

Figure 12.2 (A) A positive feedback loop (dashed curve) coupled with the R_i–R_a cycle. This loop means that the rate of production of R_a is a function of R_a as well as R_i. (R_a=active Ras, R_i=inactive Ras); (B) The steady state of R_a ($R_{a,ss}$) as a function of R_{total} (=R_i+R_a) for the case when the kinetics of the forward and reverse reactions is mass action (see Ref. [21] for more details). *Figure is modified from Ref. [21].*

of $R^\star$. As shown, $R_{a,ss}$ increases as R_{total} increases beyond $R^\star$. We emphasize that as long as R_{total} is below $R^\star$, the inactive state is the only state that exists at steady state.

The parameter that controls the Kras activation threshold is R_{total} (Figure 12.2(B)), the total Ras protein, and attention should be given to studies on the regulation of total Ras protein levels [8,22,23]. For a better understanding of Kras activity thresholds, the details of the pFBLs between Kras and its effector pathways (dashed curves in Figures 12.1 and 12.2(A)) would have to be elucidated.

KRAS EFFECTOR PATHWAYS IN PDAC DEVELOPMENT

Signals from membrane receptors (such as receptor tyrosine kinases) are transduced to Kras proteins via adapter proteins that may act as GEFs. These signals are then transmitted through cascades of protein–protein interactions that may or may not reach cellular machineries such as the cell cycle engine driven by the CDKs (cyclin-dependent kinases) or the apoptotic machinery driven by caspases. In this section, we briefly discuss a couple of the Kras effector pathways that have been implicated in pancreatic cancer. We do not give a comprehensive review of these pathways here but merely intend to give examples of the complexities in the cell-fate decision programs orchestrated by the Raf/Erk and Pi3k/Akt signaling pathways as they are currently understood (Figure 12.3).

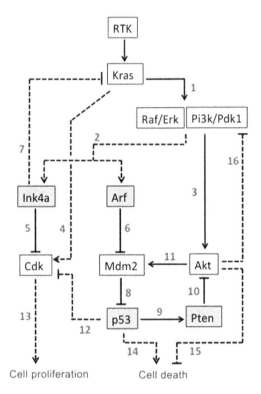

Figure 12.3 *Simplified Picture of the Kras Effector Pathways that Involve Raf/Erk and Pi3k/Akt.* Solid curves are direct interactions. Dashed curves are indirect. An arrow means "activates" or "upregulates"; a hammerhead means "inhibits" or "downregulates". See text for more details. White boxes are proto-oncogenes; gray boxes are tumor suppressor genes.

Step 1 represents processes leading to the activation of Pi3k or Raf—the initial proteins in the Pi3k/Akt pathway and Raf/Erk pathway, respectively. Pi3k (a lipid kinase and a p85/p110 heterodimer) and Pdk1 (a serine–threonine protein kinase) participate in the activation of Akt (a serine–threonine protein kinase); for a detailed review of Akt signaling, see [24]. Akt and Pdk1 are separately recruited to the plasma membrane by binding to PIP3 (phosphatidylinositol-3,4,5-trisphosphate). PIP2 (phosphatidylinositol-4,5-bisphosphate) is phosphorylated to PIP3 by Pi3k. Pdk1 phosphorylates Akt, thereby contributing to the activation of the latter. Pten, a lipid phosphatase, indirectly inhibits Akt (Step 10 in Figure 12.3) by dephosphorylating PIP3 (that is, counteracting the action of Pi3k). Akt is referred to as a survival factor because it suppresses apoptosis in various ways, including the sequence of

Steps 11, 8, and 14; other pathways that may involve suppression of pro-apoptotic factors are represented by Step 15. There also are various Akt pathways that promote cell proliferation, for example, the sequence of Steps 11, 8, and 12, and others not shown in Figure 12.3 (reviewed in Ref. [24]).

The cycle composed of Steps 8, 9, 10, and 11 effectively represents a mutual antagonism between the potentially oncogenic proteins Akt and Mdm2, on the one hand, and the tumor suppressors p53 and Pten, on the other hand [1,25,26].

As represented in Step 2, the Pi3k/Akt and Raf/Erk pathways induce the expression of the Cdkn2a gene locus that gives rise to two distinct proteins, Ink4a and Arf, by translating a common exon in alternative reading frames. Both Ink4a and Arf are tumor suppressors. In Step 5, Ink4a binds and inhibits Cdk4 and Cdk6 (cyclin-dependent kinases that drive the G1 to S phase transition of the cell cycle). Arf binds to Mdm2, thus preventing the latter's ability to downregulate p53; also, Arf arrests the cell cycle indirectly via Steps 6, 8, and 12 (net of Cdk inhibition), and can also promote apoptosis via Steps 6, 8, and 14. As indicated by Step 6, the absence of Raf would promote the Mdm2-induced degradation of p53. Pten is then expected to be downregulated, thereby increasing Akt activity. Loss of Pten has been shown to accelerate oncogenic mutant Kras-induced pancreatic cancer [27]; and combination of oncogenic Kras and Pten loss has been observed to induce NF-κB activity [28], which could further accelerate Kras activation through the positive feedback loop (dashed curve) shown in Figure 12.1.

Activation of the Pi3k/Akt pathway has been claimed to be necessary and sufficient for initiating pancreatic carcinogenesis [7,29]. A central role for the Raf-Mek-Erk pathway in generating PDAC has also been proposed [30]. Indeed, it may be necessary to inhibit multiple Kras-effector pathways in order to succeed in suppressing PDAC development.

Step 13 represents pathways that drive the cell cycle engine, including the Rb (retinoblastoma)/E2f pathway. Kras-induced senescence is believed to occur via pathways that are downstream of Ink4a and Arf, leading to inhibition of Cdk4/6. As depicted in Step 4, however, there exist possible pathways from Kras that positively regulate the cell cycle [31,32] or inhibit senescence [33]. It has been observed that increasing the activity of the Pi3k/Akt pathway dampens Ras-induced senescence [33]. This observation could be explained by the fact that there are pathways from Akt that promote Cdk activity (e.g., the sequence of Steps 11, 8, and 12).

Figure 12.3 is a schematic diagram of a more complex network. Every step of the Raf/Erk pathway has a nFBL [34]. Also, there are nFBLs in the

Pi3k/Akt pathway as shown in Step 16 in Figure 12.3 (for example, the nFBL involving mTORC1, S6K, IRS1, and Pi3k) [34,35]. It is conceivable that these nFBLs also contribute to the cell's repertoire of fine tuners and failsafe mechanisms against pathologically overactive proliferative signals. A very important negative feedback to Kras, represented by Step 7 in Figure 12.3, comes from Ink4a and will be discussed next.

NEGATIVE VERSUS POSITIVE FEEDBACK LOOPS BETWEEN KRAS AND INK4A

The Ink4a tumor suppressor is a sensor of oncogenic stress, being upregulated in response to potentially oncogenic signals such as high levels of Kras activity [36,37]. Kras-mediated induction of Ink4a is shown by Steps 1 and 2 in Figure 12.3.

Some details of the negative feedback from Ink4a to Kras (Step 7, Figure 12.3) are reported in a recent work of Rabien et al. [22]. It was shown that Ink4a suppresses Kras expression and reduces Kras protein stability. Steps 1, 2, and 7 (Figure 12.3) therefore form a nFBL (we refer to the Kras-Ink4a nFBL as the *KI-nFBL*). The significance of the KI-nFBL in the regulation of Kras activity in PDAC development is manifested in the consequences of the loss of Ink4a function in early PanINs (pancreatic intraepithelial neoplasia). The KI-nFBL may act to counterbalance the pFBLs shown in Figure 12.1 that promote runaway Kras activity.

Intriguingly, oncogenic Ras effector pathways that inhibit expression of Ink4a (Step 2 in Figure 12.4(A)) may exist. An example would be the combination of Steps 2a and 2b in Figure 12.4(B), which is a network model proposed by Ohtani et al. [37]. Kras-induced elevation of DNMT1 (DNA (Cytosine-5-)-Methyltransferase 1) causes epigenetic repression of Ink4a and subsequent proliferative burst of oncogenic Kras mutant cells; this burst generates accumulation of DNA damage and increase in ROS (reactive oxygen species), ultimately blocking DNMT1 expression. This is an example of a cross talk between the Ink4a and p53 pathways through the DNA damage response (DDR) pathway. An interesting conclusion of Ohtani et al. [37] is that the DDR pathway–induced expression of Ink4a is accelerated when p53 function is lost. Another example of Kras repressing the expression of Ink4a is provided by Lee et al. [38] who showed that a Kras-induced transcription factor, Twist, abrogates Ink4a induction.

The pFBL between Kras and Ink4a (Steps 2 and 3 in Figure 12.4(A)) is a potential source of instability in the system because suppression of Ink4a

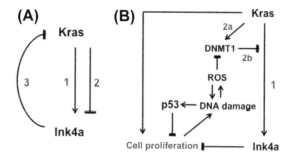

Figure 12.4 (A) Negative (edges 1,3) and positive (edges 2,3) feedback loops between Kras and Ink4a; (B) Kras can induce pathways that either inhibit or activate cell proliferation. A proliferative burst may occur with Kras-mediated upregulation of the DNMT1, which causes repression of Ink4a expression (edges 2a, 2b); the DNA damage response pathway (DDR) then downregulates DNMT1. *Figure B is modified from Ref. [37].*

could lead to runaway activation of Kras. The interplay between a nFBL (Steps 1 and 3) and a pFBL (Steps 2 and 3) is also a phenomenon observed in the interactions between Myc and p53, which we analyzed earlier [1]. Applying the same analysis, we can make the prediction that when the strength of the pFBL exceeds that of the nFBL between Kras and Ink4a, a switch to a significantly higher Kras activity occurs. The "strength" of a cycle is defined as the product of the individual strengths of the component edges (interactions) comprising the cycle [1].

INK4A AGAINST microRNAs IN THE CONTROL OF KRAS

MicroRNAs (miRs) are short (~18–24 nucleotides) endogenous noncoding RNAs that inhibit translation or induce degradation of their target mRNAs. Over half of mammalian transcripts have been predicted to be conserved targets of microRNAs [39]. MiRs play significant roles in the development of multicellular organisms, including processes that also occur during carcinogenesis. Changes in miR expression are investigated for their potential as diagnostic, prognostic, and therapeutic agents in cancer.

In this section, we focus on miRs that are differentially expressed during the early PanINs. We look at some miRs whose expressions are affected by Kras and are involved in pFBLs that amplify Kras oncogenic activity. The nFBL between Ink4a and Kras can then be viewed as acting to suppress these pFBLs. For more extensive discussions on the miRs involved in PDAC progression, see Refs [40–42].

MiRs that have been identified to target Kras include the following: let-7, miR-96, miR-143/145, miR-216b, and miR-126 [42–46]. Associated with elevated Kras activity, these miRs are observed to be downregulated in pancreatic cancer cells. Using transgenic mouse models that recapitulate PDAC progression, Ali et al. [42] report 187 miRs that significantly vary in expression between oncogenic mutant KrasG12D mice with and without Ink4a/Arf deficiency; among these, they further validated five oncogenic miRs (miR-21, miR-155, miR-221, miR-27a, miR-27b) and four tumor suppressor miRs (miR-216b, miR-216a, miR-217, miR-146a). It would be useful to elucidate the pathways that induce the expression of these miRs and how these pathways are connected to Kras.

Shown in Figure 12.5 are the Kras effector pathways that affect the expressions of miR-21 and the miR-143/145 cluster; note that the miR targets feed back to Kras and other steps in the Kras effector pathway.

MiR-21, an oncogenic miR that is elevated in early PanINs, is upregulated by Kras and EGFR, through the transcription factor AP-1 [43,47,48]. Important targets of miR-21 are the tumor suppressor Pten and the cell cycle inhibitor p21Cip1 [43,49]. MiR-21 can also drive tumorigenesis by targeting negative regulators of the MAPK (Ras/Erk) pathway such as Pdcd4, Sprouty genes, and Btg2 [50,51]. Btg2 reduces the active GTP-bound Kras state [52,53]. It has been shown that treating a panel of pancreatic cancer cell lines with antisense oligonucleotides against miR-21 arrests cell proliferation and induces apoptosis, and sensitizes cells to the effects of gemcitabine, a drug commonly used in PDAC therapy [43,54].

Loss of the miR-143/145 cluster is often observed in pancreatic cancers with oncogenic Kras mutants, and Kras activation causes downregulation of miR-143/145 in human and murine cells [45]; restoration of these miRs suppresses tumorigenesis [45]. Interestingly, it was also shown [45] that these miRs directly target RREB1 and Kras, thus, forming double-negative interactions (which are pFBLs) as shown in Figure 12.5.

The Kras-miR-21 pFBL is a double-positive loop, while that of Kras-miR-143/145 is a double-negative loop. Both are pFBLs but have different dynamics. The Kras-miR-143/145 loop acts as toggle switch that gives rise to an inverse relationship between Kras and miR levels. The Kras-miR-21 loop gives a direct relationship between Kras and miR-21 (this could act like a switch depending on the nonlinearity of the feedback interactions). Such relationships in terms of FBLs are not yet known for the miRs mentioned previously that directly target Kras, but it would be useful in the future to map the pathways between Kras and these miRs so we can have a handle on controlling their levels.

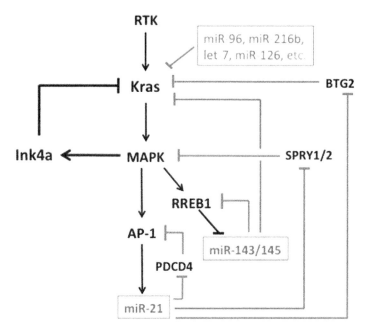

Figure 12.5 *The Kras-Ink4a Negative Feedback Loop versus the Positive Feedback Loops between Kras & miR-21, and between Kras & miR-143/145.* Figure is modified from Ref. [50].

CONCLUDING REMARKS

The concomitant Kras activating mutations and deficiencies in Ink4a/Arf in an overwhelming fraction of pancreatic cancers, especially in the early stages of PDAC development, illustrate the importance of studying the interactions between oncogenes and tumor suppressor genes that respond to these onco-genes. As with the Myc-p53 interactions [1], we have summarized here the evidence that there exists a negative feedback loop between Kras and Ink4a (KI–nFBL)—that is, activated Kras itself upregulates its downregulator, Ink4a, presumably to avoid overshooting a normal range of Kras activities. (In the language of dynamics, the KI–nFBL is a stabilizing feature of the network.) We have summarized the Kras effector pathways, Pi3k/At and Raf/Erk (Figure 12.3), to show examples of the confounding or even conflicting routes of signaling that decide whether a cell enters the cell cycle, becomes quiescent, or dies by apoptosis. We also highlighted recent reports about Kras effector pathways, especially those involving NF-κB, that induce cytokines and inflammatory mediators that then amplify Kras activity (Figure 12.1). These Kras effector pathways contribute to Kras activation thresholds (e.g., the value $R^\star$ shown in Figure 12.2(B)). Thus, the broad picture for

Kras activation involves not only the molecular-level parameters determining protein conformations but also the protein population–level kinetics and mechanisms of the nFBLs and pFBLs involving Kras effector pathways.

We have proposed the hypothesis that the KI-nFBL serves to counteract the pFBLs mediated by certain miRs (Figure 12.5) and the pFBLs induced by Kras effector pathways (Figure 12.1). If this hypothesis is valid, the disruption of KI-nFBL (due to loss or deficiency of Ink4a) would be predicted to have profound consequences on Kras activity and on all the pFBLs that Kras initiates—increasing Kras activity to pathological levels and accelerating cell transformation.

Admittedly, we have oversimplified the situation. It will be necessary to include the interactions of the Myc oncogene and p53 with Ras as depicted in Figure 12.6. Myc is overexpressed in pancreatic cancers [55], and p53 inactivating mutations show up in a majority of late PanINs and PDAC. The cooperation between Myc and Ras in cell transformation has been the subject of many papers (e.g., see Refs [56–58]). As shown in Figure 12.6, a nFBL between Ras and p53 exists (for the indirect interactions, see Ref. [59]).

To aid in the discovery of drug targets in complex pathways, it will be necessary to employ tools of mathematical network analysis and computer simulations [35]. These tools would allow us to perform network stability analysis (to discover nodes or edges that can be perturbed to elicit desired states of the cell) as well as in silico experimentation or simulations of drug dosing protocols. The reason for our focus on FBLs in this chapter is based on the results of stability analysis that cycles in qualitative networks (those with only arrows and hammerheads) are the determinants of stability [1]. We have provided an example of this stability analysis in our previous work on the Myc-p53 loop [1] where we also demonstrated how to define strengths of feedback cycles and find their relative values that destabilize the system.

It will also be necessary to deal with quantitative issues regarding Kras activity. As with Myc, and perhaps all proto-oncogenes, Ras promotes cell

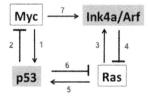

Figure 12.6 *Interactions among oncogenes (white boxes) and tumor suppressor genes (gray boxes).*

proliferation but, when overexpressed beyond a certain threshold, could trigger apoptosis [1,60]. The inhibition or insensitivity to apoptotic factors at Ras levels that would have triggered apoptosis in normal cells is a potential driver of cancer development. Thus, as with Myc, we predict that there is a range of Ras activities that lie within a "cancer zone" where the probability of initiating carcinogenesis becomes significant [1,61]

REFERENCES

[1] Aguda BD, Kim Y, Kim HS, Friedman A, Fine HA. Qualitative network modeling of the Myc-p53 control system of cell proliferation and differentiation. Biophys J 2011;101(9):2082–91.

[2] Almoguera C, Shibata D, Forrester K, Martin J, Arnheim N, Perucho M. Most human carcinomas of the exocrine pancreas contain mutant c-K-ras genes. Cell 1988;53(4):549–54.

[3] Singh SK, Ellenrieder V. Senescence in pancreatic carcinogenesis: from signalling to chromatin remodeling and epigenetics. Gut 2013;62(9):1364–72.

[4] Abramson MA, Jazag A, van der Zee JA, Whang EE. The molecular biology of pancreatic cancer. Gastrointest Cancer Res 2007;1(4 Suppl. 2):S7–12.

[5] Sharpless NE, DePinho RA. Cancer: crime and punishment. Nature 2005;436(7051): 636–7.

[6] Hezel AF, Kimmelman AC, Stanger BZ, Bardeesy N, Depinho RA. Genetics and biology of pancreatic ductal adenocarcinoma. Genes Dev 2006;20(10):1218–49.

[7] di Magliano MP, Logsdon CD. Roles for KRAS in pancreatic tumor development and progression. Gastroenterology 2013;144(6):1220–9.

[8] Daniluk J, Liu Y, Deng D, Chu J, Huang H, Gaiser S, et al. An NF-κB pathway-mediated positive feedback loop amplifies Ras activity to pathological levels in mice. J Clin Invest 2012;122(4):1519–28.

[9] Siveke JT, Crawford HC. KRAS above and beyond—EGFR in pancreatic cancer. Oncotarget 2012;3(11):1262–3.

[10] Vetter IR, Wittinghofer A. The guanine nucleotide-binding switch in three dimensions. Science 2001;294(5545):1299–304.

[11] Grant BJ, Gorfe AA, McCammon JA. Ras conformational switching: simulating nucleotide-dependent conformational transitions with accelerated molecular dynamics. PLoS Comput Biol 2009;5(3):e1000325.

[12] Hein C, Wittinghofer A, Dötsch V. How to switch a master switch. eLife 2013;2:e01159.

[13] Zhang B, Zhang Y, Shacter E, Zheng Y. Mechanism of the guanine nucleotide exchange reaction of Ras GTPase—evidence for a GTP/GDP displacement model. Biochemistry 2005;44(7):2566–76.

[14] Tian T, Plowman SJ, Parton RG, Kloog Y, Hancock JF. Mathematical modeling of K-Ras nanocluster formation on the plasma membrane. Biophys J 2010;99(2): 534–43.

[15] Marshall CB, Meiri D, Smith MJ, Mazhab-Jafari MT, Gasmi-Seabrook GM, Rottapel R, et al. Probing the GTPase cycle with real-time NMR: GAP and GEF activities in cell extracts. Methods 2012;57(4):473–85.

[16] Stites EC, Trampont PC, Ma Z, Ravichandran KS. Network analysis of oncogenic Ras activation in cancer. Science 2007;318(5849):463–7.

[17] Malumbres M, Barbacid M. RAS oncogenes: the first 30 years. Nat Rev Cancer 2003;3(6):459–65. Erratum in: Nat Rev Cancer. September 2003; 3(9):708.

[18] Downward J. Targeting RAS signalling pathways in cancer therapy. Nat Rev Cancer 2003;3(1):11–22.

[19] Ahmadian MR, Zor T, Vogt D, Kabsch W, Selinger Z, Wittinghofer A, et al. Guanosine triphosphatase stimulation of oncogenic Ras mutants. Proc Natl Acad Sci USA 1999;96(12):7065–70.

[20] Wang Z, Banerjee S, Ahmad A, Li Y, Azmi AS, Gunn JR, et al. Activated K-ras and INK4a/Arf deficiency cooperate during the development of pancreatic cancer by activation of Notch and NF-κB signaling pathways. PLoS One 2011;6(6):e20537.

[21] Aguda BD. Instabilities in phosphorylation-dephosphorylation cascades and cell cycle checkpoints. Oncogene 1999;18(18):2846–51.

[22] Rabien A, Sanchez-Ruderisch H, Schulz P, Otto N, Wimmel A, Wiedenmann B, et al. Tumor suppressor p16INK4a controls oncogenic K-Ras function in human pancreatic cancer cells. Cancer Sci 2012;103(2):169–75.

[23] Chen S, Auletta T, Dovirak O, Hutter C, Kuntz K, El-ftesi S, et al. Copy number alterations in pancreatic cancer identify recurrent PAK4 amplification. Cancer Biol Ther 2008;7(11):1793–802.

[24] Manning BD, Cantley LC. AKT/PKB signaling: navigating downstream. Cell 2007;129(7):1261–74.

[25] Mayo LD, Donner DB. The PTEN, Mdm2, p53 tumor suppressor-oncoprotein network. Trends Biochem Sci 2002;27(9):462–7.

[26] Wee KB, Aguda BD. Akt versus p53 in a network of oncogenes and tumor suppressor genes regulating cell survival and death. Biophys J 2006;91(3):857–65.

[27] Hill R, Calvopina JH, Kim C, Wang Y, Dawson DW, Donahue TR, et al. PTEN loss accelerates KrasG12D-induced pancreatic cancer development. Cancer Res 2010;70(18):7114–24.

[28] Ying H, Elpek KG, Vinjamoori A, Zimmerman SM, Chu GC, Yan H, et al. PTEN is a major tumor suppressor in pancreatic ductal adenocarcinoma and regulates an NF-κB-cytokine network. Cancer Discov 2011;1(2):158–69.

[29] Eser S, Reiff N, Messer M, Seidler B, Gottschalk K, Dobler M, et al. Selective requirement of PI3K/PDK1 signaling of Kras oncogene-driven pancreatic cell plasticity and cancer. Cancer Cell 2013;23(3):406–20.

[30] Collisson EA, Trejo CL, Silva JM, Gu S, Korkola JE, Heiser LM, et al. A central role for RAF→MEK→ERK signaling in the genesis of pancreatic ductal adenocarcinoma. Cancer Discov 2012;2(8):685–93.

[31] Fan J, Bertino JR. K-ras modulates the cell cycle via both positive and negative regulatory pathways. Oncogene 1997;14(21):2595–607.

[32] Takuwa N, Takuwa Y. Regulation of cell cycle molecules by the Ras effector system. Mol Cell Endocrinol 2001;177(1–2):25–33.

[33] Kennedy AL, Adams PD, Morton JP. Ras, PI3K/Akt and senescence: paradoxes provide clues for pancreatic cancer therapy. Small GTPases 2011;2(5):264–7.

[34] Mendoza MC, Er EE, Blenis J. The Ras-ERK and PI3K-mTOR pathways: cross-talk and compensation. Trends Biochem Sci 2011;36(6):320–8.

[35] Aguda BD. Network pharmacology of glioblastoma. Curr Drug Discov Technol 2013;10(2):125–38.

[36] Yamakoshi K, Takahashi A, Hirota F, Nakayama R, Ishimaru N, Kubo Y, et al. Real-time in vivo imaging of p16Ink4a reveals cross talk with p53. J Cell Biol 2009;186(3):393–407.

[37] Ohtani N, Yamakoshi K, Takahashi A, Hara E. Real-time in vivo imaging of p16gene expression: a new approach to study senescence stress signaling in living animals. Cell Div 2010;5:1.

[38] Lee KE, Bar-Sagi D. Oncogenic KRas suppresses inflammation-associated senescence of pancreatic ductal cells. Cancer Cell 2010;18(5):448–58.

[39] Friedman RC, Farh KK, Burge CB, Bartel DP. Most mammalian mRNAs are conserved targets of microRNAs. Genome Res 2009;19(1):92–105.

[40] Yu J, Li A, Hong SM, Hruban RH, Goggins M. MicroRNA alterations of pancreatic intraepithelial neoplasias. Clin Cancer Res 2012;18(4):981–92.

[41] Zhang L, Jamaluddin MS, Weakley SM, Yao Q, Chen C. Roles and mechanisms of microRNAs in pancreatic cancer. World J Surg 2011;35(8):1725–31.

[42] Ali S, Banerjee S, Logna F, Bao B, Philip PA, Korc M, et al. Inactivation of Ink4a/Arf leads to deregulated expression of miRNAs in K-Ras transgenic mouse model of pancreatic cancer. J Cell Physiol 2012;227(10):3373–80.

[43] Pai P, Rachagani S, Are C, Batra SK. Prospects of miRNA-based therapy for pancreatic cancer. Curr Drug Targets 2013;14(10):1101–9.

[44] Yu S, Lu Z, Liu C, Meng Y, Ma Y, Zhao W, et al. miRNA-96 suppresses KRAS and functions as a tumor suppressor gene in pancreatic cancer. Cancer Res 2010;70(14):6015–25.

[45] Kent OA, Chivukula RR, Mullendore M, Wentzel EA, Feldmann G, Lee KH, et al. Repression of the miR-143/145 cluster by oncogenic Ras initiates a tumor-promoting feed-forward pathway. Genes Dev 2010;24(24):2754–9.

[46] Jiao LR, Frampton AE, Jacob J, Pellegrino L, Krell J, Giamas G, et al. MicroRNAs targeting oncogenes are down-regulated in pancreatic malignant transformation from benign tumors. PLoS One 2012;7(2):e32068.

[47] du Rieu MC, Torrisani J, Selves J, Al Saati T, Souque A, Dufresne M, et al. MicroRNA-21 is induced early in pancreatic ductal adenocarcinoma precursor lesions. Clin Chem 2010;56(4):603–12.

[48] Talotta F, Cimmino A, Matarazzo MR, Casalino L, De Vita G, D'Esposito M, et al. An autoregulatory loop mediated by miR-21 and PDCD4 controls the AP-1 activity in RAS transformation. Oncogene 2009;28(1):73–84.

[49] Dillhoff M, Liu J, Frankel W, Croce C, Bloomston M. MicroRNA-21 is overexpressed in pancreatic cancer and a potential predictor of survival. J Gastrointest Surg 2008;12(12):2171–6.

[50] Saj A, Lai EC. Control of microRNA biogenesis and transcription by cell signaling pathways. Curr Opin Genet Dev 2011;21(4):504–10.

[51] Hatley ME, Patrick DM, Garcia MR, Richardson JA, Bassel-Duby R, van Rooij E, et al. Modulation of K-Ras-dependent lung tumorigenesis by MicroRNA-21. Cancer Cell 2010;18(3):282–93.

[52] Liu M, Wu H, Liu T, Li Y, Wang F, Wan H, et al. Regulation of the cell cycle gene, BTG2, by miR-21 in human laryngeal carcinoma. Cell Res 2009;19(7):828–37.

[53] Boiko AD, Porteous S, Razorenova OV, Krivokrysenko VI, Williams BR, Gudkov AV. A systematic search for downstream mediators of tumor suppressor function of p53 reveals a major role of BTG2 in suppression of Ras-induced transformation. Genes Dev 2006;20(2):236–52.

[54] Park JK, Lee EJ, Esau C, Schmittgen TD. Antisense inhibition of microRNA-21 or -221 arrests cell cycle, induces apoptosis, and sensitizes the effects of gemcitabine in pancreatic adenocarcinoma. Pancreas 2009;38(7):e190–9.

[55] Buchholz M, Schatz A, Wagner M, Michl P, Linhart T, Adler G, et al. Overexpression of c-myc in pancreatic cancer caused by ectopic activation of NFATc1 and the Ca^{2+}/calcineurin signaling pathway. EMBO J 2006;25(15):3714–24.

[56] Wang C, Lisanti MP, Liao DJ. Reviewing once more the c-myc and Ras collaboration: converging at the cyclin D1-CDK4 complex and challenging basic concepts of cancer biology. Cell Cycle 2011;10(1):57–67.

[57] Yancopoulos GD, Nisen PD, Tesfaye A, Kohl NE, Goldfarb MP, Alt FW. N-myc can cooperate with ras to transform normal cells in culture. Proc Natl Acad Sci USA 1985;82(16):5455–9.

[58] Ischenko I, Zhi J, Moll UM, Nemajerova A, Petrenko O. Direct reprogramming by oncogenic Ras and Myc. Proc Natl Acad Sci USA 2013;110(10):3937–42.

[59] Buganim Y, Solomon H, Rais Y, Kistner D, Nachmany I, Brait M, et al. p53 regulates the Ras circuit to inhibit the expression of a cancer-related gene signature by various molecular pathways. Cancer Res 2010;70(6):2274–84.

[60] Overmeyer JH, Kaul A, Johnson EE, Maltese WA. Active ras triggers death in glioblastoma cells through hyperstimulation of macropinocytosis. Mol Cancer Res 2008;6(6):965–77.

[61] Aguda BD, Kim Y, Piper-Hunter MG, Friedman A, Marsh CB. MicroRNA regulation of a cancer network: consequences of the feedback loops involving miR-17-92, E2F, and Myc. Proc Natl Acad Sci USA 2008;105(50):19678–83.

Systems Biology of Pancreatic Cancer Stem Cells

Ginny F. Bao[1], Philip A. Philip[2], Asfar S. Azmi[1]
[1]Department of Pathology, Wayne State University School of Medicine, Detroit, MI, USA, [2]Department of Oncology, Karmanos Cancer Institute, Detroit, MI, USA

Contents

Introduction	297
The Complexity of Pancreatic Cancer	298
Why Systems Biology is Needed for PC	302
PC Therapy Resistance and the Role of Cancer Stem Cells	307
Isolation and Biological Characterization of PC CSCs	308
Systems and Pathway Analysis of CSCs	310
Systems Analysis of PC CSC MicroRNA Network	314
Summary and Future Directions	316
References	318

INTRODUCTION

Pancreatic cancer (PC) kills ~300,000 individuals worldwide, and each year in the United States there are an estimated 43,920 new diagnoses with an annual mortality of 37,390 [1,2]. It is one of the most difficult cancers to treat, with a five-year survival (<5%) due in part to the high degree of treatment resistance leading to failure of most of the available therapies. The etiology of the disease is mostly unknown. It is suggested that PC is correlated with tobacco use, diabetes, obesity, and chronic pancreatitis [3]. There also is a genetic basis to acquiring the disease, since 5–10% of patients have a family history of PC. A major stumbling block is that PC is diagnosed at a very late stage of the disease where invasion or metastatic spreads (both micro- and macro-metastases) have already occurred, contributing to a poor prognosis. In spite of the increased understanding of the mechanisms of PC development, there is no standardized diagnostic methodology for its early detection. Many of the symptoms initially described by patients go unnoticed by physicians due to their nonspecific and variable nature, resulting in misdiagnoses. This delay in identification after the onset of some symptoms is crucial for the future prospects of PC patients. Sadly, at the time of actual diagnosis, nearly half of the patients exhibit metastasis. Typically >80% have advanced or locally advanced disease, and less than 15% of patients have organ-confined disease at the original PC site. This is partly due to the long duration of time between disease onset and diagnosis. Frequently, PC can be identified during unrelated CT scans of patients, and several studies have attempted to derive structural similarities that may alert radiologists to a malignant presence before diagnosis. Some patients were identified as having PC retrospectively about 18 months prior to diagnosis while asymptomatic. The chance observations call for urgent innovations in the areas of early diagnosis and novel development of cytotoxic agents, as well as agents for "personalized medicine". Emerging advances would likely help in early diagnosis, for example, identification of circulating tumor cells related to PC metastasis and epithelial–mesenchymal transition (EMT), as well as identification of the PC stem-like cells (CSLCs or CSCs) that are increasingly being recognized to play a role in sustaining the heterogeneous and resistant nature of the disease.

THE COMPLEXITY OF PANCREATIC CANCER

Like many other cancers, PC can be defined in terms of accumulating genetic mutations in key tumor activator and inhibitor genes such as K-ras and a myriad other regulatory molecules [4]. Analyses of upstream regulators in PC progression models have identified members of the sonic hedgehog signaling pathway (SHH and Smo) as being aberrantly expressed in the precursor PanIN lesions, which highlights the role and degree of K-ras and HER2/neu mutations and their significance in the initial appearance of PanIN lesions [5]. The significance of the SHH pathway in PC was emphasized when it was demonstrated that inhibition of this pathway strengthened the efficacy of chemotherapy in vivo [6]. Related to K-ras is the delicate balance maintained through TGF-β family molecules with dual functions, both as oncogenic and as a tumor suppressor. Smad7 was found to inhibit the function of TGFβRI from phosphorylating Smad2 or Smad3, resulting in an increased tumorigenic potential in PC by preventing nuclear localization of Smad4 [7]. Disruption of Smad4 function has been realized as an indicator of decreased survival, yet some ambiguity of results has posed problems in accurately ascertaining the role of Smad4 dependency or TGFβ resistance in PC cells [8]. Moreover, studies have shown that inhibition of hedgehog signaling had a measurable effect on the EMT that is thought to be crucial for PC invasiveness and metastasis, mediated by downstream inhibition of Snail and Slug transcription factors [9] (the role of these important signaling molecules will be further clarified when we present the PC stem cell work following). Hedgehog has also been implicated in the development of stem cells, which are normally part of the gastrointestinal (GI) tissue development [10]. Generally, progression of PC involves mutations or abnormal expression of Pdx1, hedgehog signaling, K-ras, p16, p53, DPC4, and BRCA2, as well as their interacting molecules, resulting in carcinoma [11]. Figure 13.1 is the Ingenuity Pathway Analysis (IPA)–derived pathway depicting the involvement of various signaling pathways during the different stages of PC development. In addition to frequently cited mutations and aberrant expression of the DNA sequence, epigenetic factors have been implicated whether they are methylations or dysregulations of microRNAs (miRNAs), notably a detectable hypermethylation in developing PanINs [12].

Even with extensive knowledge gained over the vast array of molecular mechanisms involved in PC, early stage identification remains problematic and at times incidental. Under ideal circumstances, the majority of patients do not possess those traits. The resectability of a PC tumor represents the initial line of defense for the treatment of PC. Detection at early stages is key, yet even with resection under ideal circumstances, the five-year survival postresection holds at 20% [13]. Mortality postresection has been a point of debate with different attempts being made to measure markers of success or failure [14]. Problems in risk stratification and availability of the surgery have contributed to many patients not being offered this course of treatment, and despite resection, adjuvant therapies such as 5-FU, FOLFIRINOX, and gemcitabine are still the standard line of care for both unresectable and resectable tumors [15]. There is high desirability of testing for PC presence and treatment progress through serum biomarkers, yet one such strategy, the testing for biomarker CA19-9, a molecule frequently observed in PC patients, has shown low sensitivity and specificity [16]. Other molecules such as HCGβ and CA-72-5 have shown higher sensitivity than CA19-9 in the laboratory setting; however, these and other markers continue to be under investigation for further clinical efficacy as efficient biomarkers in PC [17]. Interestingly, some groups have used gemcitabine as a filter for resistance or sensitivity to treatments, and at least one

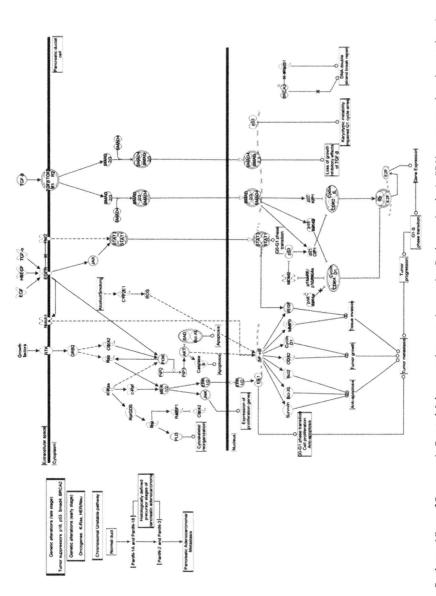

Figure 13.1 *Pathway View of Pancreatic Ductal Adenocarcinoma.* Ingenuity Pathway Analysis (IPA)–generated pathway showing different important signaling involved during the various stages of pancreatic cancer development from Normal Duct to PanIN-1A to PanIN-1B, PanIN-2, PanIN-3 to adenocarcinoma. (For color version of this figure, the reader is referred to the online version of this book.)

study was able to correlate treatment success by testing for the hENT1, a molecule that regulated gemcitabine uptake [18]. Using such a strategy, a more personalized approach was used in determining future treatment choice. The early models for studies have been aimed at precisely identifying the genetic basis of occurrence, especially of familial PC, by establishing a database to pinpoint what classifies the at-risk individuals [19]. A more generalized approach has been the use of traditional family medical histories, including diagnostic data, compared with data-based repositories to identify at-risk individuals through factors also outside genetics, such as risky behavior or environmental determinants [20]. Such a model is not new; however, it hedges a bet on the development of precise risk factors to ascertain the likelihood of PC development, some of which epidemiologically have seen a strong correlation to disease development [21]. The databases are a key step but are still in their infancy, with results anticipated in the future. Many other molecules have been characterized as possibly having high prognostic, diagnostic, or druggable values, although different studies performed have so far provided conflicting information as to their true nature in the management of PC [22]. This provides a unique problem that is only now being realized where single targets or even a small subset of related targets may not confer the expected outcome when targeted or used as biomarkers in PC.

The traditional strategies in designing treatment have centered around combination therapies as well as single-agent targeted therapies but have slowly shifted toward a multitargeted approach [23]. The identification of multiple pathways and effective targets has produced several approved inhibitors and multitarget drugs, yet a proper sequence of delivery remains a question due to the lack of comparative clinical studies [24]. One of the difficulties in the use of combination therapies is in part due to an unclear picture of precise molecular interactions between the different drugs within the used combination. In a previous study, we were able to demonstrate the delicate tug-of-war where oxaliplatin, a key component of FOLFOX and FOLFIRINOX combination therapies, participates in the activation of tumorigenic mechanisms [25]. PC is an inherently complex disease, with multiple factors influencing tumor growth, and contains very intricate genetic composition [26]. The key to better targeting and treatment depends on proper validation in the appropriate preclinical and clinical stages where accurate identification of biomarkers becomes vital in order to identify a patient population, predict efficacy in their treatment, and assess the mechanism of treatment failure [27].

WHY SYSTEMS BIOLOGY IS NEEDED FOR PC

Systems biology is the study of the interactions between different components of a biological system. It is the science that helps sieve through the complexity of interactions at multiple levels in any biological system, for example, how amino acids or DNA base pairs interact to give rise to a protein and gene, respectively. At the next level, it can help understand how different proteins interact in a single pathway. Further, using systems-based methods, one can evaluate how different pathways interact in a major signaling to give rise to a cellular phenotype. At the next level the science can help in deciphering the interaction between different cells in a tissue giving rise to the tissue phenotype, and, finally, how the different tissues interact at the organism level. Systems biology is characterized as an approach that utilizes isolated molecular and biological data and provides a macro context through "holistic" analysis, thereby providing the overall structural relationships, system dynamics, and internal interactions [28]. A number of fields have evolved from systems biology, and among them network pharmacology is increasingly being utilized in cancer research and drug discovery. Network pharmacology is the science that takes the information from biological networks and then identifies the important druggable entities within these networks that can be targeted to induce phenotypically meaningful changes in that network. Network pharmacology can allow disease stratification, biomarker identification, and other areas of cancer research that have been elaborated in our previous thematic issues and reviews [29]. A network approach to PC translational medicine has far-reaching potential in both cutting the cost and increasing accuracy of molecular understanding of the disease and in some instances delivering prognostic and diagnostic indicators [30]. The true value of these technologies in PC molecular diagnostics and therapy is due in part to obtaining meaningful data using modeling and simulation involving predictive methodologies, thereby giving conclusive and accurate results noninvasively. Additionally, through curation of available data on individual patients or from consolidated databases aggregating molecular profiles, superior diagnostics and drug combinations can be designed [31]. Data can be extracted to provide very attractive information related to the biological system-wide function of PC, providing context and discovery potential not previously seen [32]. High-throughput analysis of the proteomic profile of PC patients has established specificity and sensitivity to 100% in the identification of the disease [33].

Using such curation methodologies, evidence has surfaced from microarray analysis of a distinction in the genomic expression signatures of PC patients versus normal individuals [34]. Particularly useful is the ability to create an in silico environment improving upon the gained knowledge and observations through animal data, providing a uniquely human-databased analysis shedding light on key interactions possibly not obtainable through studies using orthotopic model alone. Evidence of this can be found through a simple comparison of genetically engineered and xenograft models, identifying the genetically engineered mice to provide more context for PC understanding in which we can infer the next logical step to be an in silico model of human PC [35]. Network and mathematical modeling have shed light on key questions of regulatory mechanisms in PC such as serine-phosphorylation of STAT1, opening up a new avenue in understanding signal transduction and regulation that may be related to specific patient subtypes [36]. Indeed, systems level analysis has provided a window of opportunity to fill the gaps of information between the xenograft model of PC and hypothesized mechanisms as well as a categorization (stratification) of data into unique patient groups [37].

Systems level analyses also provide context for the drivers of the disease that are outside the inherited genetic mutations yet frequently implicated in cancer progression. The role of microRNAs (miRNAs) has also been frequently cited as a robust and dynamic regulator of PC invasiveness and disease progression, mainly due to frequent finding of miR-21 in multiple models of tumor metastasis [38]. Through systems level analysis, these same miRNAs can be shown to harbor an acquired functional nature, either inhibiting or promoting disease formation in PC with diagnostic value [39]. Interestingly, through the systems perspective of the relationship between miRNAs and the wider network they function within, it is apparent that their ability to carry out multiple functions both good and bad while encompassing large chunks of biological pathways renders them some of the most robust class of molecules in epigenetic regulation [40]. Proper identification and analysis of miRNAs have rendered some of them capable of accurately determining disease type in the pancreas between normal pancreas tissue, pancreatitis, and PC with a hypothesized ability to ascertain prognostic outcome [41]. The presence of circulating miRNAs satisfies the noninvasive desire of any future standardized diagnostic target, and has been shown to be useful in PC diagnosis and prognosis, although it is still in the early stages of elucidation and validation [42]. Theoretically, as our understanding of miRNA interactions grow through systems study, it is not unlikely that some miRNAs might be considered candidates as biomarkers for disease development based on vast amounts of data resolving the epigenetic chain of events causing aberrant regulation or expression profiles [43].

A cornerstone of systems science is that a single factor (gene, protein, or even one pathway) alone cannot be useful as a definitive indicator as we now understand that there is a complex interaction between biological components. Early attempts have shown an acceptable initial degree of accuracy in differentiating tumor classes simply based on algorithmic analysis of gene expression in tumors [44]. The most probable scenario in the future will be a unique, patient-specific molecular signature derived from both genomic and proteomic analysis tested against epidemiological PC data or general cancer data for diagnosis, stratification, and treatment [45]. One such example was the identification of neutrophil gelatinase-associated lipocalin (NGAL), previously thought to simply function as an endocrine modulator but now seen as a dynamic component of malignancy regulation in some of the earliest predecessors to PanIN lesions, with a clear differentiation from normal, pancreatitis, and PC tissues [46].

Because the foundations of systems biology and the search for diagnostic indicators have yielded potential directions for research, a similar approach to treatment modalities has also resulted in greater insight into drug design. Subcategorizing PC into multiple types has generated common identifiable markers conserved through the disease type, and in designing compounds targeting these components, survivability and efficacy may be increased rationally [47]. Utilizing systems biology, it was shown that new efficacious combinations could be discerned from already available compounds displaying higher potency than single pathway or single target motifs in PC [48]. Not only does network modeling show chemical interactions, it also provides insight on new combinatorial possibilities, but it could also be useful in isolating key network centers eligible for targeting due to their highly active nature either in PC formation or progression [49]. The same strategy can be utilized to overcome chemoresistance, and it was shown in one in vitro model targeting Notch signaling to bypass the effect, which also partially reversed the EMT, a characteristic of metastatic and invasive cells [50]. The use of neutraceutical (naturally found biologically active compounds in diet and diet-derived agents) compounds within this context, although controversial, represents a prime opportunity in the era of new treatment strategies as well as identifying previously unseen network players in PC [51]. Although natural agents may not work in the most targeted manner, many have shown potency in preclinical PC models with minimal toxicity compared to traditional cytotoxic chemotherapeutic agents. Therefore, identification of key active molecules within such entities in combination with a network-based strategy for PC treatment should yield not just single target goals but also multinodal targeting objectives through capitalizing on the promiscuity of such compounds against the complex cancer networks. Identifiable promiscuity thus becomes an asset; it was demonstrated by Keiser et al., in 2009 through analysis of 3665 FDA-approved chemical entities that yielded 23 novel associations, five of which showed remarkable potency against novel and unrelated pathways at submicromolar concentrations [52]. It is well recognized that PC research has benefited immensely from the development of transgenic mice models that mimic the disease very closely. Such transgenic mice models have allowed deeper evaluations of PC microenvironment as these animals harbor desmoplastic stroma, which replicates that present in human carcinoma. Specifically, the PDX-1-Cre;LSL-KRAS^{G12D} (KPC) model has played a pivotal role in understanding the early forms of PC [53]. However, computational biology analysis, particularly systems and network biology, has not been fully exploited on these models. This remains an uncharted area of research that can immensely benefit from systems and network technologies. In all likelihood, future directions of diagnosis will combine such factors, including miRNA expression profiling, protein and gene expression profiling, as well as the traditional phenotypic (e.g., histologic) indicators of malignancy for a complete picture of PC development, like a full painting with many colors placed in the right context.

It is quite possible that the most effective combination treatments are currently on the market yet have not been evaluated for their efficacy against PC. Considering that new chemical entities for cancers in general have so far experienced >80% failure rate, especially during phase II and phase III trials, it would be both economically valuable and time saving to validate efficacies in proper cellular and animal models prior to the advanced stages of treatment development for PC [54]. Current data and evidence highlight the strong need to better model strategies in PC for both drug design and patient stratification [55]. By analyzing such association from a network pharmacology perspective, more reliable predictive models can be created for PC with molecularly driven and patient-specific personalization tracking the success of any given treatment [56]. Vitally, an in silico model for targeting potential, synergy, and combination design represents an asset in drug identification, the same model in one instance identifying 52 drug targets, half of which already exist as approved drugs for targeting them [57].

This methodology has seen success in determining the most relevant bioactive ingredients in some neutraceuticals and will most likely expand to PC models for efficacy identification [58]. Furthermore, elaborated statistical and computational methods can build upon already identified patterns of interaction and could predict drug-target dynamics in PC through in silico analyses and a highly efficient possibility for high-throughput chemical screening [59].

One of the major challenges in treatment of PC that can be suitably addressed by systems science is the early assessment of toxicity and treatment failure of any novel regimen. During the drug selection process, PC patients are typed into a one-size-fits-all category that is based on the targeted molecule or a phenotypic characteristic. This is the primary reason for high failure rates, which could be due in part to either ineffectiveness of the drugs being used or the associated toxicity in phase III clinical development, where sometimes there is an unclear endpoint for assessing treatment outcome due to unreliable biomarkers [60]. Just as the search for versatile and reliable biomarkers is important in preclinical studies, they serve much the same purpose in assessing treatment success. Utilizing the same mechanisms of analysis and understanding in drug targeting and perturbation effects, similar information and methods can be extracted to predict toxicity and its mechanism relevant to whole organ systems [61]. As the PC-specific perturbations can be explained mechanistically and systematically, the same drug-based perturbations can be correlated to markers already known physiologically related to toxicity [62]. One of the most basic methods has been the extrapolation of genetic polymorphisms on a patient-specific scale rendering them susceptible to adverse reactions from one compound or another [63]. By combining preexisting omics data with other cursory metabolite response data, information can be derived from perturbations that not only serve a biomarker function but also a macro-scale survey of the intricate metabolic balance [64]. Access to large databases and high-throughput analytics provides a widespread network of raw information that would allow a systematically analyzed and statistically validated approach to provide a full global picture of chemical function, uptake, and metabolism [65]. Systems of this nature are already in place and have seen an inclusion in translational research as a predictive risk management and patient selection tool with reliable dosage selection in clinical trials, rendering them scalable to clinical-level monitoring during treatment duration [66]. Rationally chosen combinations of targeted agents may improve therapeutic outcome by overcoming drug resistance.

However, the lack of molecular biomarkers for patient selection and current reductionist clinical trial methodologies limit successful drug development for PC. Application of new research tools including systems and network biology is expected to assist in the design of effective drug combinations in PC.

In spite of these advances, there is little data available on mid-trial analyses on PC patient tissue samples that are undergoing first-round therapies. We propose that systems and network-based analyses should be performed midway in PC clinical trials to influence decision making, i.e., incorporating newer and optimal drugs or their combinations. This would depend on the proper selection of time points as to when the test material should be collected for mRNA expression, central gene analysis, gene enrichment analysis, and pathway network analysis. Ideally, once the advanced cancer is selected through molecular profiling, the patients undergo first biopsy for gene expression and systems analysis. In this case the drug selection is dependent on a single or combination regimen that has shown preclinical efficacy. However, in systems-based clinical trial design, we propose that once treated, the patient should undergo a second biopsy that is again subjected to gene expression and systems analysis to evaluate whether the drugs were effective in eliminating the intended target and their network. Depending on the outcome of the second biopsy, clinicians can either continue treatment or optimize it to enhance the efficacy by incorporating newer drugs. It should be noted that such studies have their own restrictions that have statistical limitations. In the end, the success of such tailored trials depends heavily on the close interaction between laboratory researcher, clinician, and computational biologist. Therapies that have undergone rigorous lab–clinic and lab evaluations and are supported by systems level sciences are expected to drive the future of clinical trials for PC.

PC THERAPY RESISTANCE AND THE ROLE OF CANCER STEM CELLS

The high drug resistance observed in PC significantly contributes to the low prognosis of the disease and represents the biggest barrier to effective treatment. Thus, improving our understanding of the mechanisms underlying drug resistance in PC may contribute to new strategies in combating the disease. Although much of the mechanism is still under investigation, there has been increasing evidence over the past decade that points to the critical role of cancer stem cells (CSCs) in regulating drug resistance [67]. CSCs, similar to normal stem cells, have the ability to self-regenerate, replicate heterogeneously, and resist apoptosis. They were first discovered in human leukemia cells in 1997, and further investigations have identified CSCs in numerous solid tumors including breast, brain, colon, prostate, lung, and PC tumors [68,69]. Even though CSCs represent only a small subpopulation of the tumor cells (0.05–1%), current evidence suggests that they are responsible for producing the complex, differentiated tumor cell lineages present in highly malignant tumors. CSCs share many characteristics with EMT cells, including CD44 and CD24 cell surface marker expression, vimentin upregulation, and cadherin 1 downregulation [70]. Further clinical theories suggest that the presence of CSCs contributes to the low efficacy of chemoradiation therapy. Even though chemoradiation may reduce tumor mass by killing differentiated cell progenies, the continued existence of CSCs has been suggested to result in recurring PC tumors. The molecular mechanism of CSC tumorigenic regulation and signaling pathways is currently being investigated in order to find more effective therapies for patients. miRNAs have been shown to support the pathways that maintain gastric CSCs [71,72]. Further studies with PC also suggest that suppression of these CSC sustaining miRNAs decrease the aggressive phenotype of the tumors [73].

PC stem cells (or stem-like cells) have been identified through various cellular and animal models as a small subset of malignant cells capable of initiating new tumor tissue either through metastatic spread or at the original site [74]. Evidence suggests that these CSCs play a critical role in cell proliferation/migration, metastasis, and chemotherapy resistance, thus resulting in high mortality rates. Inhibiting CSCs and their downstream effects may provide a novel, effective strategy in treating pancreatic and other malignant cancers. However, the challenges lie in the identification and mechanism of inhibiting CSCs.

ISOLATION AND BIOLOGICAL CHARACTERIZATION OF PC CSCS

Using flow-sorting methodologies, our laboratory has recently identified triple-positive (CD44+/CD133+/EpCAM+) CSCs from human PC cell lines MiaPaCa-2 and AsPC-1 (Figure 13.2(A)). The CSCs have the ability to self-regenerate (spheroid formation assay), which replicates increased

(A)

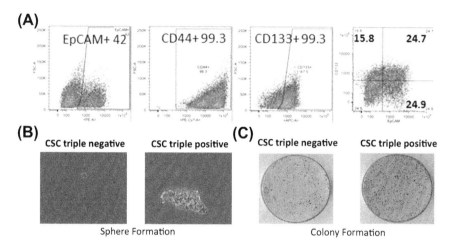

(B)

CSC triple negative   CSC triple positive

Sphere Formation

(C)

CSC triple negative   CSC triple positive

Colony Formation

Figure 13.2 *Isolation and Biological Analysis of Pancreatic Cancer Stem-Like Cells.* MiaPaCa-2 cells were flow sorted for CD44+CD133+EpCAM+ cells using FACs analysis (A). The propensity of cells to form colonies was evaluated using colonogenic and sphere forming assays. Briefly, 1000 single suspended cells were plated on ultra-low attachment wells of Costar six-well plates (Corning Inc., Corning, NY) in 2 ml of sphere formation medium. After seven days of incubation, the sphere cells were collected by centrifuge (300× g for 5 min), and the number of pancreatospheres was counted under a microscope (B). Colony formation was performed according to established protocols (C). (For color version of this figure, the reader is referred to the online version of this book.)

clonogenicity that is a characteristic of CSCs obtained in breast, colon, and other tumor models (Figure 13.2(B) and (C)).

These triple-positive PC CSC cells have increased cell migratory capabilities (as analyzed through scratch assay), which attests to their plasticity and invasive potential (Figure 13.3(A)). The flow-sorted markers in these CSCs could be validated using confocal microscopy where we observed enhanced expression of CD44, CD133, and EpCAM (Figure 13.3(B)). Confirming their stem-like characteristics, few triple positive CSCs could give rise to tumors at subcutaneous and orthotopic sites in SCID mice. This is unlike regular PC cell lines that need more than a million cells to grow at subcutaneous and orthotopic sites. Furthermore, we evaluated the expression of the above markers in xenograft-derived tumors using immunohistochemistry (Figure 13.3(C)). Our findings could replicate that of flow-sorted cells where we observed enhanced expression of Notch1, CD44, and CD133. These multiple lines of evidence support our hypothesis attesting to the stem-like characteristics, although these experiments do not provide

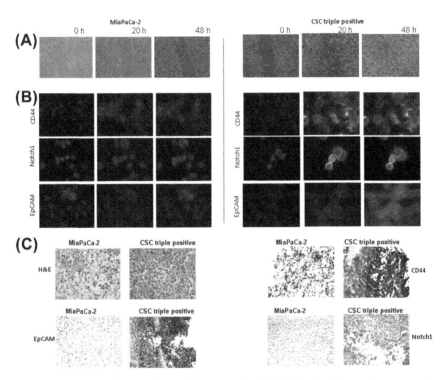

Figure 13.3 *Molecular Analysis of Pancreatic CSCs.* The invasive and metastatic potential of the FACs sorted CSCs was evaluated using wound healing (scratch assay) (A). The markers for CSCs were evaluated using immunofluorescence. Cells were grown on chambered slides and stained, immunofluorescence assay was performed using previously published methods [75]. (B) 40× immunofluorescence images showing comparative staining of triple negative vs. triple positive cells using EVOS imaging system. Note: enhancement of CD44, CD133, and EpCAM in triple positive population. (C) FACs sorted cells were grown in subcutaneous site, tumors were harvested, and IHC was performed to evaluate the expression of CSC markers. As can be seen, CSC-derived tumors showed higher expression of stemness markers, CD44, CD133, and Notch, which was not found in parent MiaPaCa-2–derived tumors. (For color version of this figure, the reader is referred to the online version of this book.)

information on the signaling networks that support their resistant nature for which we exploited systems level analyses.

SYSTEMS AND PATHWAY ANALYSIS OF CSCS

While the evaluation of recognized CSC markers can be useful in isolating these resistant cells among the general PC cell population, such reductionist analysis cannot provide information on the molecular networks that sustain their unique characteristics. It is logical that deeper evaluations of the CSCs sustaining signaling will help identify the drivers of stemness, which in turn can help design effective strategies that can eliminate these resistant cells. However, the intricate cross talk among the CSC sustaining pathways cannot be gleaned through isolationist approaches. Rather, systems biology methodologies that take a holistic view of the different signaling molecules involved in CSC sustenance need to be applied. Therefore, we undertook a computational approach to study these CSCs as presented following.

In order to validate the differences between (−−−) and (+++) cells, the mRNA microarray assay was conducted for gene expression profiling analysis. Differential gene expression analysis was used to compare parent cell line vs. triple negative cells vs. triple positive cells, which revealed some striking results. A total of 1653 mRNAs were identified to be differentially expressed in CSLCs (+++) vs. (−−−) (Figure 13.4(A)). Among these genes, 753 mRNAs were upregulated and 900 mRNAs were downregulated in the CSLCs (triple positive cells), compared to triple negative cells; 1,581 mRNAs were identified to be differentially expressed in CSLCs (triple positive) vs. its parental MiaPaCa-2 cells. There was a 1216 differentially expressed gene overlap between the CSLCs (triple positive cells) vs. triple negative or MiaPaCa-2 cells. The pathway enrichment analysis shows that the differentially expressed genes are involved in 21 (top 10 shown here) of the major biological function groups including cell cycle, polo–like kinase, tight junction, cell–cell junction, IGF-1, PI3K/Akt, ERK/MAPK, and VEGF signaling (Figure 13.4(B)). Notably, FoxQ1 (forkhead box Q1) was found to be elevated in CSCs, which is a member of the forkhead transcription factor family that is recognized to be critically involved in the regulation of gene expression during early development, metabolism, and immune function [76,77]. Emerging evidence suggest that FoxQ1 may have an important function during tumorigenesis and tumor progression mediated by deregulation of several signaling pathways such as EMT, a biological process known to be associated with drug resistance and metastasis, and also known to be linked with CSC characteristics [78]. Recent clinical studies have shown high levels of FoxQ1 expression in breast, gastric cancer, colorectal cancer and non-small cell lung cancer [79]. Moreover, several in vitro and in vivo experimental studies have shown that FoxQ1 expression increases cell growth/proliferation, migration/invasion, angiogenesis, tumorigenicity, and metastasis, which was found to be mediated by the upregulation of NRXN3 (neurexin 3, a tumor prognostic marker), ZEB1/2, VEGF, Wnt, and BCL in different tumor cells such as breast, liver, glioma,

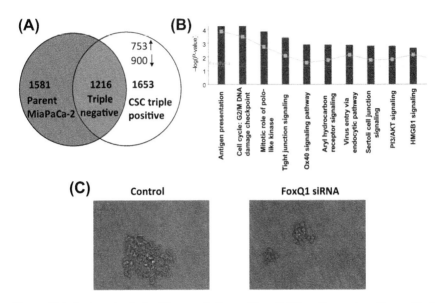

Figure 13.4 *Systems Analysis of Pancreatic Cancer Stem Cell Gene Expression.* The purified total RNAs from parent MiaPaCa-2, triple negative MiaPaCa-2, and triple positive MiaPaCa-2 were isolated by using Vana mRNA Isolation kit (Ambion Inc., Austin, TX), following the manufacturer's instructions. Total RNA quantity and quality was examined by analysis using the NanoDrop and Agilent Bioanalyzer (Agilent Technologies). All the RNA samples had RIN scores equal or above seven. The whole genome expression profiling was analyzed by a two-color microarray-based approach. The RNA samples were hybridized to Agilent 4 x 44K human arrays and scanned with the Agilent G2505B scanner system. All the data were analyzed by Agilent Feature Extraction software that generated expression data parameters including LogRatio expression levels, LogRatio error, and p values LogRatio. The features included in further analysis were annotated, gene level that passed a p value LogRatio cutoff equal or less than 0.001. ANOVA analysis and multiple test correction (Benjamin-Hochberg $p \le 0.05$) was conducted using Partek software to compare the two sets of four two-color arrayed replicates for the identification of the gene expression level changes (≥ 2 fold changes). (A) Venn diagram showing the number of differentially expressed genes in parent, triple negative, and triple positive cells. (B) The pathway enrichment analysis shows that differential expression of selected genes are involved in 21 (top 10 shown here) of the major biological function groups, including cell cycle, polo-like kinase, tight junction, cell–cell junction, IGF-1, PI3K/Akt, ERK/MAPK, and VEGF signaling. (C) siRNA silencing of FoxQ1 suppresses spheroid forming ability of triple positive CSCs indicating their role in stem cell sustenance. (For color version of this figure, the reader is referred to the online version of this book.)

colorectal, and ovarian cancers [80]. In addition, the expression of FoxQ1 is regulated by TGF-β, which suggests that TGF-β–mediated overexpression of FoxQ1 may lead to the acquisition of EMT, a process that is reminiscent of CSC (CSLC) characteristics [81]. The blockage of FoxQ1 by its siRNA inhibitor has been found to inhibit cell invasion and metastasis in vitro through the reversal of EMT in bladder cancer cells [82]. However, the role of FoxQ1 in the regulation of CSC phenotypes and functions during PC tumorigenesis and tumor progression has not been clearly elucidated. In our systems analysis, we demonstrate for the first time that higher expression of FoxQ1 is associated with CSC signatures/markers and functions in triple positive cells isolated from PC cells. Further analysis of FoxQ1 and other identified markers is ongoing and is the subject of another article. Most importantly, the knockdown of FoxQ1 by its siRNA inhibitor resulted in the attenuation of spheroid forming ability (Figure 13.4(C)), aggressive CSC phenotypes, consistent with the inhibition in the expression of EpCAM and Snail in triple positive cells. These data clearly suggest that FoxQ1 plays a key role in the regulation of CSC phenotypes and functions in PC. We also found overexpression of bone morphogenic proteins (BMPs) such as BMP4, which belongs to a class of important extracellular signaling transducer proteins and is part of the transforming growth factor-β (TGF-β) superfamily, and have been considered to exhibit a critical role in early tissue development [83]. There is available clinical data showing that alterations in the expression of BMP4 in various tumors including PC are associated with poor overall prognosis [84]. There is a large body of in vitro and in vivo evidence supporting the important role of BMP4 in tumorigenesis and tumor progression mediated by promoting cell growth/proliferation and migration/invasion via several different signaling pathways/networks including apoptosis and PI3K/Akt, Wnt, hedgehog, and EMT in different cancers including PC [85]. However, there are some controversial reports showing an inhibitory effect of BMP4 on tumor cell growth in vitro and in vivo [86]. Therefore, the biological function of BMP4 appears to be tumor context dependent. Nevertheless, the exact role of BMP4 in the regulation of PC CSC phenotypes has not been molecularly investigated. There are some limited studies that suggest that BMP4 may be involved in the regulation of CSC phenotypes and functions [87]. For example, BMP4 could decrease cell growth and proliferation in CSC-like CD133+ cells of glioblastoma in vitro and in vivo. It has also been noted that Lin-28 and Oct4, two recognized stem cell factors, work together to upregulate the expression of BMP4 at the posttranscriptional level, which contributes to the modulation of ovarian tumor microenvironment [88]. In our present study, we found that CSLCs (triple positive cells) exhibit aggressive tumor cell phenotypes and functions, which was consistent with overexpression of BMP4 and other stem cell markers, suggesting that BMP4 may have an important role in the regulation of PC CSC characteristics. However, further mechanistic studies are needed for determining the role of BMP4 in CSLCs of PC.

We were able to validate the top-ranked differentially expressed genes in (+++) CSCs using molecular assays such as western blotting, confocal microscopy, and RT-PCR. Interestingly, knockdown of some of the top-ranked differentially expressed genes could reverse stemness and sensitivity to chemotherapeutic drugs (data for FoxQ1 shown here). These studies prove that systems and pathway analysis–identified genes can help not only characterize the PC CSCs but can also help in defining key CSC drivers that can be used as therapeutic markers for targeted therapies and their combinations.

SYSTEMS ANALYSIS OF PC CSC microRNA NETWORK

Aside from differential gene expression analysis, we also performed differential miRNA analysis to analyze the role of different miRNAs in sustaining the PC CSC signaling. For these studies, miRNA microarray assay was performed. The miRNA expression profiling analysis was performed by miRBase version 16 (LC Sciences). The values of log (2) of each miRNA from data comparisons were used to represent fold change, and the data were normalized by using selected housekeeping genes. Systems and pathway analysis was performed by using the Web-based bioinformatics tool IPA (Ingenuity Systems, Redwood, CA) for predicting functional network. Microarray analysis was performed to examine the differential expression of miRNAs of CSLCs (triple positive cells), compared to either the parental MiaPaCa-2 cells or triple negative cells. Our results showed 438 miRNAs to be differentially expressed in CSLCs (triple positive) vs. triple negative cells. Among these miRNAs, 191 miRNAs were upregulated and 247 miRNAs were downregulated in CSLCs (triple positive cells), compared to triple negative cells. Moreover, we found 486 miRNAs that were differentially expressed between CSLCs (triple positive) and the parental MiaPaCa-2 cells. Among those miRNAs, 243 miRNAs were upregulated and 243 miRNAs were downregulated. However, there were only 180 differentially expressed miRNAs between triple negative cells and the parental MiaPaCa-2 cells. Among those miRNAs, 108 miRNAs were upregulated and 72 miRNAs were downregulated (Figure 13.5 (A)).

We further subjected the differentially expressed miRNAs to IPA miRNA target filter to better understand the miRNA target pathways that are involved and how they influence their target genes. The algorithms of

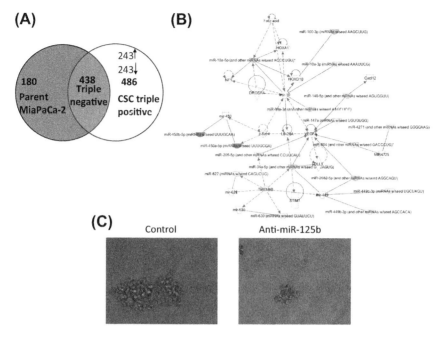

Figure 13.5 *Systems Analysis of miRNA Microarrays in Pancreatic Cancer Stem Cells.* Purified total RNAs were isolated by using mirVana miRNA Isolation kit (Ambion Inc., Austin, TX), following the manufacturer's instructions. The miRNA microarray assay was performed by LC Sciences (Houston, TX). The miRNA expression profiling analysis was performed by miRBase version (LC Sciences). The values of log (2) of each miRNA from data comparisons were used for the fold change levels. Data were normalized by using selected housekeeping genes. (A) Venn diagram depicting differentially expressed genes. (B) Pathway analysis of mirs that were found differentially expressed in CSCs compared to triple negative cells. System network analysis was performed by using the Web-based bioinformatics tool IPA software (Ingenuity Systems, Redwood, CA) for predicting functional networks. (C) Silencing of mir125b results in abrogation of spheroid forming ability of triple positive CSCs. (For color version of this figure, the reader is referred to the online version of this book.)

networks of selected miRNAs that are involved were generated based on their pathway connectivity. Our pathway enrichment analysis of CSCs (triple positive) vs. triple negative cells was found to be similar to that of CSCs (triple positive) vs. the parental MiaPaCa-2 cells. There are 10 biological functional groups that showed such connectivity, including cancer, GI disease, and genetic disorder. These results suggest that differential expression of miRNAs in CSCs (triple positive cells) is highly associated with the development and progression of tumors, including GI tumors. The network analysis of selected miRNAs in CSCs (triple positive) vs. triple

Table 13.1 List of Differentially Expressed miRNAs Identified through miRNA Microarray Analysis

miRNAs	CSC Triple +ve vs. Parent (Fold Change)	CSC Triple +ve vs. Parent (p Value)
Let-7f	−0.33	9.78E-05
Let7i	−4.00	2.54E-07
miR-30a	−5.12	2.59E-06
miR-30c	−0.71	1.12E-05
miR-125b-5p	6.87	3.01E-07
miR-335-5p	2.13	4.61E-04

negative cells is similar to that of CSCs (triple positive) vs. MiaPaCa-2 cells (Figure 13.5(B)). Furthermore, our network analysis showed that many miRNAs were intricately regulated by each other either directly or indirectly, which were also further regulated by several target genes, indicating a very complex interaction system. We found changes in a number of miRNAs in CSCs (triple positive cells), compared to MiaPaCa-2 and triple negative cells including let-7f,i, miR-30a,b, miR-125b, and miR-335, compared to its parental MiaPaCa-2 cells and triple negative cells (Table 13.1). The knockdown of miR-125b by transfecting siRNA inhibitor reduced spheroid forming ability (Figure 13.5(C)), clonogenicity, cell migration, and self-renewal capacity. These experiments validated their role in sustaining CSCs networks. Collectively, these systems studies identified key miRNAs that promote CSC signaling that could not have been pinpointed using traditional molecular biology.

SUMMARY AND FUTURE DIRECTIONS

PC is a deadly and by far incurable disease harboring a signaling circuitry as complex as that present in super computers. It is logical that such complex circuitry cannot be fully evaluated using traditional biology and a computational component in our analyses system is needed. This is especially critical knowing the heterogeneous nature of PC tumors that are composed of different types of cells, each emanating unique signatures that form the very complex tumor microenvironment. It has now been well accepted that CSCs (or cancer stem-like cells) hold a major place in this heterogeneous tumor microenvironment and play an important role during PC tumorigenesis. Such rare populations of CSCs comprise less than 1% of the PC tumor cells and have been implicated in therapy resistance and poorer clinical outcomes such as reduced disease-free survival rate and increased mortality [89]. The CSLC subpopulations exhibit distinct features such as superior self-renewal capacity, prolonged survival potential, and enhanced ability to differentiate into multiple different cell types of tumor cells or tumor-associated cells. Most of the chemotherapeutics used in the clinic can eliminate the bulk of the tumor cells. However, it is this distinct sub population of cells that do not respond to standard chemotherapeutics, and such residual population has been attributed to giving rise to recurring tumors. Therefore, understanding and targeted killing of these CSCs would, in principle, provide an effective therapeutic approach for the treatment of aggressive PC. However, the regulation of CSC characteristics during tumorigenesis and tumor progression has not been clearly elucidated, especially in PC. Therefore, further characterization of CSCs may lead to the discovery of genes that could be targeted for therapy. As shown here, such understanding requires holistic molecular characterization that is coupled with systems level approaches that look at the entire set of CSC-associated pathways, both genetic and epigenetic, and their cross talk and the ensuing signaling. The molecular biology allowed isolation of a highly purified fraction of cells from PC cell lines that were CD44+/CD133+/EpCAM+ and behaved like CSCs/CSLCs. These triple positive CSCs have aggressive phenotypes and functions, which is consistent with overexpression of CSC signatures/markers. In the next phase that involved holistic characterization, the systems level analysis demonstrated the differential expression of large numbers of genes unique to triple positive CSC fraction. Targeted elimination of these differentially expressed genes could suppress CSC signaling networks, resulting in their elimination.

In relation to miRNA signatures, our systems analysis revealed that the aggressive phenotypes displayed by CSCs and functions such as increased cell growth, clonogenicity, cell migration, and self-renewal capacity are supported by a large number of miRNAs, including let-7f,i, miR-30a,b, miR-125b, and miR-335, compared to its parental MiaPaCa-2 cells and triple negative cells. The knockdown of miR-125b by transfecting siRNA inhibitor reduced clonogenicity, cell migration, and self-renewal capacity, which was consistent with downregulation of CSC signatures/mediators such as CD44, EpCAM, EZH2, and Snail, strongly indicating that miRNA-targeted approach could become a novel therapeutic strategy for the successful elimination of PC.

In the future, more rigorous systems level analysis of CSCs from a larger number of sources such as cell lines, primary tumors, and genetic model–derived cells will bring forward the hidden players supporting stemness in PC tumors. Such exercises are expected to drive the discovery of CSC-targeted therapies that will shape future personalized medicine for better treatment outcomes in patients suffering from this devastating disease.

ACKNOWLEDGMENT

We acknowledge Dr Fazlul Sarkar for providing the necessary reagents (CSCs) to conduct the studies described in this chapter.

REFERENCES

[1] Siegel R, Naishadham D, Jemal A. Cancer statistics, 2013. CA Cancer J Clin 2013;63:11–30.
[2] Jemal A. Global burden of cancer: opportunities for prevention. Lancet 2012;380:1797–9.
[3] Hezel AF, Kimmelman AC, Stanger BZ, Bardeesy N, DePinho RA. Genetics and biology of pancreatic ductal adenocarcinoma. Genes Dev 2006;20:1218–49.
[4] Li D, Xie K, Wolff R, Abbruzzese JL. Pancreatic cancer. Lancet 2004;363:1049–57.
[5] Thayer SP, di Magliano MP, Heiser PW, Nielsen CM, Roberts DJ, Lauwers GY, et al. Hedgehog is an early and late mediator of pancreatic cancer tumorigenesis. Nature 2003;425:851–6.
[6] Olive KP, Jacobetz MA, Davidson CJ, Gopinathan A, McIntyre D, Honess D, et al. Inhibition of Hedgehog signaling enhances delivery of chemotherapy in a mouse model of pancreatic cancer. Science 2009;324:1457–61.
[7] Kleeff J, Ishiwata T, Maruyama H, Friess H, Truong P, Buchler MW, et al. The TGF-beta signaling inhibitor Smad7 enhances tumorigenicity in pancreatic cancer. Oncogene 1999;18:5363–72.
[8] Bardeesy N, DePinho RA. Pancreatic cancer biology and genetics. Nat Rev Cancer 2002;2:897–909.
[9] Hao K, Bosse Y, Nickle DC, Pare PD, Postma DS, Laviolette M, et al. Lung eQTLs to help reveal the molecular underpinnings of asthma. PLoS Genet 2012;8:e1003029.
[10] Ghaneh P, Costello E, Neoptolemos JP. Biology and management of pancreatic cancer. Postgrad Med J 2008;84:478–97.
[11] Maitra A, Kern SE, Hruban RH. Molecular pathogenesis of pancreatic cancer. Best Pract Res Clin Gastroenterol 2006;20:211–26.
[12] Cleary-Wheeler AL, Lomberk GA, Weiss FU, Schneider G, Fabbri M, Poshusta TL, et al. Insights into the epigenetic mechanisms controlling pancreatic carcinogenesis. Cancer Lett 2013;328:212–21.
[13] Tempero MA, Berlin J, Ducreux M, Haller D, Harper P, Khayat D, et al. Pancreatic cancer treatment and research: an international expert panel discussion. Ann Oncol 2011;22:1500–6.
[14] varo-Meca A, Akerkar R, varez-Bartolome M, Gil-Prieto R, Rue H, de Miguel AG. Factors involved in health-related transitions after curative resection for pancreatic cancer. 10-years experience: a multi state model. Cancer Epidemiol 2013;37:91–6.
[15] Witkowski ER, Smith JK, Tseng JF. Outcomes following resection of pancreatic cancer. J Surg Oncol 2013;107:97–103.
[16] Poruk KE, Firpo MA, Adler DG, Mulvihill SJ. Screening for pancreatic cancer: why, how, and who? Ann Surg 2013;257:17–26.

[17] Louhimo J, Alfthan H, Stenman UH, Haglund C. Serum HCG beta and CA 72-4 are stronger prognostic factors than CEA, CA 19-9 and CA 242 in pancreatic cancer. Oncology 2004;66:126–31.

[18] Ansari D, Tingstedt B, Andersson R. Pancreatic cancer – cost for overtreatment with gemcitabine. Acta Oncol 2013;52:1146–51.

[19] Petersen GM, de Andrade M, Goggins M, Hruban RH, Bondy M, Korczak JF, et al. Pancreatic cancer genetic epidemiology consortium. Cancer Epidemiol Biomarkers Prev 2006;15:704–10.

[20] Klein AP. Identifying people at a high risk of developing pancreatic cancer. Nat Rev Cancer 2013;13:66–74.

[21] Lynch HT, Smyrk T, Kern SE, Hruban RH, Lightdale CJ, Lemon SJ, et al. Familial pancreatic cancer: a review. Semin Oncol 1996;23:251–75.

[22] Garcea G, Neal CP, Pattenden CJ, Steward WP, Berry DP. Molecular prognostic markers in pancreatic cancer: a systematic review. Eur J Cancer 2005;41:2213–36.

[23] Petrelli A, Giordano S. From single- to multi-target drugs in cancer therapy: when aspecificity becomes an advantage. Curr Med Chem 2008;15:422–32.

[24] Naraev BG, Strosberg JR, Halfdanarson TR. Current status and perspectives of targeted therapy in well-differentiated neuroendocrine tumors. Oncology 2012; 83:117–27.

[25] Alian OM, Azmi AS, Mohammad RM. Network insights on oxaliplatin anti-cancer mechanisms. Clin Transl Med 2012;1:26.

[26] Hoelder S, Clarke PA, Workman P. Discovery of small molecule cancer drugs: successes, challenges and opportunities. Mol Oncol 2012;6:155–76.

[27] Floyd E, McShane TM. Development and use of biomarkers in oncology drug development. Toxicol Pathol 2004;32(Suppl. 1):106–15.

[28] Kitano H. Systems biology: a brief overview. Science 2002;295:1662–4.

[29] Azmi AS. Network pharmacology: an emerging field in cancer drug discovery. Curr Drug Discov Technol 2013;10:93–4.

[30] Thongboonkerd V. The promise and challenge of systems biology in translational medicine. Clin Sci (Lond) 2013;124:389–90.

[31] Bhattacharya S, Mariani TJ. Systems biology approaches to identify developmental bases for lung diseases. Pediatr Res 2013;73:514–22.

[32] Roukos DH. Novel clinico-genome network modeling for revolutionizing genotype-phenotype-based personalized cancer care. Expert Rev Mol Diagn 2010; 10:33–48.

[33] Bhattacharyya S, Siegel ER, Petersen GM, Chari ST, Suva LJ, Haun RS. Diagnosis of pancreatic cancer using serum proteomic profiling. Neoplasia 2004;6:674–86.

[34] Li Y, St John MA, Zhou X, Kim Y, Sinha U, Jordan RC, et al. Salivary transcriptome diagnostics for oral cancer detection. Clin Cancer Res 2004;10.8442–50.

[35] Zhang Y, Chen L, Yang J, Fleming JB, Chiao PJ, Logsdon CD, et al. Study human pancreatic cancer in mice: how close are they? Biochim Biophys Acta 2013; 1835:110–8.

[36] Kossow C, Jose D, Jaster R, Wolkenhauer O, Rateitschak K. Mathematical modelling unravels regulatory mechanisms of interferon-gamma-induced STAT1 serine-phosphorylation and MUC4 expression in pancreatic cancer cells. IET Syst Biol 2012;6:73–85.

[37] Gadaleta E, Cutts RJ, Kelly GP, Crnogorac-Jurcevic T, Kocher HM, Lemoine NR, et al. A global insight into a cancer transcriptional space using pancreatic data: importance, findings and flaws. Nucleic Acids Res 2011;39:7900–7.

[38] Zhu S, Wu H, Wu F, Nie D, Sheng S, Mo YY. MicroRNA-21 targets tumor suppressor genes in invasion and metastasis. Cell Res 2008;18:350–9.

[39] Calin GA, Croce CM. MicroRNA signatures in human cancers. Nat Rev Cancer 2006;6:857–66.

[40] Azmi AS, Beck FW, Bao B, Mohammad RM, Sarkar FH. Aberrant epigenetic grooming of miRNAs in pancreatic cancer: a systems biology perspective. Epigenomics 2011;3:747–59.

[41] Bloomston M, Frankel WL, Petrocca F, Volinia S, Alder H, Hagan JP, et al. MicroRNA expression patterns to differentiate pancreatic adenocarcinoma from normal pancreas and chronic pancreatitis. JAMA 2007;297:1901–8.

[42] Kosaka N, Iguchi H, Ochiya T. Circulating microRNA in body fluid: a new potential biomarker for cancer diagnosis and prognosis. Cancer Sci 2010;101:2087–92.

[43] Croce CM. Causes and consequences of microRNA dysregulation in cancer. Nat Rev Genet 2009;10:704–14.

[44] Ramaswamy S, Tamayo P, Rifkin R, Mukherjee S, Yeang CH, Angelo M, et al. Multiclass cancer diagnosis using tumor gene expression signatures. Proc Natl Acad Sci USA 2001;98:15149–54.

[45] Yee NS. Toward the goal of personalized therapy in pancreatic cancer by targeting the molecular phenotype. Adv Exp Med Biol 2013;779:91–143.

[46] Moniaux N, Chakraborty S, Yalniz M, Gonzalez J, Shostrom VK, Standop J, et al. Early diagnosis of pancreatic cancer: neutrophil gelatinase-associated lipocalin as a marker of pancreatic intraepithelial neoplasia. Br J Cancer 2008;98:1540–7.

[47] Weinstein IB, Joe AK. Mechanisms of disease: oncogene addiction – a rationale for molecular targeting in cancer therapy. Nat Clin Pract Oncol 2006;3:448–57.

[48] Azmi AS, Wang Z, Philip PA, Mohammad RM, Sarkar FH. Proof of concept: network and systems biology approaches aid in the discovery of potent anticancer drug combinations. Mol Cancer Ther 2010;9:3137–44.

[49] Azmi AS, Banerjee S, Ali S, Wang Z, Bao B, Beck FW, et al. Network modeling of MDM2 inhibitor-oxaliplatin combination reveals biological synergy in wt-p53 solid tumors. Oncotarget 2011;2:378–92.

[50] Wang Z, Li Y, Ahmad A, Azmi AS, Banerjee S, Kong D, et al. Targeting Notch signaling pathway to overcome drug resistance for cancer therapy. Biochim Biophys Acta 2010;1806:258–67.

[51] Azmi AS, Mohammad RM, Sarkar FH. Can network pharmacology rescue neutraceutical cancer research? Drug Discov Today 2012;17:807–9.

[52] Keiser MJ, Setola V, Irwin JJ, Laggner C, Abbas AI, Hufeisen SJ, et al. Predicting new molecular targets for known drugs. Nature 2009;462:175–81.

[53] Hingorani SR, Petricoin EF, Maitra A, Rajapakse V, King C, Jacobetz MA, et al. Preinvasive and invasive ductal pancreatic cancer and its early detection in the mouse. Cancer Cell 2003;4:437–50.

[54] Walker I, Newell H. Do molecularly targeted agents in oncology have reduced attrition rates? Nat Rev Drug Discov 2009;8:15–6.

[55] Straehle C, Cardoso F, Azambuja E, Dolci S, Meirsman L, Vantongelen K, et al. Better translation from bench to bedside: breakthroughs in the individualized treatment of cancer. Crit Care Med 2009;37:S22–9.

[56] Benson JD, Chen YN, Cornell-Kennon SA, Dorsch M, Kim S, Leszczyniecka M, et al. Validating cancer drug targets. Nature 2006;441:451–6.

[57] Folger O, Jerby L, Frezza C, Gottlieb E, Ruppin E, Shlomi T. Predicting selective drug targets in cancer through metabolic networks. Mol Syst Biol 2011;7:501.

[58] Tao W, Xu X, Wang X, Li B, Wang Y, Li Y, et al. Network pharmacology-based prediction of the active ingredients and potential targets of Chinese herbal radix curcumae formula for application to cardiovascular disease. J Ethnopharmacol 2013;145:1–10.

[59] Yamanishi Y. Chemogenomic approaches to infer drug-target interaction networks. Methods Mol Biol 2013;939:97–113.

[60] Rowinsky EK. Curtailing the high rate of late-stage attrition of investigational therapeutics against unprecedented targets in patients with lung and other malignancies. Clin Cancer Res 2004;10:4220s–6s.

[61] Bai JP, Abernethy DR. Systems pharmacology to predict drug toxicity: integration across levels of biological organization. Annu Rev Pharmacol Toxicol 2013;53: 451–73.

[62] Jack J, Wambaugh J, Shah I. Systems toxicology from genes to organs. Methods Mol Biol 2013;930:375–97.

[63] Harrill AH, Rusyn I. Systems biology and functional genomics approaches for the identification of cellular responses to drug toxicity. Expert Opin Drug Metab Toxicol 2008;4:1379–89.

[64] Nicholson JK, Lindon JC. Systems biology: metabonomics. Nature 2008;455:1054–6.

[65] Penrod NM, Cowper-Sal-lari R, Moore JH. Systems genetics for drug target discovery. Trends Pharmacol Sci 2011;32:623–30.

[66] Gibbs JP. Prediction of exposure-response relationships to support first-in-human study design. AAPS J 2010;12:750–8.

[67] Wang Z, Ahmad A, Li Y, Azmi AS, Miele L, Sarkar FH. Targeting notch to eradicate pancreatic cancer stem cells for cancer therapy. Anticancer Res 2011;31:1105–13.

[68] Azmi AS, Sarkar FH. Prostate cancer stem cells: molecular characterization for targeted therapy. Asian J Androl 2012;14:659–60.

[69] Bao B, Ahmad A, Azmi AS, Ali S, Sarkar FH. Overview of cancer stem cells (CSCs) and mechanisms of their regulation: implications for cancer therapy. Curr Protoc Pharmacol 2013. Chapter 14, Unit 14, 25.

[70] Hermann PC, Huber SL, Herrler T, Aicher A, Ellwart JW, Guba M, et al. Distinct populations of cancer stem cells determine tumor growth and metastatic activity in human pancreatic cancer. Cell Stem Cell 2007;1:313–23.

[71] Bao B, Azmi AS, Li Y, Ahmad A, Ali S, Banerjee S, et al. Targeting CSCs in tumor microenvironment: the potential role of ROS-associated miRNAs in tumor aggressiveness. Curr Stem Cell Res Ther 2014;9(1):22–35.

[72] Bao B, Li Y, Ahmad A, Azmi AS, Bao G, Ali S, et al. Targeting CSC-related miRNAs for cancer therapy by natural agents. Curr Drug Targets 2012;13:1858–68.

[73] Bao B, Ali S, Ahmad A, Azmi AS, Li Y, Banerjee S, et al. Hypoxia-induced aggressiveness of pancreatic cancer cells is due to increased expression of VEGF, IL-6 and miR-21, which can be attenuated by CDF treatment. PLoS One 2012;7:e50165.

[74] Hermann PC, Bhaskar S, Cioffi M, Heeschen C. Cancer stem cells in solid tumors. Semin Cancer Biol 2010;20:77–84.

[75] Azmi AS, Aboukameel A, Bao B, Sarkar FH, Philip PA, Kauffman M, et al. Selective inhibitors of nuclear export block pancreatic cancer cell proliferation and reduce tumor growth in mice. Gastroenterology 2013;144:447–56.

[76] Wotton KR, Mazet F, Shimeld SM. Expression of FoxC, FoxF, FoxL1, and FoxQ1 genes in the dogfish Scyliorhinus canicula defines ancient and derived roles for Fox genes in vertebrate development. Dev Dyn 2008;237:1590–603.

[77] Mazet F, Luke GN, Shimeld SM. The amphioxus FoxQ1 gene is expressed in the developing endostyle. Gene Expr Patterns 2005;5:313–5.

[78] Qiao Y, Jiang X, Lee ST, Karuturi RK, Hooi SC, Yu Q. FOXQ1 regulates epithelial-mesenchymal transition in human cancers. Cancer Res 2011;71:3076–86.

[79] Abba M, Patil N, Rasheed K, Nelson LD, Mudduluru G, Leupold JH, et al. Unraveling the role of FOXQ1 in colorectal cancer metastasis. Mol Cancer Res 2013;11:1017–28.

[80] Gao M, Shih I, Wang TL. The role of forkhead box q1 transcription factor in ovarian epithelial carcinomas. Int J Mol Sci 2012;13:13881–93.

[81] Zhang H, Meng F, Liu G, Zhang B, Zhu J, Wu F, et al. Forkhead transcription factor foxq1 promotes epithelial-mesenchymal transition and breast cancer metastasis. Cancer Res 2011;71:1292–301.

[82] Zhu Z, Zhu Z, Pang Z, Xing Y, Wan F, Lan D, et al. Short hairpin RNA targeting FOXQ1 inhibits invasion and metastasis via the reversal of epithelial-mesenchymal transition in bladder cancer. Int J Oncol 2013;42:1271–8.

[83] Pregizer S, Mortlock DP. Control of BMP gene expression by long-range regulatory elements. Cytokine Growth Factor Rev 2009;20:509–15.

[84] Hamada S, Satoh K, Hirota M, Fujibuchi W, Kanno A, Umino J, et al. Expression of the calcium-binding protein S100P is regulated by bone morphogenetic protein in pancreatic duct epithelial cell lines. Cancer Sci 2009;100:103–10.

[85] Hamada S, Satoh K, Hirota M, Kimura K, Kanno A, Masamune A, et al. Bone morphogenetic protein 4 induces epithelial-mesenchymal transition through MSX2 induction on pancreatic cancer cell line. J Cell Physiol 2007;213:768–74.

[86] Tsuchida R, Osawa T, Wang F, Nishii R, Das B, Tsuchida S, et al. BMP4/Thrombospondin-1 loop paracrinically inhibits tumor angiogenesis and suppresses the growth of solid tumors. Oncogene 2013.

[87] Topic I, Ikic M, Ivcevic S, Kovacic N, Marusic A, Kusec R, et al. Bone morphogenetic proteins regulate differentiation of human promyelocytic leukemia cells. Leuk Res 2013;37:705–12.

[88] Ma W, Ma J, Xu J, Qiao C, Branscum A, Cardenas A, et al. Lin28 regulates BMP4 and functions with Oct4 to affect ovarian tumor microenvironment. Cell Cycle 2013;12:88–97.

[89] Altaner C. Glioblastoma and stem cells. Neoplasma 2008;55:369–74.

CHAPTER 14

Characterizing the Metabolomic Effects of Pancreatic Cancer

Oliver F. Bathe

Departments of Surgery and Oncology, University of Calgary, Calgary, AB, Canada

Contents

Introduction   323
  Metabolic Derangements Associated with Pancreatic Cancer   324
    Metabolic Derangements in Tumor Cells   324
    Metabolic Alterations Accompanying Pathogenic Processes Leading to Pancreatic Cancer 328
    Metabolic Alterations Originating in Host Tissues   328
  Metabolomic Characterization of Pancreatic Cancer   329
  Biological Insights Derived from Metabolomic Studies   332
  Development of Metabolomics-Based Diagnostic Testing   333
  Development of Therapeutics Targeting Disordered Metabolism   336
Conclusion   337
References   338

INTRODUCTION

Pancreatic cancer is the fourth most common cause of cancer death in North America. The five-year survival rate is only 5.1% [1]. The high lethality related to pancreatic cancer is due to a number of factors. It is biologically aggressive, it has profound effects on the host, and it is resistant to most cytotoxic agents. Moreover, early diagnosis is infrequent, and so resection (which represents the only chance for long-term control of this devastating disease) can be performed only in a minority of patients. Because of the limited success in diagnosing and treating pancreatic cancer, it is timely to consider alternative approaches to understanding the underlying pathophysiology. Pancreatic cancer is known to have metabolic effects on the host, and the tumor itself contains genetic aberrations with a number of metabolic consequences. Enhancing our understanding of the metabolic sequelae of pancreatic cancer therefore may lead to the development of new methods for diagnosis, as well as novel approaches to treatment.

Molecular Diagnostics and Treatment of Pancreatic Cancer

With advances in technologies capable of the multiparametric interrogation of the metabolome, a more comprehensive view of the metabolic alterations that characterize pancreatic cancer is now possible. A number of groups have initiated such an effort. Some novel biological observations have been derived from metabolomics studies, although there is considerable potential to leverage on those initial observations. Metabolomic studies also have provided a foundation for development of novel diagnostic tests.

Metabolic Derangements Associated with Pancreatic Cancer

The metabolic derangements observed in any individual with pancreatic cancer are related to a multitude of factors. The diseased tissue (i.e., tumor cells and stroma) displays aberrant metabolism. Environmental and host factors that have predisposed the individual to pancreatic cancer in the first place also will be evident. Finally, established disease induces bioenergetic changes in adjacent and remote host tissues (Figure 14.1).

Metabolic Derangements in Tumor Cells

One of the hallmarks of a cancer cell is the reprogramming of energy metabolism [2]. Large amounts of adenosine triphosphate (ATP) and substrate are required to support rapidly proliferating cells. Adaptations in metabolic pathways that typify cancer cells produce sufficient ATP as well as carbohydrates, proteins, lipids, and nucleotides to sustain the high metabolic demand. The classic example of metabolic reprogramming is the Warburg effect, described decades ago [3]. In normal cells, in the presence of sufficient oxygen, glucose is processed through oxidative phosphorylation, generating a maximal amount of ATP. Glycolysis, a less efficient means to produce ATP, only becomes a primary means to metabolize glucose in hypoxic conditions. In contrast, in cancer cells, glycolysis is the dominant pathway for glucose metabolism regardless of oxygen supply. Although glycolysis is not as efficient as oxidative phosphorylation at generating ATP, it is a much more rapid means of ATP production, necessary to support multiple cellular divisions. This phenomenon of increased glucose processing in cancer cells forms the basis of using ^{18}F-fluorodeoxyglucose positron emission tomography (FDG-PET) to detect and monitor tumors [4,5]. In addition to accelerated glycolysis, tumor cells have other characteristic features of metabolic reprogramming, each functioning to support the rapidly expanding

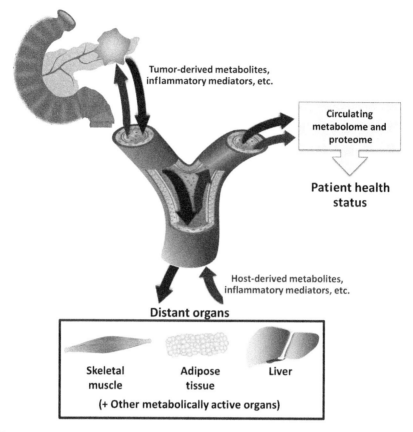

Figure 14.1 *Schematic representation of tissues contributing to the circulating pool of metabolites, in individuals with cancer.* In addition to cancer cells, tumors consist of an assortment of cells, including vascular endothelial cells, fibroblasts, and various inflammatory cells—forming the tumor microenvironment. Thus, not only do cancer cells affect the circulating metabolome; other (stromal) cells forming the tumor microenvironment contribute as well. Tumors have metabolic effects on adjacent normal tissue, as well as distant tissues, including muscle, fat, and liver. The metabolic response derived from the host also contributes to the circulating metabolome and may further modify tumor biology. The inflammatory and metabolic behavior of tumor and host tissues together contribute to the health of the pancreatic cancer patient. (For color version of this figure, the reader is referred to the online version of this book.)

biomass within the tumor. For example, glutamine uptake is enhanced, to replenish the tricarboxylic acid cycle; glutaminolysis also contributes to the production of acetyl coenzyme A for subsequent lipid biosynthesis, and increased fatty acid and lipid synthesis sustain synthesis of cell membranes and lipid derivatives.

The metabolic phenotype of cancer cells is regulated by both onco-genes and tumor suppressor genes (reviewed in [6]). In pancreatic cancer, mutations in the *KRAS* oncogene are found in more than 90% of pan-creatic cancers [7,8].Tumors with *KRAS* mutations express high levels of glucose transporter-1 (GLUT1), providing the ability for enhanced glu-cose uptake and glycolysis, enabling survival in low glucose conditions [9]. High levels of *c-MYC* expression are seen in almost 80% of pancreatic cancers [10]. *c-MYC* overexpression accelerates glutaminolysis by several mechanisms, including increased expression of mitochondrial glutamin-ase (GLS) [6,11–13]. Interestingly, *c-MYC* transcriptionally represses microRNAs mIR23a and mIR23b, resulting in increased expression of mitochondrial GLS [12]. One additional effect of *c-MYC* overexpression is increased synthesis of acetyl-CoA in mitochondria, which subsequently increases histone acetylation and fatty acid biosynthesis [13,14]. Hypoxia-inducible factor (HIF)-1α protein expression is seen in about half of pan-creatic cancers [15] as a result of intratumoral hypoxia and paracrine insulin [16]; hypoxia stabilizes the transcription factor and the protein [6]. HIF-1 transcription factor activates numerous target genes (reviewed in [17]). HIF-1 transcription factor not only is a pivotal regulator of oxygen homeostasis but also encourages glycolysis, contributes to the metabolism of nucleotides and iron, and exerts additional effects on cellular bioener-getics through its mitogenic effects. Both *c-MYC* and HIF-1α increase the rate of transcription of some of the GLUT transporters (increasing glu-cose uptake by the cell) and hexokinase-2 [6].Thus, genetic alterations in the tumor can contribute to the metabolic phenotype of tumor cells and subsequently disturb host energy homeostasis (Figure 14.2).

The metabolic phenotype of tumor cells can be influenced further by events at the transcriptional and protein levels. One example of this is the enzyme pyruvate kinase (PK), the enzyme that catalyzes the last step of glycolysis. In cancer cells, the M2-PK isoform (normally found in embry-onic tissue) is the predominant PK isoform. Selective binding of M2-PK to tyrosine-phosphorylated peptides causes inhibition of M2-PK enzymatic activity [18], causing a shift in cellular metabolism to aerobic metabolism (the Warburg effect) [19]. Impaired PK activity also leads to an accumula-tion of metabolites, preceding PK in the glycolytic pathway, which act as precursors for nucleic acids, amino acids, and phospholipids.This metabolic switch has been shown to provide a selective growth advantage to tumor cells [19].

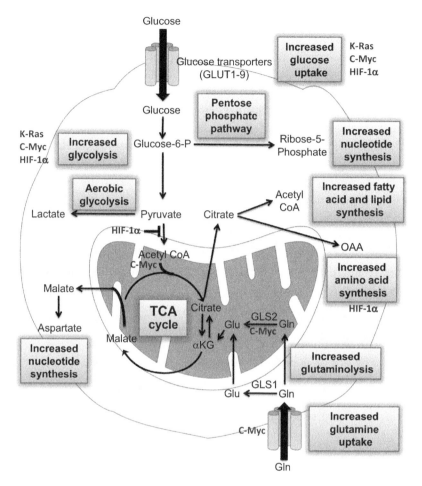

Figure 14.2 *General features of the reprogrammed energy metabolism that characterizes pancreatic cancer cells.* Generally, the metabolic changes that typify cancer cells support cell growth and proliferation. Glucose uptake is increased, and glycolysis is accelerated. Lactic acid fermentation is prominent, even in the presence of high oxygen levels. Glutamine (Gln) uptake is markedly enhanced, then converted to glutamate (Glu). Glutamate replenishes the tricarboxylic acid (TCA) cycle, which is essential because metabolites of the TCA cycle are required for synthesis of lipids, nonessential amino acids, and nucleotides. Fatty acid and lipid synthesis are increased, which provides the necessary products to sustain synthesis of cell membranes and other lipid derivatives. Overexpression of *KRAS, c-MYC* and HIF-1α frequently occur in pancreatic cancer; known metabolic effects are summarized. (aKG = a-ketoglutarate; GLS = glautaminase; GLUT = glucose transporter.) (For color version of this figure, the reader is referred to the online version of this book.)

Metabolic Alterations Accompanying Pathogenic Processes Leading to Pancreatic Cancer

It has become clear that the pathogenesis of pancreatic cancer is promoted by environmental and host factors, which may contribute to the overall metabolic milieu of the patient with established pancreatic cancer. Obesity increases the risk of gastrointestinal cancers [20], including pancreatic cancer [21]. Similarly, diabetes is a risk factor for pancreatic cancer. These conditions have clear metabolic consequences. Inflammation also may be an important factor in the pathogenesis; chronic pancreatitis predisposes to pancreatic cancer [22,23]. Experimentally, interactions between dietary factors, inflammation, and genetic predisposition have been shown. In mice with pancreas-specific activation of oncogenic *KRAS*, a high-fat diet accelerates development of pancreatic intraepithelial neoplasm (the lesion preceding development into malignancy) [24]. In that model, obesity-related promotion of pancreatic malignancy is mediated by tumor necrosis factor (TNF), as abrogation of TNF signaling inhibits this effect. In this same model, inflammation and tissue damage are essential to the development of pancreatic cancer [22]. Thus, in addition to the aberrant metabolism of pancreatic cancer cells, the environmental and host factors that have predisposed an individual to pancreatic cancer will contribute to the many metabolic derangements seen in pancreatic cancer patients.

Metabolic Alterations Originating in Host Tissues

Pancreatic cancer is known to have profound effects on key metabolic pathways in host tissues, with detrimental effects on the health of the host and further adding to the eccentric metabolic milieu. Jaundice frequently accompanies tumors in the head of the pancreas, with gross effects on fat absorption and coagulation factors, as well as more subtle effects on mentation (lethargy, fatigue, anorexia), presumably influenced by metabolic mediators. Diabetes mellitus (DM) and cachexia are frequent sequelae of pancreatic cancer.

The prevalence of DM in pancreatic cancer is reported as 40–47%, of which the majority of cases are new onset (i.e., within two years of the diagnosis of pancreatic cancer) [25–27]. It has been suggested that pancreatic cancer causes DM due to secretion of diabetogenic factors by tumor [28], although these factors have not yet been identified. Hyperinsulinemia and peripheral insulin resistance is the prevailing trait in pancreatic cancer, which distinguishes it from the diabetes that typifies chronic pancreatitis, which is accompanied by islet cell destruction and impaired insulin production [29,30]. Yet the diabetes of pancreatic cancer is also atypical for type II DM. Family history is often noncontributory, there is an absence of obesity, and there is a rapid progression to insulin dependence [31]. Although it is known that different mechanisms of DM have variable metabolic consequences, such as different effects on lipid metabolism [32,33], the full range of metabolic effects of different causes of DM are unknown. Moreover, the underlying metabolic effects of the tumor are poorly understood.

Cachexia involves weight loss, skeletal muscle wasting (sarcopenia), and loss of adipose tissue. Unlike simple malnutrition (lack of food), this tumor-associated syndrome is characterized by hypermetabolism, activation of catabolic processes (including lipolysis and proteolysis), and systemic endocrine and metabolic alterations. Cachexia is especially apparent in pancreatic cancer and portends a worse prognosis [34,35]. Muscle wasting in cachexia occurs as a result of depressed protein synthesis and increased protein degradation [36]. Fat metabolism also appears to be altered markedly. There is depletion of circulating phospholipids and deficits of essential fatty acids [37–39]. Lipolysis at the level of the adipocyte is accelerated and loss of fat accelerates as patients approach death [38,40] In all, the higher metabolic rates seen with cachexia increase demand for energy substrates; a 40% increase in metabolic rate would require approximately 600 additional calories per day if no change in dietary intake occurred to accommodate metabolic need.

Metabolomic Characterization of Pancreatic Cancer

Given the multiplicity of cancer-derived, environmental, and host-derived factors that can influence the metabolic milieu in a whole cancer patient, it is clear that understanding the overall impact of each of these factors will require a systems biology approach. That is, a more comprehensive picture of the metabolome is required in tumor and host tissues, factors that influence their interactions will need to be elucidated, and effects on the health of the whole patient will need to be delineated. The field of metabolomics represents a tool for developing this understanding.

Metabolomics is the multiparametric characterization of low-molecular-weight metabolites in a biological system, including in the pathophysiologic state. The metabolome can be evaluated in a multiplexed fashion using two primary technologies: nuclear magnetic resonance (NMR) spectroscopy and mass spectrometry (MS). These two technologies are complementary, as metabolites detectable in one technology are not necessarily detectable in the other. Moreover, the methodology is now well established for combining data obtained from the two technologies [41].

Proton nuclear magnetic resonance (^{1}H-NMR) spectroscopy exploits the magnetic properties of protons (i.e., the ^{1}H nucleus). The sample is exposed to radiofrequency (RF) radiation generated from a magnetic field, and an NMR spectrum is produced by the emission of absorbed RF energy by a compound at a particular magnetic field strength. This analytical method is particularly useful for investigating abnormal body fluid compositions, as a wide range of metabolites can be quantified simultaneously, with no sample preparation or sample destruction [42,43].

MS represents a means of obtaining more comprehensive multivariate metabolic data, useful for the analysis of clinical samples [44]. Mass spectra are generated by the mass-to-charge ratio of various compounds. MS is analytically more sensitive than NMR, but differential ionization suppression can make pattern quantification difficult [43], particularly in a complex mixture such as serum. Combining MS with a separation technique (e.g., gas chromatography, liquid chromatography) reduces the complexity of the mass spectra, and delivers additional information on the physicochemical properties of the metabolites [45]. Alternatively, tandem MS, in which some form of fragmentation occurs between multiple steps of MS, is a means to perform a focused analysis of amino acids [46].

Currently, no single analytical technology is capable of detecting all metabolites in a biological sample. ^{1}H-NMR spectroscopy is excellent for the nontargeted analysis of metabolites, but it lacks the sensitivity to detect metabolites present at lower levels. Gas chromatography–MS (GC–MS) is useful for the detection of volatile organic compounds as well as a number of metabolites made amenable to detection by chemical derivatization [45]. Liquid chromatography–MS does not require chemical derivatization, it is sensitive, and it is useful for the detection of a large variety of metabolite classes, including lipids and fatty acids because of its high resolution [47,48].

From a biological perspective, understanding the metabolome as it relates to malignancy has a number of advantages. Metabolites represent the end product of transcription and translation, providing functional insight. Analytical platforms are sensitive and high throughput, allowing the study of real-time metabolic perturbations that result from events such as cancer initiation, progression, and metastasis.

From a biomarker perspective, metabolomic biomarkers have a number of advantages over transcriptomic and proteomic biomarkers. First, changes in the metabolome are amplified relative to changes in the transcriptome and proteome [49]. Therefore, metabolites may change even when protein levels do not; changes in physiology are relatively immediately associated with metabolomic perturbations. Second, metabolomic profiling is cheaper, easier, and higher throughput than proteomic and transcriptomic profiling. Thus, a test based on metabolomics could be implemented easily in the clinic, even in mass screening. Third, changes in metabolism result in alterations of the abundance of *groups* of metabolites. Therefore, identification of the patterns of changes in metabolites would provide insight on the functional changes that occur because of any given condition. The metabolomic profile therefore represents a biomarker (or metabiomarker) of considerable interest, albeit one that has been studied relatively little so far.

The metabolome can be studied using practically any biofluid, including serum, plasma, and urine, as well as tissues, including tumor and normal tissue. So far, no attempts have been made to evaluate the metabolome of tumor tissue in pancreatic cancer, although other tumor types have been studied in this fashion [50–52]. Because a large component of pancreatic cancer is composed of nontumor (stromal) cells, there may be challenges in the interpretation of data from this type of analysis.

A number of groups have analyzed circulating metabolites in pancreatic cancer, as well as excreted (urinary) metabolites [46,53–60]. Most studies have consisted of small groups of patients. In some studies, disease-free controls were used as comparators; and, in others, patients with benign pancreatic disease were used as comparators. The heterogeneity of study design, differences in analytical modalities, and reports on small groups of patients make it difficult to derive consistent observations, although some metabolic features are reported on repeated occasions.

Studies on the serum metabolome using ^{1}H-NMR spectroscopy have been reported by several groups [53 55,57]. Increased glucose, decreased lactate, increased triglycerides, increased leucine and isoleucine, decreased proline and asparagine, and decreased urea have been observed. Analysis of serum by GC–MS in a small group of patients demonstrated a reduction phenylalanine, tryptamine, and inosine [56]. A larger study [59] revealed decreased valine, methionine, asparagine, histidine, tyrosine, and uric acid in pancreatic cancer compared with healthy controls. Decreased glutamine and increased glutamate frequently have been reported by studies utilizing various analytical platforms.

The urine metabolome has been studied using ^{1}H-NMR spectroscopy [60]. Cancer-specific increases in a number of amino acids and amino acid derivatives were noted. Elevations of hypoxanthine, choline, trimethyl-amine-N-oxide, o-acetylcarnitine, and acetone also were seen.

Biological Insights Derived from Metabolomic Studies

Interrogating circulating and excreted metabolites provides some insight on the biological effects of pancreatic cancer. On the other hand, blood and urine metabolites may originate from the tumor or the host, and the challenge remains to dissect how metabolomic perturbations reflect processes originating in the tumor microenvironment or in normal host tissues. Despite that caveat, some metabolomic features of pancreatic cancer can be extrapolated from available data.

Pancreatic cancer is associated with disordered carbohydrate metabolism as manifested by impaired glycemic control. 1,5-anhydro-D-glucitol, a serum biomarker of short-term glycemic control [61], is decreased in pancreatic cancer [59]. In our interrogation of the metabolome associated with pancreatic cancer, we have observed that even in patients without overt DM, changes in carbohydrate metabolism congruent with latent diabetes were seen [54]. Galactose, a glucose substitute, is increased for reasons that are not understood.

In pancreatic cancer, there are decreases in serum levels of amino acids. At the same time, excreted amino acids are increased. Serum urea, a nitrogenous waste product generated with protein and nucleic acid catabolism, can be increased. This pattern may be reflective of muscle protein breakdown, during which all constituent amino acids enter oxidative pathways. This is perhaps reflective of cachexia, which is common in pancreatic cancer.

Glutamine is decreased and glutamate is increased. This pattern often is seen in other malignancies, likely reflecting accelerated glutaminolysis, which is known to be an important source of fuel in tumor cells [62–64]. Oxidative metabolism of glucose and glutamine produces citrate, and citrate subsequently is metabolized to acetyl-coenzyme A for lipid synthesis, as well as intermediates that contribute to the tricarboxylic acid (TCA) cycle. Thus far, this has not been reported in metabolomics studies. Moreover, little is known about the lipidomic changes associated with pancreatic cancer.

To better understand the host contribution of changes in circulating and excreted metabolites in pancreatic cancer, further studies are required. Specifically, it will be important to understand exactly how the metabolome of pancreatic cancer-associated DM differs from type I and type II DM, the effects of jaundice must be further delineated, and the effects of pancreatic cancer-associated cachexia must be understood. It is becoming clear that the overall health of the patient with pancreatic cancer is not only a function of tumor biology but also of the host response to tumor. Understanding the range of host responses to pancreatic cancer and the effects on clinical outcomes will perhaps provide novel opportunities for therapeutic intervention.

Once we have improved knowledge of the contributions of tumor and host to the circulating metabolome and once the implications of each of these changes are understood, the genetic basis of these phenomena as well as the proteomic correlates can be dissected. The multiplexed metabolomic information derived from metabolomic studies provides a means to identify pathways putatively affected by pancreatic cancer using bioinformatic approaches [65,66]. Pathways so extrapolated from metabolomic data generate hypotheses, allowing interrogation of metabolomic changes associated with tumor or host genotype. Alternatively, multiplexed genomic, transcriptomic, proteomic, and metabolomic data sets can be derived in parallel to catalog linkages in genotype and phenotype. Some attempts have been made to integrate "omics" information [67–69]. Even alterations in the activity of a single metabolic enzyme, however, can affect multiple cellular signaling pathways [70]. Therefore, such an approach would be challenging from a bioinformatics perspective and little mechanistic insight would be derived, except in discreet experimental systems. So far, few studies linking genotype and metabolic phenotype have been done, and this represents an important direction in the field.

Interestingly, we also have seen that the metabolomic profile of pancreatic cancer differs slightly from that of other periampullary adenocarcinomas (i.e., bile duct cancer, duodenal cancer, and ampullary cancer) (unpublished data). Our studies so far suggest that the disordered carbohydrate metabolism that typifies pancreatic cancer is much less pronounced in nonpancreatic periampullary adenocarcinomas. Nonpancreatic periampullary adenocarcinomas generally have a better prognosis related to a less aggressive biology. Further studies will be required to understand how differences in metabolism might contribute to these different biologies.

Development of Metabolomics-Based Diagnostic Testing

Biomarkers may be defined as any biomolecule or panel of biomolecules that can aid in the diagnosis of disease, prognostication, prediction of biology, or prediction of sensitivity to specific therapies. For pancreatic cancer, biomarkers may be clinically useful in a number of instances. A biomarker that aids in diagnosing pancreatic cancer would be useful. Biomarkers that identify prognostic subsets of patients with pancreatic cancer may be useful, perhaps to refine selection of operative candidates. One subset of patients that may be particularly important to identify is the subset that is susceptible to cancer cachexia, for it may be possible to inhibit progression of that condition if detected early. Predictive biomarkers may become more important as better (and more diverse) systemic therapy options become available. In the setting of pancreatic cancer, the serum or plasma and urine represent the biofluids of greatest interest, as they are most convenient to collect.

Clinically, one difficult diagnostic dilemma is whether any pancreatic mass or biliary stricture is benign or malignant. None of the clinical features or radiographic findings is pathognomonic. Obtaining a tissue diagnosis is difficult. Bile duct brushings (in the event of a biliary stricture) only have a yield of 23–41% [71,72]. The diagnostic rate of endoscopic ultrasound (EUS)-guided biopsies for pancreatic masses is only about 71% [73]. Although their sensitivity is about 85%, the negative predictive value is only about 64% [74]. Percutaneous biopsies have similar sensitivities and negative predictive values [75]. Therefore, negative biopsies are not particularly informative and do not aid in clinical decision making [76].

Serum tumor markers, such as the carbohydrate antigen CA19-9 and carcinoembryonic antigen (CEA), also have been utilized to aid in the diagnosis of pancreatic and other periampullary malignancies [77–82]. Unfortunately, neither of these markers is particularly sensitive or specific. CA19-9 has been best characterized in this context because it is more frequently elevated in pancreatic and periampullary cancers. Unfortunately, a number of related benign conditions cause elevated CA19-9 levels [77,79,83]. In most series, the sensitivity of serum CA19-9 is 50–80% and the specificity is about 90% [77,78,81,82]. This implies that very high levels of CA19-9 strongly support the diagnosis of malignancy, but normal or slightly elevated levels of these tumor markers do not rule out malignancy. CEA levels have a similar diagnostic value.

The inherent difficulty in distinguishing benign and malignant lesions has a number of consequences. First, gastroenterologists and other referring physicians are reluctant to refer patients to a surgeon without convincing evidence that there is a cancer. This may lead to treatment delays, perhaps even resulting in growth of the tumor beyond resectability. Second, surgeons often are faced with deciding whether to resect a suspicious (but undiagnosed) mass. This is not a trivial decision, as pancreatic resections are extensive operations associated with high morbidity and mortality rates [84–86]. In the United States, the overall in-hospital mortality rate for pancreatic resections is 7.6% [87]. In surgical series, 7–16% (and as high as 25%) of patients who undergo a Whipple procedure or a radical pancreatectomy are found on final pathology to have benign lesions [88–92]. In our center, 26% of patients who have major pancreatic resections ultimately are found to have benign disease [93]. Third, even in patients with advanced disease, a tissue diagnosis is sometimes not possible, and decisions related to chemotherapy must be made based on best clinical evidence. Clearly, there is a substantial need for an improved means of distinguishing benign and malignant pancreatic lesions.

A metabolomics-based test represents one potential solution to enhance the clinician's capability to distinguish benign and malignant pancreatic and periampullary lesions. Our group has demonstrated the feasibility of using ^{1}H-NMR spectroscopy to derive metabolomics profiles that distinguish benign and malignant lesions [54]. In that series, which did not include an external validation set, the area under the receiver operating curve (AUROC) for identifying pancreatic cancer was 0.8372. Further studies are required to validate the metabolomic profile diagnostic for pancreatic cancer. GC–MS similarly has been shown to identify a metabolomic profile diagnostic for pancreatic cancer with an AUROC of 0.76 on an external validation cohort [59]. Our experience is that combining GC–MS and ^{1}H-NMR spectroscopy does not add to diagnostic power, despite the more comprehensive interrogation of the metabolome (unpublished data). More studies are required to determine the clinical utility of metabolomics-based tests, which reflects to what degree such tests could affect clinical decision making.

Cancer cachexia, a prominent sequela of pancreatic cancer, is known to be associated with poor clinical outcomes. Although additional studies are required to understand what tumor or host-derived factors predispose to cachexia, the metabolic disturbances that accompany cachexia are becoming apparent. Therefore, potentially useful therapeutic interventions can be devised in the hopes that the pathogenesis of cachexia can be halted to the patient's benefit. Clinical trials of therapies require accurate identification of the subgroup that has cachexia. Cross-sectional imaging (using *computed tomography* [CT] scan) demonstrating muscle wasting (sarcopenia) is useful for identifying patients who have advanced cachexia [94,95]. Using ^{1}H-NMR spectroscopy, the profile of urine metabolites associated with the CT scan-evident sarcopenia has been described [95]. It may be possible, using longitudinal studies in which the trajectory of muscle wasting is known, to identify earlier metabolomic changes that characterize a precachectic state. Earlier identification of individuals susceptible to cachexia may enhance the likelihood that any given therapeutic intervention would provide benefit.

Development of Therapeutics Targeting Disordered Metabolism

Systemic agents presently used to treat pancreatic cancer (gemcitabine, 5-fluoropyrimidine, capecitabine) employ metabolic strategies to impair nucleic acid synthesis. Unfortunately, they have minimal impact on survival, although there is some benefit to quality of life. Therefore, there is a need for novel strategies to treat pancreatic cancer. Information derived from metabolomics studies may point the way to improved ways of targeting the disordered metabolism seen in pancreatic cancer.

The most obvious means to target metabolism is to direct interventions at the disordered carbohydrate metabolism that characterizes pancreatic cancer. Small molecule metabolic inhibitors such as oxythiamine, a transketolase inhibitor, have been shown to inhibit pancreatic cancer cell proliferation [96] and therefore may have some therapeutic potential. Oral hypoglycemics used to treat diabetes are being investigated, and retrospective studies have demonstrated reductions in cancer-related mortality in diabetics taking metformin [97,98], although this has not been shown in pancreatic cancer [99]. Interestingly, metformin is toxic to cancer stem cells [100], including some populations of pancreatic cancer stem cells [101]. In breast cancer patients, metformin is associated with higher response rates to cytotoxic chemotherapy [102]. Metformin is known to inhibit pancreatic cancer cell growth in vitro and in vivo [103,104]. Thus, further studies are required to understand how targeting carbohydrate metabolism may improve clinical outcomes in pancreatic cancer.

Tumors with *KRAS* and MYC mutations may be particularly susceptible to such interventions. Oncogenic MYC promotes glutaminolysis and addiction to glucose and glutamine; cells with *c-MYC* overexpression die in the absence of glucose or glutamine [11]. *KRAS* transformed fibroblasts lose their proliferative ability with glutamine deprivation [105]. In preclinical models, targeting metabolic enzymes to disrupt glucose metabolism is effective in the treatment of tumors driven by *KRAS* and *c-MYC* [9,106,107]. Glutaminolysis is catalyzed by GLS, which has two major isoforms, GLS1 and GLS2. Mitochondrial GLS (GLS2) is a downstream effector of MYC, encouraging entry of glutamine into the

TCA cycle [11,12]. Therefore, in pancreatic cancer, inhibition of gluta-minolysis, perhaps by interference with GLS2 represents one potential therapeutic strategy.

The main challenge in designing agents that target metabolism will be to avoid toxicity related to targeting metabolic pathways in normal prolif-erating cells. Therefore, it will be imperative to identify pathways that are redundant in normal cells but absent in cancer cells. Identification of such a therapeutic window may be facilitated by comprehensive analysis of the metabolome in cancer cells and normal cells.

Finally, clinical outcomes may be enhanced if the metabolic and inflam-matory features of the host response to pancreatic cancer could be ablated. For example, if the early metabolic changes of cachexia were recognized and cachexia could be anticipated, nutritional or pharmacologic interven-tion could be instituted. A number of agents for the treatment of cachexia are in clinical development, including anabolic agents, but none have yet been approved for this indication [94].

CONCLUSION

Pancreatic cancer has long been known to have metabolic consequences, including DM, obstructive jaundice, and any attending liver dysfunction, as well as cachexia. Multiplexed analysis of the metabolome in normal and malignant tissues using ^{1}H-NMR spectroscopy and MS has the potential to provide a more comprehensive picture of the metabolic changes associated with pancreatic cancer. This will yield an improved understanding of the biology of pancreatic cancer, particularly when metabolomic data are linked with genomic and proteomic data. The practical implications of this information will become apparent when these data are linked with data on clinical outcomes. With the develop-ment of systemic therapies that can target tumor metabolism or that can moderate any adverse host responses to cancer, there will be a need to catalog the specific metabolic alterations associated with pancreatic can-cer. In addition, with properly designed biomarker studies, analysis of the circulating or urinary metabolome will allow identification of bio-markers, which could enhance the diagnosis and subcategorization of pancreatic cancer. Progress in the field will require meaningful collabo-rations between clinicians, basic scientists, experts in metabolomics, and biostatisticians.

REFERENCES

[1] Ries LAG MD, Krapcho M, Stinchcomb DG, Howlader N, Horner MJ, Mariotto A, et al. *SEER cancer statistics review, 1975–2005.* Bethesda, MD: National Cancer Institute; 2007. [updated November, 2007; cited 2008 June 21, 2008]; Available from: http://seer.cancer.gov/csr/1975_2005/.

[2] Hanahan D, Weinberg RA. Hallmarks of cancer: the next generation. Cell 2011;144(5):646–74.

[3] Warburg O. On the origin of cancer cells. Science 1956;123(3191):309–14.

[4] Liu T, Zhang J, Wang X, Yang J, Tang Z, Lu J. Radiolabeled glucose derivatives for tumor imaging using SPECT and PET. Curr Med Chem 2013. [Epub 2013/09/03].

[5] Tamm EP, Bhosale PR, Vikram R, de Almeida Marcal LP, Balachandran A. Imaging of pancreatic ductal adenocarcinoma: state of the art. World J Radiol 2013;5(3): 98–105.

[6] Levine AJ, Puzio-Kuter AM. The control of the metabolic switch in cancers by oncogenes and tumor suppressor genes. Science 2010;330(6009):1340–4.

[7] Jones S, Zhang X, Parsons DW, Lin JC, Leary RJ, Angenendt P, et al. Core signaling pathways in human pancreatic cancers revealed by global genomic analyses. Science 2008;321(5897):1801–6.

[8] Collins MA, Brisset JC, Zhang Y, Bednar F, Pierre J, Heist KA, et al. Metastatic pancreatic cancer is dependent on oncogenic Kras in mice. PLoS One 2012;7(12):e49707.

[9] Yun J, Rago C, Cheong I, Pagliarini R, Angenendt P, Rajagopalan H, et al. Glucose deprivation contributes to the development of KRAS pathway mutations in tumor cells. Science 2009;325(5947):1555–9.

[10] He C, Jiang H, Geng S, Sheng H, Shen X, Zhang X, et al. Expression of c-Myc and Fas correlates with perineural invasion of pancreatic cancer. Int J Clin Exp Pathol 2012;5(4):339–46.

[11] Wise DR, DeBerardinis RJ, Mancuso A, Sayed N, Zhang XY, Pfeiffer HK, et al. Myc regulates a transcriptional program that stimulates mitochondrial glutaminolysis and leads to glutamine addiction. Proc Natl Acad Sci USA 2008;105(48):18782–7.

[12] Gao P, Tchernyshyov I, Chang TC, Lee YS, Kita K, Ochi T, et al. c-Myc suppression of miR-23a/b enhances mitochondrial glutaminase expression and glutamine metabolism. Nature 2009;458(7239):762–5.

[13] Miller DM, Thomas SD, Islam A, Muench D, Sedoris K. c-Myc and cancer metabolism. Clin Cancer Res 2012;18(20):5546–53.

[14] Morrish F, Noonan J, Perez-Olsen C, Gafken PR, Fitzgibbon M, Kelleher J, et al. Myc-dependent mitochondrial generation of acetyl-CoA contributes to fatty acid biosynthesis and histone acetylation during cell cycle entry. J Biol Chem 2010;285(47):36267–74.

[15] Kasuya K, Tsuchida A, Nagakawa Y, Suzuki M, Abe Y, Itoi T, et al. Hypoxia-inducible factor-1alpha expression and gemcitabine chemotherapy for pancreatic cancer. Oncol Rep 2011;26(6):1399–406.

[16] Wang F, Li SS, Segersvard R, Strommer L, Sundqvist KG, Holgersson J, et al. Hypoxia inducible factor-1 mediates effects of insulin on pancreatic cancer cells and disturbs host energy homeostasis. Am J Pathol 2007;170(2):469–77.

[17] Semenza GL. Targeting HIF-1 for cancer therapy. Nat Rev Cancer 2003;3(10): 721–32.

[18] Christofk HR, Vander Heiden MG, Wu N, Asara JM, Cantley LC. Pyruvate kinase M2 is a phosphotyrosine-binding protein. Nature 2008;452(7184):181–6.

[19] Christofk HR, Vander Heiden MG, Harris MH, Ramanathan A, Gerszten RE, Wei R, et al. The M2 splice isoform of pyruvate kinase is important for cancer metabolism and tumour growth. Nature 2008;452(7184):230–3.

[20] Calle EE, Rodriguez C, Walker-Thurmond K, Thun MJ. Overweight, obesity, and mortality from cancer in a prospectively studied cohort of U.S. adults. New Engl J Med 2003;348(17):1625–38.

[21] Isaksson B, Jonsson F, Pedersen NL, Larsson J, Feychting M, Permert J. Lifestyle factors and pancreatic cancer risk: a cohort study from the Swedish Twin Registry. Int J Cancer 2002;98(3):480–2.

[22] Guerra C, Schuhmacher AJ, Canamero M, Grippo PJ, Verdaguer L, Perez-Gallego L, et al. Chronic pancreatitis is essential for induction of pancreatic ductal adenocarcinoma by K-Ras oncogenes in adult mice. Cancer Cell 2007;11(3):291–302.

[23] Huggett MT, Pereira SP. Diagnosing and managing pancreatic cancer. Pract 2011; 255(1742):21–5, 2–3.

[24] Khasawneh J, Schulz MD, Walch A, Rozman J, Hrabe de Angelis M, Klingenspor M, et al. Inflammation and mitochondrial fatty acid beta-oxidation link obesity to early tumor promotion. Proc Natl Acad Sci USA 2009;106(9):3354–9.

[25] Pannala R, Leirness JB, Bamlet WR, Basu A, Petersen GM, Chari ST. Prevalence and clinical profile of pancreatic cancer-associated diabetes mellitus. Gastroenterology 2008;134(4):981–7.

[26] Chari ST, Leibson CL, Rabe KG, Timmons LJ, Ransom J, de Andrade M, et al. Pancreatic cancer-associated diabetes mellitus: prevalence and temporal association with diagnosis of cancer. Gastroenterology 2008;134(1):95–101.

[27] Chari ST, Leibson CL, Rabe KG, Ransom J, de Andrade M, Petersen GM. Probability of pancreatic cancer following diabetes: a population-based study. Gastroenterology 2005;129(2):504–11.

[28] Katsumichi I, Pour PM. Diabetes mellitus in pancreatic cancer: is it a causal relationship? Am J Surg 2007;194(Suppl. 4):S71–5.

[29] Meisterfeld R, Ehehalt F, Saeger HD, Solimena M. Pancreatic disorders and diabetes mellitus. Exp Clin Endocrinol Diabetes 2008;116(Suppl. 1):S7–12.

[30] Larsen S. Diabetes mellitus secondary to chronic pancreatitis. Dan Med Bull 1993;40(2):153–62.

[31] Noy A, Bilezikian JP. Clinical review 63: diabetes and pancreatic cancer: clues to the early diagnosis of pancreatic malignancy. J Clin Endocrinol Metab 1994;79(5):1223–31.

[32] Muoio DM, Newgard CB. Mechanisms of disease: molecular and metabolic mechanisms of insulin resistance and beta-cell failure in type 2 diabetes. Nat Rev Mol Cell Biol 2008;9(3):193–205.

[33] Muoio DM, Newgard CB. Fatty acid oxidation and insulin action: when less is more. Diabetes 2008;57(6):1455–6.

[34] Fearon KC, Baracos VE. Cachexia in pancreatic cancer: new treatment options and measures of success. HPB (Oxford) 2010;12(5):323–4.

[35] Tan BH, Birdsell LA, Martin L, Baracos VE, Fearon KC. Sarcopenia in an overweight or obese patient is an adverse prognostic factor in pancreatic cancer. Clin Cancer Res 2009;15(22):6973–9.

[36] Tisdale MJ. Cancer cachexia. Curr Opin Gastroenterol 2010;26(2):146–51.

[37] Murphy RA, Mourtzakis M, Chu QS, Reiman T, Mazurak VC. Skeletal muscle depletion is associated with reduced plasma (n-3) fatty acids in non-small cell lung cancer patients. J Nutr 2010;140(9):1602–6.

[38] Murphy RA, Wilke MS, Perrine M, Pawlowicz M, Mourtzakis M, Lieffers JR, et al. Loss of adipose tissue and plasma phospholipids: relationship to survival in advanced cancer patients. Clin Nutr 2010;29(4):482–7.

[39] Murphy RA, Mourtzakis M, Chu QS, Baracos VE, Reiman T, Mazurak VC. Nutritional intervention with fish oil provides a benefit over standard of care for weight and skeletal muscle mass in patients with nonsmall cell lung cancer receiving chemotherapy. Cancer 2011;117(8):1775–82.

[40] Ryden M, Agustsson T, Laurencikiene J, Britton T, Sjolin E, Isaksson B, et al. Lipolysis—not inflammation, cell death, or lipogenesis—is involved in adipose tissue loss in cancer cachexia. Cancer 2008;113(7):1695–704.

[41] Crockford DJ, Holmes E, Lindon JC, Plumb RS, Zirah S, Bruce SJ, et al. Statistical heterospectroscopy, an approach to the integrated analysis of NMR and UPLC-MS data sets: application in metabonomic toxicology studies. Anal Chem 2006;78(2): 363–71.

[42] Nicholson JK, Lindon JC, Holmes E. 'Metabonomics': understanding the metabolic responses of living systems to pathophysiological stimuli via multivariate statistical analysis of biological NMR spectroscopic data. Xenobiotica 1999;29(11):1181–9.

[43] Nicholson JK, Connelly J, Lindon JC, Holmes E. Metabonomics: a platform for studying drug toxicity and gene function. Nat Rev Drug Discov 2002;1(2):153–61.

[44] Denkert C, Budczies J, Kind T, Weichert W, Tablack P, Sehouli J, et al. Mass spectrometry-based metabolic profiling reveals different metabolite patterns in invasive ovarian carcinomas and ovarian borderline tumors. Cancer Res 2006;66(22):10795–804.

[45] Dettmer K, Aronov PA, Hammock BD. Mass spectrometry-based metabolomics. Mass Spectrom Rev 2007;26(1):51–78.

[46] Leichtle AB, Ceglarek U, Weinert P, Nakas CT, Nuoffer JM, Kase J, et al. Pancreatic carcinoma, pancreatitis, and healthy controls: metabolite models in a three-class diagnostic dilemma. Metabolomics 2013;9(3):677–87.

[47] Roberts LD, McCombie G, Titman CM, Griffin JL. A matter of fat: an introduction to lipidomic profiling methods. J Chromatogr B Analyt Technol Biomed Life Sci 2008;871(2):174–81.

[48] Forcisi S, Moritz F, Kanawati B, Tziotis D, Lehmann R, Schmitt-Kopplin P. Liquid chromatography-mass spectrometry in metabolomics research: mass analyzers in ultra high pressure liquid chromatography coupling. J Chromatogr A 2013;1292:51–65.

[49] Kell DB. Metabolomic biomarkers: search, discovery and validation. Expert Rev Mol Diagn 2007;7(4):329–33.

[50] Denkert C, Budczies J, Weichert W, Wohlgemuth G, Scholz M, Kind T, et al. Metabolite profiling of human colon carcinoma–deregulation of TCA cycle and amino acid turnover. Mol Cancer 2008;7:72.

[51] Chan EC, Koh PK, Mal M, Cheah PY, Eu KW, Backshall A, et al. Metabolic profiling of human colorectal cancer using high-resolution magic angle spinning nuclear magnetic resonance (HR-MAS NMR) spectroscopy and gas chromatography mass spectrometry (GC/MS). J Proteome Res 2009;8(1):352–61.

[52] Cheng LL, Burns MA, Taylor JL, He W, Halpern EF, McDougal WS, et al. Metabolic characterization of human prostate cancer with tissue magnetic resonance spectroscopy. Cancer Res 2005;65(8):3030–4.

[53] Fang F, He X, Deng H, Chen Q, Lu J, Spraul M, et al. Discrimination of metabolic profiles of pancreatic cancer from chronic pancreatitis by high-resolution magic angle spinning 1H nuclear magnetic resonance and principal components analysis. Cancer Sci 2007;98(11):1678–82.

[54] Bathe OF, Shaykhutdinov R, Kopciuk K, Weljie AM, McKay A, Sutherland FR, et al. Feasibility of identifying pancreatic cancer based on serum metabolomics. Cancer Epidemiol Biomarkers Prev 2011;20(1):140–7.

[55] Tesiram YA, Lerner M, Stewart C, Njoku C, Brackett DJ. Utility of nuclear magnetic resonance spectroscopy for pancreatic cancer studies. Pancreas 2012;41(3):474–80.

[56] Urayama S, Zou W, Brooks K, Tolstikov V. Comprehensive mass spectrometry based metabolic profiling of blood plasma reveals potent discriminatory classifiers of pancreatic cancer. Rapid Commun Mass Spectrom 2010;24(5):613–20.

[57] OuYang D, Xu J, Huang H, Chen Z. Metabolomic profiling of serum from human pancreatic cancer patients using 1H NMR spectroscopy and principal component analysis. Appl Biochem Biotechnol 2011;165(1):148–54.

[58] Zhang H, Wang Y, Gu X, Zhou J, Yan C. Metabolomic profiling of human plasma in pancreatic cancer using pressurized capillary electrochromatography. Electrophoresis 2011;32(3–4):340–7.
[59] Kobayashi T, Nishiumi S, Ikeda A, Yoshie T, Sakai A, Matsubara A, et al. A novel serum metabolomics-based diagnostic approach to pancreatic cancer. Cancer Epidemiol Biomarkers Prev 2013;22(4):571–9.
[60] Davis VW, Schiller DE, Eurich D, Bathe OF, Sawyer MB. Pancreatic ductal adenocarcinoma is associated with a distinct urinary metabolomic signature. Ann Surg Oncol 2012.
[61] Yamanouchi T, Akanuma Y. Serum 1,5-anhydroglucitol (1,5 AG): new clinical marker for glycemic control. Diabetes Res Clin Pract 1994;(Suppl. 24):S261–8.
[62] Turowski GA, Rashid Z, Hong F, Madri JA, Basson MD. Glutamine modulates phenotype and stimulates proliferation in human colon cancer cell lines. Cancer Res 1994;54(22):5974–80.
[63] Wasa M, Bode BP, Abcouwer SF, Collins CL, Tanabe KK, Souba WW. Glutamine as a regulator of DNA and protein biosynthesis in human solid tumor cell lines. Ann Surg 1996;224(2):189–97.
[64] Lobo C, Ruiz-Bellido MA, Aledo JC, Marquez J, Nunez De Castro I, Alonso FJ. Inhibition of glutaminase expression by antisense mRNA decreases growth and tumourigenicity of tumour cells. Biochem J 2000;348(Pt 2):257–61.
[65] Xia J, Psychogios N, Young N, Wishart DS. MetaboAnalyst: a web server for metabolomic data analysis and interpretation. Nucleic Acids Res 2009;37(Web Server Issue):W652–60.
[66] Ingenuity Systems Pathway Analysis. 2013; Available from: http://www.ingenuity.com.
[67] Kanani H, Dutta B, Klapa MI. Individual vs. combinatorial effect of elevated CO_2 conditions and salinity stress on Arabidopsis thaliana liquid cultures: comparing the early molecular response using time-series transcriptomic and metabolomic analyses. BMC Syst Biol 2010;4:177.
[68] Grimplet J, Cramer GR, Dickerson JA, Mathiason K, Van Hemert J, Fennell AY. Vitis-Net: "Omics" integration through grapevine molecular networks. PLoS One 2009;4(12):e8365.
[69] Oberbach A, Bluher M, Wirth H, Till H, Kovacs P, Kullnick Y, et al. Combined proteomic and metabolomic profiling of serum reveals association of the complement system with obesity and identifies novel markers of body fat mass changes. J Proteome Res 2011;10(10):4769–88.
[70] Wang J, Zhang X, Ma D, Lee WN, Xiao J, Zhao Y, et al. Inhibition of transketolase by oxythiamine altered dynamics of protein signals in pancreatic cancer cells. Exp Hematol Oncol 2013;2(1):18.
[71] Fogel EL, deBellis M, McHenry L, Watkins JL, Chappo J, Cramer H, et al. Effectiveness of a new long cytology brush in the evaluation of malignant biliary obstruction: a prospective study. Gastrointest Endosc 2006;63(1):71–7.
[72] Mahmoudi N, Enns R, Amar J, AlAli J, Lam E, Telford J. Biliary brush cytology: factors associated with positive yields on biliary brush cytology. World J Gastroenterol 2008;14(4):569–73.
[73] Savides TJ, Donohue M, Hunt G, Al-Haddad M, Aslanian H, Ben-Menachem T, et al. EUS-guided FNA diagnostic yield of malignancy in solid pancreatic masses: a benchmark for quality performance measurement. Gastrointest Endosc 2007; 66(2):277–82.
[74] Ross WA, Wasan SM, Evans DB, Wolff RA, Trapani LV, Staerkel GA, et al. Combined EUS with FNA and ERCP for the evaluation of patients with obstructive jaundice from presumed pancreatic malignancy. Gastrointest Endosc 2008;68(3):461–6.
[75] Clarke D, Clarke B, Thomson S, Garden O, Lazarus N. The role of preoperative biopsy in pancreatic cancer. HPB (Oxford) 2004;6(3):144–53.

[76] Members NPP, editor. NCCN clinical practice guidelines in oncology: pancreatic adenocarcinoma. Version 1.2008. Fort Washington, PA: National Comprehensive Cancer Network, Inc; 2007.

[77] Steinberg W. The clinical utility of the CA 19-9 tumor-associated antigen. Am J Gastroenterol 1990;85:350–5.

[78] Ni XG, Bai XF, Mao YL, Shao YF, Wu JX, Shan Y, et al. The clinical value of serum CEA, CA19-9, and CA242 in the diagnosis and prognosis of pancreatic cancer. Eur J Surg Oncol 2005;31:164–9.

[79] Kim HJ, Kim MH, Myung SJ, Lim BC, Park ET, Yoo KS, et al. A new strategy for the application of CA19-9 in the differentiation of pancreaticobiliary cancer: analysis using a receiver operating characteristic curve. Am J Gastroenterol 1999;94: 1941–6.

[80] Kau SY, Shyr YM, Su CH, Wu CW, Lui WY. Diagnostic and prognostic values of CA 19-9 and CEA in periampullary cancers. J Am Coll Surg 1999;188:415–20.

[81] Kim HJ, Lee KT, Kim SH, Lee JK, Lim SH, Paik SW, et al. Differential diagnosis of intrahepatic bile duct dilatation without demonstrable mass on ultrasonography or CT: benign versus malignancy. J Gastroenterol Hepatol 2003;18:1287–92.

[82] Patel AH, Harnois DM, Klee GG, LaRusso NF, Gores GJ. The utility of CA 19-9 in the diagnoses of cholangiocarcinoma in patients without primary sclerosing cholangitis. Am J Gastroenterol 2000;95:204–7.

[83] Nehls O, Gregor M, Klump B. Serum and bile markers for cholangiocarcinoma. Semin Liver Dis 2004;24:139–54.

[84] Crist DW, Sitzmann JV, Cameron JL. Improved hospital morbidity, mortality, and survival after the Whipple procedure. Ann Surg 1987;206:358–65.

[85] Bathe OF, Caldera H, Hamilton KL, Franceschi D, Sleeman D, Livingstone AS, et al. Diminished benefit from resection of cancer of the head of the pancreas in patients of advanced age. J Surg Oncol 2001;77(2):115–22.

[86] Bathe OF, Caldera H, Hamilton-Nelson K, Franceschi D, Sleeman D, Levi JU, et al. Influence of Hispanic ethnicity on outcome after resection of carcinoma of the head of the pancreas. Cancer 2001;91(6):1177–84.

[87] Meguid RA, Ahuja N, Chang DC. What constitutes a "high-volume" hospital for pancreatic resection? J Am Coll Surg 2008;206(4):e1–9.

[88] van Heerden JA, McIlrath DC, Dozois RR, Adson MA. Radical pancreatoduodenectomy—a procedure to be abandoned? Mayo Clin Proc 1981;56(10):601–6.

[89] Abraham SC, Wilentz RE, Yeo CJ, Sohn TA, Cameron JL, Boitnott JK, et al. Pancreaticoduodenectomy (Whipple resections) in patients without malignancy: are they all 'chronic pancreatitis'? Am J Surg Pathol 2003;27(1):110–20.

[90] Kennedy T, Preczewski L, Stocker SJ, Rao SM, Parsons WG, Wayne JD, et al. Incidence of benign inflammatory disease in patients undergoing Whipple procedure for clinically suspected carcinoma: a single-institution experience. Am J Surg 2006;191(3): 437–41.

[91] Hoshal Jr VL, Benedict MB, David LR, Kulick J. Personal experience with the Whipple operation: outcomes and lessons learned. Am Surg 2004;70(2):121–5.

[92] Aranha GV, Hodul PJ, Creech S, Jacobs W. Zero mortality after 152 consecutive pancreaticoduodenectomies with pancreaticogastrostomy. J Am Coll Surg 2003;197(2): 223–31.

[93] McLean SR, Karsanji D, Wilson J, Dixon E, Sutherland FR, Pasieka J, et al. The effect of wait times on oncological outcomes from periampullary adenocarcinomas. J Surg Oncol 2013;107(8):853–8.

[94] Dodson S, Baracos VE, Jatoi A, Evans WJ, Cella D, Dalton JT, et al. Muscle wasting in cancer cachexia: clinical implications, diagnosis, and emerging treatment strategies. Annu Rev Med 2011;62:265–79.

[95] Stretch C, Eastman T, Mandal R, Eisner R, Wishart DS, Mourtzakis M, et al. Prediction of skeletal muscle and fat mass in patients with advanced cancer using a metabolomic approach. J Nutr 2012;142(1):14–21.

[96] Zhang H, Cao R, Lee WN, Deng C, Zhao Y, Lappe J, et al. Inhibition of protein phosphorylation in MIA pancreatic cancer cells: confluence of metabolic and signaling pathways. J Proteome Res 2010;9(2):980–9.

[97] Evans JM, Donnelly LA, Emslie-Smith AM, Alessi DR, Morris AD. Metformin and reduced risk of cancer in diabetic patients. BMJ 2005;330(7503):1304–5.

[98] Bowker SL, Majumdar SR, Veugelers P, Johnson JA. Increased cancer-related mortality for patients with type 2 diabetes who use sulfonylureas or insulin. Diabetes Care 2006;29(2):254–8.

[99] Hwang AL, Haynes K, Hwang WT, Yang YX. Metformin and survival in pancreatic cancer: a retrospective cohort study. Pancreas 2013;42(7):1054–9.

[100] Hirsch HA, Iliopoulos D, Tsichlis PN, Struhl K. Metformin selectively targets cancer stem cells, and acts together with chemotherapy to block tumor growth and prolong remission. Cancer Res 2009;69(19):7507–11.

[101] Gou S, Cui P, Li X, Shi P, Liu T, Wang C. Low concentrations of metformin selectively inhibit CD133(+) cell proliferation in pancreatic cancer and have anticancer action. PLoS One 2013;8(5):e63969.

[102] Jiralerspong S, Palla SL, Giordano SH, Meric-Bernstam F, Liedtke C, Barnett CM, et al. Metformin and pathologic complete responses to neoadjuvant chemotherapy in diabetic patients with breast cancer. J Clin Oncol 2009;27(20):3297–302.

[103] Nair V, Pathi S, Jutooru I, Sreevalsan S, Basha R, Abdelrahim M, et al. Metformin inhibits pancreatic cancer cell and tumor growth and downregulates Sp transcription factors. Carcinogenesis 2013.

[104] Karnevi E, Said K, Andersson R, Rosendahl AH. Metformin-mediated growth inhibition involves suppression of the IGF-I receptor signalling pathway in human pancreatic cancer cells. BMC Cancer 2013;13:235.

[105] Gaglio D, Soldati C, Vanoni M, Alberghina L, Chiaradonna F. Glutamine deprivation induces abortive s-phase rescued by deoxyribonucleotides in k-ras transformed fibroblasts. PLoS One 2009;4(3):e4715.

[106] Clem B, Telang S, Clem A, Yalcin A, Meier J, Simmons A, et al. Small-molecule inhibition of 6-phosphofructo-2-kinase activity suppresses glycolytic flux and tumor growth. Mol Cancer Ther 2008;7(1):110–20.

[107] Le A, Cooper CR, Gouw AM, Dinavahi R, Maitra A, Deck LM, et al. Inhibition of lactate dehydrogenase A induces oxidative stress and inhibits tumor progression. Proc Natl Acad Sci USA 2010;107(5):2037–42.

CHAPTER 15

Prioritizing Diagnostic, Prognostic, and Therapeutic MicroRNAs in Pancreatic Cancer: Systems and Network Biology Approaches

Osama M. Alian[1], Shadan Ali[1], Ramzi M. Mohammad[1,2],
Asfar S. Azmi[3], Fazlul H. Sarkar[1,3]

[1]Department of Oncology, Karmanos Cancer Institute, Wayne State University, Detroit, MI, USA, [2]Hamad Medical Corporation, Doha, Qatar, [3]Department of Pathology, Wayne State University, Detroit, MI, USA

Contents

An Introduction and Brief Overview of MicroRNAs	345
MicroRNAs and Disease Priming and Progression	346
Diagnostic, Prognostic, and Therapeutic Value of miRNAs in Pancreatic Cancer	349
Prioritizing miRNAs from Pancreatic Biospecimens Using Pathway Tools	352
Clinical Targeting of miRNAs	352
Implications—New Hope or Wild-Goose Chase?	357
Conclusion	359
References	359

AN INTRODUCTION AND BRIEF OVERVIEW OF MicroRNAs

MicroRNAs (miRNAs) are short noncoding RNAs 22 nucleotides in length that carry out complex regulatory functions through post-transcriptional targeting and modification. Initially, these miRNAs were discovered through analyses of *Caenorhabditis elegans* development, in which it was shown that the *lin-4* and *let-7* antisense RNAs exhibited developmental regulatory function in the organism post-transcriptionally [1]. The miRNAs are exported from the nucleus and undergo processing from larger to smaller segments via various endonucleases [2]. For a time, their role relative to or within cellular function was largely unknown, yet with increasing analyses of sequence complementarity, mounting evidence suggested that miRNAs function as a family formed of RNA duplexes directly capable of gene regulation post-transcriptionally [3].

Given the remarkable placement of miRNAs in the regulatory chain, it makes sense that a corresponding expression variance could be ascertained through different cell types or cell states. Indeed this is the case, wherein various specific types of miRNAs are found exclusively in specific cellular systems in a context-dependent manner. An example of this is the highly concentrated presence of miR-122 in the liver or miR-223 in mouse bone marrow granulocytes and macrophages [4]. Such nuanced differences in expression levels also could be seen in stem versus differentiated cells in animal models. Recently, an experiment demonstrated the use of miR-291-3p, miR-294, and miR-295 in the enhancement of induced pluripotency, highlighting the valuable role of these molecules in normal development [5].

Logic stands that, given the delicate placement of miRNAs within the post-transcriptional regulatory pathway, disease development and progression could be correlated closely to aberrant miRNA function. Indeed, this is the case because erroneous expression (deregulated expression) or depletion of this class of molecules results in a concurrent defect in cellular function, ranging from contrasting phenotypic changes, such as developmental aberrations, to physiological abnormalities, such as degenerative conditions linked to malignancies [6].

This chapter thus explores the significance of miRNAs in disease and the various facets surrounding their relevance clinically and experimentally as well as their future implications in the ever-changing omics paradigms.

MicroRNAs AND DISEASE PRIMING AND PROGRESSION

Because of the intricate links of miRNAs in genetic post-transcriptional control, their aberrant behavior can be analogous to "disease priming" whereby a fine homeostatic balance is effectively disturbed, initiating the development of a disease state. Key within this fact is the very basis of many clinically presented malignancies essentially being deregulated cells, no longer able to carry out apoptosis. The miRNAs have presented themselves as regulators of many aspects of cell function, and when their mechanisms fail, they contribute to cancer development [7]. Healthy cells thus require a cascade of events to take place dissociating the cell from its regulatory mechanisms. The miRNAs contribute to this cascade as a form of a switch that functions to activate or deactivate pathways or "microcircuits" within the regulatory schematic [8]. These control points vary in location and function both regulating the progression and timing of cellular events as well as disrupting them in a highly regulated context-dependent fashion.

If we subdivide the process of cancer development according to the Hallmarks of Cancer scheme of Hanahan and Weinberg, then we arrive at six distinct phases of cellular function that must be analyzed synergistically: proliferative signaling, evasion, invasiveness and metastasis, replicative immortality, angiogenesis, and resisting cell death (Figure 15.1) [9]. Each of

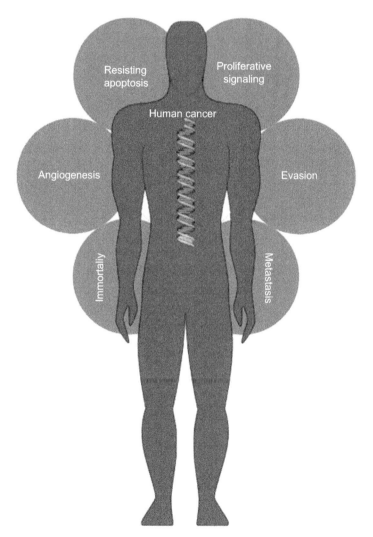

Figure 15.1 *A Representative Diagram of the Interrelated Drivers of Human Cancer.* (For color version of this figure, the reader is referred to the online version of this book.)

these has had miRNAs implicated in one form or another either as direct interacting partners with molecules or as part of larger feedback loops for regulatory control.

A search through any article database will yield thousands of articles highlighting the many thousands of possible mechanisms miRNAs use to exert their regulatory control over physiology. Generally, under normal conditions, many miRNAs have been shown to provide oversight, earlier characterized as microswitches. This regulatory oversight has been implicated in multiple pathways, one of which is progenitor cell proliferation and downstream function [10]. Placed in the context of the well-studied epithelial-to-mesenchymal transition (EMT) exhibited in highly malignant cells, many of the same miRNAs were shown to exert a concerted control over crucial signaling pathways—for example, Hedgehog signaling leading to concurrent proliferation of the cells [11]. It then becomes readily apparent that aberrations in miRNA signaling stimulate a breakdown of the regulatory cascade of cellular function from a genetic perspective. One telling example is reduced expression of the *let*-7 tumor suppressor miRNA through phosphorylating the human miRNA-generating complexes, which in turn mediate the mitogen-activated protein kinase/extracellular signal-regulated kinase (MAPK/ERK) signaling pathway [12]. MAPK/ERK is particularly important because of its involvement in maintaining stem cell pluripotency [13]. From this can be inferred further the maintenance of cancer stem cell populations contributing to the later proliferative phases of cancer but still sharing the same signaling malfunctions expressed earlier in the cell cycle [14]. This signaling motif contributes to the self-sustainability of the cancer cells, which also enhances their ability to evade the body's regulatory policing by responding to various stimuli. In glioma cells, an interesting relationship was established between glucose levels and the expression of miR-451 [15]. When glucose is present, miR-451 exists at elevated levels, but when the reverse takes place, a concurrent decrease in miR-451 results in slowed proliferation but enhanced evasion in terms of migration and survival. Thus, miR-451 was established as a possible regulator of the liver kinase B1/adenosine monophosphate-activated protein kinase signaling pathway. A similar mechanism was elucidated for the PI3K/AKT pathway also in gliomas where miR-451 was downregulated, causing inhibition of cell growth and initiation of apoptosis [16]. Interestingly, an upregulation of miR-451 expression (albeit without glucose starvation) elicited a different response in esophageal carcinoma, whereby apoptosis was initiated, and cell invasiveness and proliferation were diminished in the EC9706 cell line [17].

Many examples could be found in which miRNAs present themselves as important components of key regulatory pathways related to cellular communication and function [18]. In some pathways, miRNAs exert a direct and stringent function on downstream regulators. Some of these very mechanisms are inherently important for basic physiological functions; when they are aberrant, however, they become the root causes of cancer development even when no outright phenotypic patterns are demonstrated [19]. The same pathways involving miRNAs in their chain of function also regularly are perturbed when analyzed in patients, such as the forkhead box protein M1 transcription factor [20]. Representing some of the complexities arising from dynamic miRNA function, it has been shown that some cancer cells have even evolved through a scheme of deleting miRNA recognition sequences evading regulation by the molecules in B-cell lymphomas [21]. The perturbations can vary and the family of miRNA can be quite different in function, depending on their location in the body [22]. One malfunctioning miRNA, implicated in one disease model in fact may be benign in another, and several seemingly unrelated benign miRNAs together may interact to form a disease phenotype [23].

DIAGNOSTIC, PROGNOSTIC, AND THERAPEUTIC VALUE OF miRNAs IN PANCREATIC CANCER

Pancreatic cancer (PC) is one of the leading causes of cancer mortality in the United States, with an estimated 43,920 new diagnoses and 37,390 resulting mortalities in 2012 [24]. Despite many advances in targeted drug discovery, progress on the five-year survival averages remains horrifically dismal at 5–6% [25]. PC continues to be an invasive and aggressive disease, combined with the late stages of discovery and diagnosis, ultimately resulting in low life expectancy. Multiple factors have been known to contribute to PC development and progression, ranging from environmental and genetic predisposition to epigenetic regulation and lifestyle habits, which collectively are increasing the risk for PC, such as through chronic pancreatitis [26].

One of the key elements making a dramatic entrance into PC research has been the presence of miRNA within several regulatory pathways of the disease, either contributing to the development or playing an important role in tumor aggressiveness. In a general survey of miRNA presence in cell lines and surgical specimens, Zhang et al. identified eight miRNAs (miR-296a, miR-190, miR-186, miR-221, miR-222, miR-200b, miR-15b, and miR-95) previously unidentified as components of the PC disease network [27]. Similarly, expression profiling of cancer cells led to the identification of miRNA signatures capable of discriminating between tumors and healthy tissues [28]. Within this same study, interestingly, many of the small number of identified perturbed miRNAs also were the same miRNAs initially uncovered as regulators of growth and development, such as the *let-7* family of miRNAs. A key question that inevitably is asked is can miRNAs be used to correctly identify and distinguish cancer types? Collins et al. in a recent study were able to utilize a reasonably small number of miRNAs (8 miRNAs) to distinguish distinct signatures of cholangiocarcinoma and pancreatic adenocarcinoma [29]. Critically, miRNAs have been implicated in the regulation or bolstering of cancer stem cells (CSCs) circulating in the body [30]. Targeting these CSCs through regulation of miRNA expression was demonstrated repeatedly. Furthermore, it has shown great promise in the creation of targeted synergistic combinations inhibiting or reversing the much-described EMT that is known to be a key phenotype of aggressive or metastatic behavior of cancer cells [31].

A large part of the high mortality and low five-year survival rate for PC result from its inability to be diagnosed at an early enough stage, rendering it a high priority to uncover early strategies for diagnosis [32]. Often, no obvious symptoms present themselves to direct diagnostic tests, and thus identification frequently is incidental to a search for another illness. Unfortunately, at this stage of identification, the disease usually has progressed aggressively into the surrounding tissues if not metastasized (locally advanced nonmetastatic disease). Additionally, a subset of patients with metastatic disease have tumors that are unresectable (80% of patients are not surgical candidates).

Within the scope of diagnosis and prognostic biomarkers, computational analysis of high-throughput data has shed some light on previously obscured genetic or epigenetic regulators of disease in PC. Computational analyses of these same pathways has shed light on the precise involvement and the level of control carried out by miRNAs, which can exert different functions depending on their partnered molecules. These relationships without sophisticated statistical analysis are hidden within the functions of the partnered molecules, which often are masked. The short life of miRNAs also contributes to their ability to fleetingly affect many cellular components, with many of the more highly studied miRNAs typically exhibiting prolonged and sustained levels of their concentrations during the biological function. Systems biology and computational analyses are able to derive relationships between seemingly unrelated networks of molecules, which are some of the characteristic nature of miRNA and their function. This was vividly implicated within the heavily studied p53 tumor-suppressing network as one of the key components of dysregulation in terms of the regulatory role of miR-34 [33]. Network analyses of 377 microarrays of pancreatic ductal adenocarcinoma (PDAC), chronic pancreatitis, and normal pancreas tissues were able to home in on 26 miRNAs highlighted in perturbation within PDAC [34]. The same study also was able to confirm the characteristic miRNA signature of miR-216/miR-217 expression, while lacking the expression of miR-133a. Multiple studies either in the form of direct analysis or meta-analysis have been able to link multiple miRNAs between different cancers, conserved along developmental aberration phenotypes that eventually lead to the development of cancer. Without systems analysis, an miRNA in one location with its direct partners can on the surface appear to exert a form of feedback control on a seemingly disconnected network unrelated to it without a contextual understanding of this relationship. Mathematical analysis of high-throughput data, such as that previously described, was able to discern expression correlations between what appear to be disconnected networks through biological analysis, and through that, it was determined that miRNAs exert orders of magnitude levels of control through this motif of regulation by interacting with binding partners and initiating both downstream effects and feedback loops within the scope of post-transcriptional regulation [35]. In this particular study, Gusev and colleagues, using the combinatorial target prediction algorithm miRgate and a two-step data reduction procedure, determined Gene Ontology categories as well as biological functions, disease categories, toxicological categories, and signaling pathways that are targeted by multiple miRNAs, statistically significantly enriched with target genes, and known to be affected in specific cancers (especially pancreatic cancer). Their global analysis of predicted miRNA targets suggested that coexpressed miRNAs collectively provide systemic compensatory response to the abnormal phenotypic changes in cancer cells by targeting a broad range of functional categories and signaling pathways known to be affected in PC. Such systems biology–based approaches provides new avenues for biological interpretation of miRNA profiling data and generation of experimentally testable hypotheses regarding collective regulatory functions of miRNA in cancer.

The same procedures and information potentially can be used for the identification of prognostic biomarkers to both stratify patients by their individual cancer subtype as well as to determine treatment efficacy down to the patient's own molecular level. Many such miRNAs have been uncovered and studied as candidates for prognosis [36]. One such example, the identification of miR-21 as a possible prognostic indicator in resectable PDAC, showed a marked ability to stratify success with adjuvant therapy [37]. The miR-21 in another study also was able to show as a good indicator of success with gemcitabine therapy or an indicator of gemcitabine resistance, which was able to predict for better treatment efficacy [38]. This is a highly important aspect of miRNA involvement in clinical diagnosis and prognosis as it provides a measurable molecular marker for predicting possible chemoresistance, a recurring problem in clinical treatment, as well as determination of suitable combination therapy tailored to the patient phenotype.

PRIORITIZING miRNAs FROM PANCREATIC BIOSPECIMENS USING PATHWAY TOOLS

To prioritize pancreatic miRNAs, our group evaluated large-scale PDAC patient samples. Using serum and paraffin-embedded tissue from fine-needle aspirate (FNA) biopsies, we were able to selectively pinpoint the differential expression of a number of miRNAs in tumor versus normal tissue. Among the major miRNAs discovered, the levels of mirR-21, miR-155, and miR-205 were found to be higher in tumors compared with normal tissue (Figure 15.2(A)). On the other hand, *let-7b* mir-146a, and *miR-185* were consistently lower in patient tumor samples compared with normal counterparts (Figure 15.2(B)).

Evaluation of the differentially expressed miRNAs using pathway analysis demonstrated that the lower expression of mir-146 led to the activation of prosurvival signaling NF-κB and related pathway (Figure 15.2(C)). These studies provide insights into how pathway analysis can help prioritize PDAC-related miRNAs that can further be incorporated in therapeutic strategies.

CLINICAL TARGETING OF miRNAs

Because of the many miRNAs uncovered throughout the past decade of research and the focus on their relationship to cancer and disease, a tremendous amount of work has been done to examine the viability of miRNAs

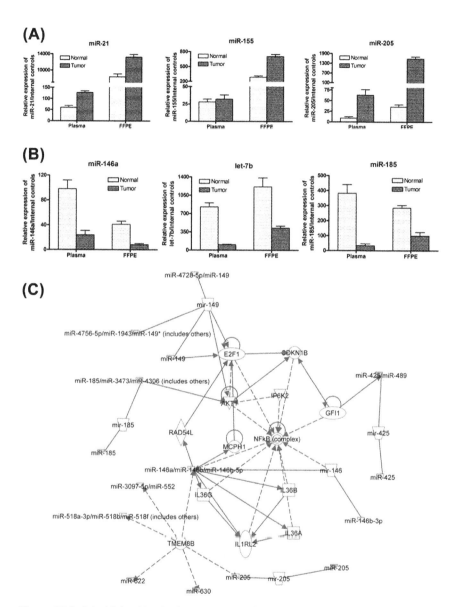

Figure 15.2 *Prioritizing PDAC miRNAs Using Differential Expression and Pathway Analyses in Patient Derived Samples.* Serum and FNA biopsies from 22 patients and 7 normal healthy individuals were compared for differences in expression of miRNAs. (A) The expression of miR-21, miR-155 and miR-205 was higher in tumor samples compared with normal. (B) On the other hand, miR-146, let-7b and miR-185 were found to be downregulated. (C) Pathway analysis demonstrated a direct link to activation of prosurvival signaling by lowering of miR-145 expression. (For color version of this figure, the reader is referred to the online version of this book.)

as both biomarkers of disease and treatable targets. It has been reported that in ovarian cancer, miR-200, miR-100, miR-141, miR-200b, and miR-200c presented themselves as suitable candidates as prognostic biomarkers in patients with distinct differential expression levels [39]. Similar screening of miRNA expression profiles yielded another closely linked set of molecules from the same family (e.g., miR-141) as a clinical diagnostic and prognostic indicator of bladder cancer [40]. The value of such miRNAs is in their ability to control function at a post-transcriptional genetic level, essentially cutting off the disease at its start [41]. Some may be targeted for upregulation as antagomiRs, antagonizing the misregulated expression of oncogenic miRNAs or oncomiRs, and others can be targeted for knockout or inhibition. This concept in a colorectal cancer model was explored by Akao et al., in which miR-143 was modified chemically yielding a greater inhibitory effect in what is believed to be tumor initiation than with endogenous miR-143 [42]. Many studies were carried out demonstrating the clinical potential of miRNA-based therapies yet one of the unique scientific potentials in miRNAs clinically relies on the ability to better quantify disease data. Many of these studies have been based on thorough analysis of high-throughput data in a large number of samples for statistical reliability. Some of the studies yielded new miRNA targets for clinical potential whether diagnostic or treatment markers, but their reliability requires further validation and wet-lab testing [43].

In the omics era, clinical medicine is moving toward a more computational approach of disease management, from the search for biomarkers in early diagnosis to unique high-throughput signatures of individual patient and population disease characteristics [44,45]. Initially, these studies were based on proteomics or genomics alone in terms of the central dogma of biology (DNA > RNA > Protein). Yet as our knowledge increased and with the discovery of miRNAs as key regulators of cellular function, which represent hundreds if not thousands of individual functioning miRNAs, their relationship to each other as well as the physiological system as a whole became a highly dynamic and complicated network of interactions [46]. These interactions also fail to be standard in the normal sense, but rather they are unique to each individual's physiology and environment, responding to their homeostatic needs. The goal essentially then becomes a question of being able to properly quantify disease characteristics as they change from patient to patient and how this heterogeneity of functional interactions can be utilized in both diagnosis and treatment [47]. The traditional methods of diagnosis and treatment thus are no longer adequate when compared with the amount of fine-tuned cellular regulation uncovered and its variability between patients. Because miRNAs function at a regulatory level, their analysis is crucial within the framework of dynamic genetic networks displaying such interaction and stochasticity [48]. This stochasticity and variability in theory can be used to categorize both populations of patients as well as subpopulations of disease in concert with genetic and protein partners, thereby specifying treatment modalities for better clinical outcomes [49]. Understanding these complex interactions is a feat that can be accomplished only through mathematical modeling along with the traditional biological tools of research. This is a basic tenet of computational biology and a key goal of personalized medicine as further knowledge is gained.

How do miRNAs fit in this paradigm? A distinction needs to be made between the older antiquated reductionist approach to cancer and the current evolving holistic approach. Understanding a tremendous amount of the detailed workings of molecular biology, we still lack a true understanding of how complex systems function or interact with other systems [50]. With the continuous development of sophisticated molecular tools for the analysis and understanding of molecular biology, there is highly anticipated hope that with the discovery and mapping of genes and proteins, a disease such as cancer could be wiped out through the targeting of a unique protein or gene. This goal has been met with strategic setbacks because of the incredibly dynamic nature of genes and their regulatory components either in dosage or transcriptional control [51]. Much of the research focused on the development and testing of highly specific compounds aimed at targeting either genetic function or protein products. Such was the excitement over the introduction of the highly targeted receptor tyrosine kinases, but increasing problems of relapse have demonstrated the insufficiency of such a single target-oriented treatment modality [52]. Over the past several decades, however, although other new classes of drugs were introduced, there were only modest increases in survival with relatively steady if not increasing drug attrition rates [53].

Then came the development of computational models to analyze the role of molecular networks in disease to ask a fundamental question of why some of these highly discriminating drugs failed [54]. The reality of our physiology, either normal or aberrant, is that no one magic molecule or gene is responsible for success or failure [55]. A disease such as cancer represents a series of compounding failures of the cellular regulatory chain that ultimately results in the disease. By working backward from disease to genes to understand the makeup of the malignancy, much of the evidence over-whelmingly was based on the most consistently expressed aberrant proteins, and then mutated genes and gene products, whereby each successive discov-ery was touted as the answer to defeating cancer. Unfortunately, this has created an environment of false hope surrounding much research as it is translated into the media [56]. The advent of network science as a means to bring mathematical sense to high-throughput data in step with the increas-ingly attractive realm of miRNA research leads us to the logical next phase of cancer research within the omics methodologies and that is not just characterizing erroneous expression but also the level or aberrant relation-ship between regulatory components [57]. Indeed, sophisticated analyses have been carried out such as the mirDREM (MIRna Dynamic Regula-tory Events Miner) method for determining computationally and mathe-matically the interactive relationships of miRNAs and their targets [58]. By establishing these relationships and following up with biological validation in a lung-development model, Schulz et al. were able to, within a reasonable degree of certainty, quantify the depth of regulatory interaction taking place between several previously unpredicted associated miRNAs (miR-466d, miR-466a, miR-23b, miR-30a, miR-30d, miR-125a) in addition to the already established miR-337 and miR-476c in development.

It is believed that miRNAs in humans, which are nearly a thousand or possibly more unique molecules, are capable of manipulating almost 60% of human genes [59]. This is in addition to their interactions with one another and the various feedback regulatory loops existing within their relationships [60]. Here we end up with an elegant example of nature's efficiency in which case a small number of molecules through dense and layered interac-tions exert orders of magnitude greater influence on their targets than their original number [61]. This is where the earlier presented microswitch anal-ogy really shines, as miRNAs indeed present themselves as sophisticated microswitches within a highly interactive system. The only reasonable way to analyze this role is through an in silico to in vitro to in vivo approach coupled with a reasonable analytical platform to bring about better contex-tual understanding of data [62].

Many of miRNA placements within functional regulation are strategic in nature, providing first, second, third, or more degrees of interactions which is a basic mechanism of signal amplification in biology and is the only logical explanation for such an extensive control of human genes [63]. Computational studies have shown indeed that the level of control exerted by miRNAs goes far into the traditional signaling networks extensively studied in all aspects of biology, such development, cell cycle control, proliferation, metastasis, and invasiveness [64]. At times, some key questions in canonical pathways or disease models were not answered until miRNA placement in the chain, sometimes many molecules away in relationship or perceived interaction [65].

IMPLICATIONS—NEW HOPE OR WILD-GOOSE CHASE?

There is a striking reality to the ubiquity of miRNAs and that is simply because of their *ubiquitous* nature in feedback or feed-forward regulation [66]. In a chemical study aimed at determining miRNA concentrations within various body fluids, Weber et al. found that detectable numbers of molecules can range from 204 in urine to 458 in saliva [67]. This begs a simple question of statistical viability (and variability)—that is, given the propensity of miRNAs to have many targets, sometimes unaccountable, do they represent enough of a fine-tuned platform of experimental or clinical significance? Table 15.1(A–C) represents a simple example of the difficulties posed with miRNAs as targets for either biomarkers or therapy. Utilizing a selected set of candidate miRNAs compiled from literature, each was run through an algorithmic database (miRanda) to determine target probabilities [68]. The results, although theoretical and statistical in nature, perfectly illustrate the tremendously complex dynamic interactions among miRNAs. Furthermore, does intervention via miRNAs and their relevant mechanisms present a reliable approach to disease fighting that does not threaten the body's own homeostatic balance or its omic ecosystem, given their remarkable and intricate involvement in nearly all facets of function? This remains one of the questions to be answered by researchers considering the fragility of the pathways within which miRNAs function. It becomes a dangerous scenario wherein manipulation of one chain of miRNA function inadvertently results in the collapse of another, causing yet another problem requiring intervention [69]. Intriguing examples exist; however, the lack of efficacious response to miRNA targeting is biological. Torrisani et al. were able to restore *let*-7 levels in pancreatic cancer cells that aberrantly expressed it, but contrary to expectation, while relevant gene expression was deregulated (e.g., K-Ras and MAPK), tumors still grew at a measurable rate [70]. This is much the same dilemma facing standard chemotherapeutic treatments since their inception and that is the balance between benefit to the system, no effect and harm. The one-size-fits-all methodology of medical treatment is no longer viable, and it is well recognized by the medical community, which

Table 15.1 Selected Candidate miRNAs

miRNA	Number of Predicted Gene Targets
A: Selected Candidate miRNAs in Bladder Cancer and Their Predicted Number of Target Genes	
miR–20a	9156
miR–106b	9046
miR–130b	7771
miR–141	7721
miR–200a	7645
miR–200a★	5770
B: Selected Candidate miRNAs in Gastric Cancer and Their Predicted Number of Target Genes	
miR–21	5203
miR–27a	9154
miR–106b	9046
miR–146a	6798
miR–148a	7402
miR–433	6659
C: Selected Candidate miRNAs in Cervical Squamous Cell Carcinoma and Their Predicted Number of Target Genes	
miR–1246	5983
miR–20a	9156
miR–3147	5839
miR–3162–5p	5521

in response has been hesitant in the adoption of gene therapies and highly novel experimental treatments [71]. Currently, extensive studies and clinical trials have been focused on determining whether there is a suitable combination of highly potent and highly targeted compounds capable of working on multiple targets to halt various aspects of cancer. Indeed, it has been seen that a promiscuous drug indeed may be more efficacious in a treatment modality than a highly specific compound [72]. This is the new paradigm in translational medicine where, fundamentally, all the tools of science inherently are combined to both uncover disease and target it on multiple fronts with as little side effect to the patient as possible.

A suitable treatment will not only target miRNAs or genes or aim at increasing or decreasing protein expression alone. Instead, it will entail a host of strategies to both return the patient to a state of physiological health and maintain a personalized approach to the methodology. Several examples exist of a highly dynamic team of both clinicians and researchers applying the latest knowledge to patient treatment [73]. Treatments cannot solely rely on targeting one component for mass effect, and they will be based on the nuanced differences between patient populations and disease subtypes, a stratification strategy that is still under development for reliable use [74]. Key strategies should utilize computational–network pharmacology and biology for more targeted drug delivery and disease monitoring that eventually will lead to better treatment outcomes of cancer patients, especially for patients diagnosed with PC.

CONCLUSION

Pancreatic cancer, along with other cancers, inherently is due to the loss of entire systems of regulation and control. These system are connected intricately through multiple layers of both genetic and epigenetic regulation, which require sophisticated analyses to provide insight into their dynamic actions. In the omics era, it is no longer feasible to simply examine both miRNAs and their relevant counterparts solely in terms of the reductionist biochemical principles, of which over many years we have elucidated some of the most nuanced biochemical and physiological mechanisms. The reality is that this entire system contains layer upon layer of fine control that at times can be redundant and seemingly unrelated to the disease in question. By bridging the vast science of network analysis with the various basic science disciplines as well as with the clinical application of basic science tools, an incredible detailed and versatile picture of cancer can be ascertained, targeted, and manipulated to better fight the disease. Through this very same mechanism, truly personalized treatments can be created that both more efficiently target patients' cancer cells as well as limit the harm caused to their healthy cells. It thus only makes sense to increase our knowledge of miRNA function, its relationship to the larger physiological system, and its greater implication in patient health and treatment outcome.

REFERENCES

[1] Lee RC. An extensive class of small RNAs in *Caenorhabditis elegans*. Science 2001; 294:862–4.
[2] Lund E. Nuclear export of microRNA precursors. Science 2004;303:95–8.
[3] Lai EC, Micro RNAs are complementary to 3' UTR sequence motifs that mediate negative post-transcriptional regulation. Nat Genet 2002;30:363–4.
[4] Bartel DP. MicroRNAs: genomics, biogenesis, mechanism, and function. Cell 2004; 116:281–97.

[5] Judson RL, Babiarz JE, Venere M, Blelloch R. Embryonic stem cell–specific microRNAs promote induced pluripotency. Nat Biotechnol 2009;27:459–61.

[6] Bushati N, Cohen SM. microRNA functions. Annu Rev Cell Dev Biol 2007;23: 175–205.

[7] Jovanovic M, Hengartner MO. miRNAs and apoptosis: RNAs to die for. Oncogene 2006;25:6176–87.

[8] Sotiropoulou G, Pampalakis G, Lianidou E, Mourelatos Z. Emerging roles of microRNAs as molecular switches in the integrated circuit of the cancer cell. RNA 2009;15:1443–61.

[9] Hanahan D, Weinberg RA. Hallmarks of cancer: the next generation. Cell 2011; 144:646–74.

[10] Johnnidis JB, Harris MH, Wheeler RT, Stehling-Sun S, Lam MH, Kirak O, et al. Regulation of progenitor cell proliferation and granulocyte function by microRNA-223. Nature 2008;451:1125–9.

[11] Ferretti E, De Smaele E, Miele E, Laneve P, Po A, Pelloni M, et al. Concerted microRNA control of Hedgehog signalling in cerebellar neuronal progenitor and tumour cells. EMBO J 2008;27:2616–27.

[12] Paroo Z, Ye X, Chen S, Liu Q. Phosphorylation of the human microRNA-generating complex mediates MAPK/Erk signaling. Cell 2009;139:112–22.

[13] Armstrong L. The role of PI3K/AKT, MAPK/ERK and NF signalling in the maintenance of human embryonic stem cell pluripotency and viability highlighted by transcriptional profiling and functional analysis. Hum Mol Genet 2006;15:1894–913.

[14] Singh SR. Cancer stem cells: recent developments and future prospects. Cancer Lett 2013;338:1–2.

[15] Godlewski J, Nowicki MO, Bronisz A, Nuovo G, Palatini J, et al. MicroRNA-451 regulates LKB1/AMPK signaling and allows adaptation to metabolic stress in glioma cells. Mol Cell 2010;37:620–32.

[16] Tian Y, Nan Y, Han L, Zhang A, Wang G, Jia Z, et al. MicroRNA miR-451 downregulates the PI3K/AKT pathway through CAB39 in human glioma. Int J Oncol 2012;40:1105–12.

[17] Wang T, Zang W, Li M, Wang N, Zheng Y, Zhao G. Effect of miR-451 on the biological behavior of the esophageal carcinoma cell line EC9706. Dig Dis Sci 2013;58:706–14.

[18] Xiong L, Jiang W, Zhou R, Mao C, Guo Z. Identification and analysis of the regulatory network of Myc and microRNAs from high-throughput experimental data. Comput Biol Med 2013;43:1252–60.

[19] Leal JA, Lleonart ME. MicroRNAs and cancer stem cells: therapeutic approaches and future perspectives. Cancer Lett 2013;338:174–83.

[20] Shi M, Cui J, Xie K. Signaling of miRNAs-FOXM1 in cancer and potential targeted therapy. Curr Drug Targets 2013;14:1192–202.

[21] Shaffer AL, Young RM, Staudt LM. Pathogenesis of human B cell lymphomas. Annu Rev Immunol 2012;30:565–610.

[22] Lundstrom K. Micro-RNA in disease and gene therapy. Curr Drug Discov Technol 2011;8:76–86.

[23] Sioud M, Cekaite L. RNA therapeutics, methods in molecular biology, vol. 629. Totowa, NJ: Humana Press; 2010. p. 255–69.

[24] Siegel R, Naishadham D, Jemal A. Cancer statistics, 2012. CA Cancer J Clin 2012; 62:10–29.

[25] Oberstein PE, Olive KP. Pancreatic cancer: why is it so hard to treat? Therap Adv Gastroenterol 2013;6:321–37.

[26] Pinho AV, Chantrill L, Rooman I. Chronic pancreatitis: a path to pancreatic cancer. Cancer Lett 2013. http://dx.doi.org/10.1016/j.canlet.2013.08.015.

[27] Zhang Y, et al. Profiling of 95 microRNAs in pancreatic cancer cell lines and surgical specimens by real-time PCR analysis. World J Surg 2008;33:698–709.

[28] Lee EJ, Baek M, Gusev Y, Brackett DJ, Nuovo GJ, Schmittgen TD. Expression profiling identifies microRNA signature in pancreatic cancer. Int J Cancer 2006;120:1046–54.

[29] Collins AL, Wojcik S, Liu J, Frankel WL, Alder H, Yu L, et al. A differential microRNA profile distinguishes cholangiocarcinoma from pancreatic adenocarcinoma. Ann Surg Oncol 2014;21:133–8.

[30] Bhardwaj A, Arora S, Prajapati VK, Singh S, Singh AP. Cancer "stemness"-regulating microRNAs: role, mechanisms and therapeutic potential. Curr Drug Targets 2013; 14:1175–84.

[31] Wang Z, Li Y, Ahmad A, Azmi AS, Kong D, Banerjee S, et al. Targeting miRNAs involved in cancer stem cell and EMT regulation: an emerging concept in overcoming drug resistance. Drug Resist Updat 2010;13:109–18.

[32] Ghatnekar O, Andersson R, Svensson M, Persson U, Ringdahl U, Zeilon P, et al. Modelling the benefits of early diagnosis of pancreatic cancer using a biomarker signature. Int J Cancer 2013;133:2392–7.

[33] He L, He X, Lim LP, de Stanchina E, Xuan Z, Liang Y, et al. A microRNA component of the p53 tumour suppressor network. Nature 2007;447:1130–4.

[34] Szafranska AE, Davison TS, John J, Cannon T, Sipos B, et al. MicroRNA expression alterations are linked to tumorigenesis and non-neoplastic processes in pancreatic ductal adenocarcinoma. Oncogene 2007;26:4442–52.

[35] Gusev Y, Schmittgen TD, Lerner M, Postier R, Brackett D. Computational analysis of biological functions and pathways collectively targeted by co-expressed microRNAs in cancer. BMC Bioinformatics 2007;8(Suppl. 7):S16.

[36] Schetter AJ, Leung SY, Sohn JJ, Zanetti KA, Bowman ED, et al. MicroRNA expression profiles associated with prognosis and therapeutic outcome in colon adenocarcinoma. JAMA 2008;299:425–36.

[37] Hwang J-H, Voortman J, Giovannetti E, Steinberg SM, Leon LG, et al. Identification of microRNA-21 as a biomarker for chemoresistance and clinical outcome following adjuvant therapy in resectable pancreatic cancer. PLoS One 2010;5:e10630.

[38] Giovannetti E, Funel N, Peters GJ, Del Chiaro M, Erozenci LA, et al. MicroRNA-21 in pancreatic cancer: correlation with clinical outcome and pharmacologic aspects underlying its role in the modulation of gemcitabine activity. Cancer Res 2010;70:4528–38.

[39] Chen Y, Zhang L, Hao Q. Candidate microRNA biomarkers in human epithelial ovarian cancer: systematic review profiling studies and experimental validation. Cancer Cell Int 2013;13:86.

[40] Ratert N, et al. miRNA profiling identifies candidate miRNAs for bladder cancer diagnosis and clinical outcome. J Mol Diagn 2013;15:695–705.

[41] Hobert O. Gene regulation by transcription factors and microRNAs. Science 2008; 319:1785–6.

[42] Akao YY, et al. Role of anti-oncomirs miR-143 and -145 in human colorectal tumors. Cancer Gene Ther 2010;17:398–408.

[43] Markou A, Sourvinou I, Vorkas PA, Yousef GM, Lianidou E. Clinical evaluation of microRNA expression profiling in non small cell lung cancer. Lung Cancer 2013; 81:388–96.

[44] Rosenblum D, Peer D. Omics-based nanomedicine: the future of personalized oncology. Cancer Lett 2013. http://dx.doi.org/10.1016/j.canlet.2013.07.029.

[45] Gray JAM. The shift to personalised and population medicine. Lancet 2013;382: 200–1.

[46] Azmi AS, Wang Z, Philip PA, Mohammad RM, Sarkar FH. Proof of concept: network and systems biology approaches aid in the discovery of potent anticancer drug combinations. Mol Cancer Ther 2010;9:3137–44.

[47] Koutsogiannouli E, Papavassiliou AG, Papanikolaou NA. Complexity in cancer biology: is systems biology the answer? Cancer Med 2013;2:164–77.

[48] Macneil LT, Walhout AJM. Gene regulatory networks and the role of robustness and stochasticity in the control of gene expression. Genome Res 2011;21:645–57.

[49] Rosenfeld S. Mathematical descriptions of biochemical networks: stability, stochasticity, evolution. Prog Biophys Mol Biol 2011;106:400–9.

[50] Mazzocchi F. Complexity in biology. Exceeding the limits of reductionism and determinism using complexity theory. EMBO Rep 2008;9:10–4.

[51] Weber GF. Gene therapy–why can it fail? Med Hypotheses 2013;80:613–6.

[52] Giordano S, Petrelli A. From single- to multi-target drugs in cancer therapy: when aspecificity becomes an advantage. Curr Med Chem 2008;15:422–32.

[53] Moreno LL, Pearson ADA. How can attrition rates be reduced in cancer drug discovery? Expert Opin Drug Discov 2013;8:363–8.

[54] Alian OM, Shah M, Mohammad M, Mohammad RM. Network pharmacology: reigning in drug attrition? Curr Drug Discov Technol 2013;10:155–9.

[55] Goh K-I, Choi I-G. Exploring the human diseasome: the human disease network. Brief Funct Genomics 2012;11:533–42.

[56] Cooper CP, Yukimura D. Science writers' reactions to a medical 'breakthrough' story. Soc Sci Med 2002;54:1887–96.

[57] Iskar M, Zeller G, Zhao X-M, van Noort V, Bork P. Drug discovery in the age of systems biology: the rise of computational approaches for data integration. Curr Opin Biotechnol 2012;23:609–16.

[58] Schulz MH, Pandit KV, Lino Cardenas CL, Ambalavanan N, Kaminski N, Bar-Joseph Z. Reconstructing dynamic microRNA-regulated interaction networks. Proc Natl Acad Sci USA 2013;110:15686–91.

[59] Friedman RC, Farh KKH, Burge CB, Bartel DP. Most mammalian mRNAs are conserved targets of microRNAs. Genome Res 2008;19:92–105.

[60] Libri V, Miesen P, van Rij RP, Buck AH. Regulation of microRNA biogenesis and turnover by animals and their viruses. Cell Mol Life Sci 2013;70:3525–44.

[61] Lim LP, Lau NC, Garrett-Engele P, Grimson A, Schelter JM, Castle J, et al. Microarray analysis shows that some microRNAs downregulate large numbers of target mRNAs. Nature 2005;433:769–73.

[62] Horvát E-Á, Zhang JD, Uhlmann S, Sahin O, Zweig KA. A network-based method to assess the statistical significance of mild co-regulation effects. PLoS One 2013;8:e73413.

[63] Nilsen TW. Mechanisms of microRNA-mediated gene regulation in animal cells. Trends Genet 2007;23:243–9.

[64] Gurtan AM, Sharp PA. The role of miRNAs in regulating gene expression networks. J Mol Biol 2013;425:3582–600.

[65] Li Z, et al. Exploring the role of human miRNAs in virus-host interactions using systematic overlap analysis. Bioinformatics 2013;29:2375–9.

[66] de Souza N. microRNAs—subtler than you think. Nat Methods 2008;5:753.

[67] Weber JA, Baxter DH, Zhang S, Huang DY, Huang KH, Lee MJ, et al. The microRNA spectrum in 12 body fluids. Clin Chem 2010;56:1733–41.

[68] John B, Enright AJ, Aravin A, Tuschl T, Sander C, et al. Human microRNA targets. PLoS Biol 2004;2:e363.

[69] Garzon R, Marcucci G, Croce CM. Targeting microRNAs in cancer: rationale, strategies and challenges. Nat Rev Drug Discov 2010;9:775–89.

[70] Torrisani J, Bournet B, du Rieu MC, Bouisson M, Souque A, et al. let-7 MicroRNA transfer in pancreatic cancer-derived cells inhibits in vitro cell proliferation but fails to alter tumor progression. Hum Gene Ther 2009;20:831–44.

[71] Scanlon KJ. Cancer gene therapy: challenges and opportunities. Anticancer Res 2004;24:501–4.

[72] Mencher SK, Wang LG. Promiscuous drugs compared to selective drugs (promiscuity can be a virtue). BMC Clin Pharmacol 2005;5:3. BMC Pharmacology and Toxicology.

[73] Heinemann V, Douillard JY, Ducreux M, Peeters M. Targeted therapy in metastatic colorectal cancer – an example of personalised medicine in action. Cancer Treat Rev 2013;39:592–601.

[74] West M, Ginsburg GS, Huang AT, Nevins JR. Embracing the complexity of genomic data for personalized medicine. Genome Res 2006;16:559–66.

SECTION *V*

Systems Approaches to Pancreatic Cancer Therapeutics

Integration of Protein Network Activation Mapping Technology for Personalized Therapy: Implications for Pancreatic Cancer

Mariaelena Pierobon, Julie Wulfkuhle, Lance A. Liotta, Emanuel F. Petricoin III
Center for Applied Proteomics and Molecular Medicine, George Mason University, Manassas, VA, USA

Contents

Introduction	367
Defective Protein Signaling Networks Underpin Tumorigenesis	368
Phosphoproteins as Critical CDx Markers	368
Reverse Phase Protein Microarrays as a Tool for Personalized Cancer Therapy	371
Pre-Analytical Factors Influence Phosphoprotein Pathway Activation Mapping	374
Case Studies in Pathway Activation Mapping of Human Cancer	375
Generation of a Cellular Circuit Diagram for Patient Management: A Summary	377
References	379

INTRODUCTION

The underpinning and ultimate promise of personalized therapy is that the molecular fingerprint of a patient's tumor becomes the rationale for targeted and patient-tailored therapy. Until recently, this fingerprint has been a genomics-centered analysis using exome panels, whole genome sequencing, and/or RNA sequencing comprising the details that most scientists and treating oncologists consider when considering a "precision medicine"–based approach. Stratification and selection of patients for certain targeted therapies based on genomics analysis has certainly been successful in a number of instances such as with non-small cell lung cancer (NSCLC), where EGFR mutations [1] and ROS/ALK translocations [2] can be highly predictive for therapeutic response, or HER2 amplification in breast cancer [3], BRAFV600E mutations in melanoma [4], etc., but these approaches have imperfect sensitivity and specificity and often show little to no predictive value [5,6].

However, while these examples show the potential for genomic-based therapy prediction, not every NSCLC patient that harbors an EGFR mutation responds to EGFR-directed therapy, not every HER2+ breast cancer responds to Herceptin™, etc., thus genomic derangement analysis alone is unable to completely explain all targeted therapeutic response even in an enriched population. Cancer is certainly causally determined by specific genomic derangements, but in fact cancer is a proteomic disease. It is the proteins that are the "software" of the cell and do nearly all the work of the cell. More practically, the mechanism of action of most cancer therapies works at the protein level and protein enzymatic level (e.g., kinase inhibitors). It is proteins that are the drug targets and make up the signaling circuitry and biochemical networks of the cell. When scientists refer to aberrant signaling "pathways" or targeting cellular "networks", it is the proteins, not genes that make up these pathways and networks.

Molecularly targeted agents for cancer treatment are now being cleared by the FDA on a regular basis, and thus the era of personalized therapy for cancer treatment has begun in earnest. In the near future, the oncologist will have a large number of FDA-approved agents to select from for any given patient, along with a compendium of molecular profiling–based companion diagnostic tests (CDx) that would be used for drug selection. However, based on these molecular profiling technologies, while drugs such as imatinib, sunitinib, traztuzumab, etc. have had a dramatic impact on GIST, CML renal cancer, and c-erbB2+ breast cancers, respectively, the emphasis will shift from the specific therapies themselves to the CDx biomarkers that will be used to stratify and select the right therapy for each patient. The new CDx biomarkers will serve as the gatekeepers to the drugs. Thus, CDx marker discovery is under intense current investigation because of their elevated status within the treatment selection process, and the near-future CDx will not be single markers but panels of dozens or hundreds of markers that are the gateways to dozens to hundreds of targeted therapies.

DEFECTIVE PROTEIN SIGNALING NETWORKS UNDERPIN TUMORIGENESIS

Phosphoproteins as Critical CDx Markers

Aberrantly activated protein signaling networks are the key central feature in tumorigenesis and metastatic progression [7–14], and posttranslational modifications, such as phosphorylation, play the dominant role in orchestrating and regulating cell signaling processes. Thus, phosphoprotein pathway biomarkers may be among the most important class CDx markers [10,14–16]. As discussed previously, EGFR mutations can identify NSCLC patients that respond to EGFR-directed therapy, however, recent findings point to the fact that EGFR activation/phosphorylation may be much more predictive for response to EGFR-targeted therapy than any other measurement [17], even in EGFR wild-type NSCLC patients [18]. The hope that gene transcription profiling will effectively predict ongoing protein signaling events and provide an effective molecular surrogate for protein pathway biomarkers has not come to pass as recent studies have revealed little example correlation between gene expression and protein expression [19,20]. Indeed, measurement of total protein expression levels of a given protein often do not correlate with the phosphorylation levels of a given protein since cellular signaling works by rapid phosphorylation of a large substrate pool, and total levels of a protein often do not predict therapy response whereas the phosphorylation level carries the weight of response prediction [17]. Very recently, a series of papers that utilize a systems level analysis of genomic and functional protein activation analysis of drug response prediction in breast cancer models revealed the advantages provided by phosphoprotein analysis over a genomics oriented approach [21]. Consequently, there is a critical need for technologies that can directly assess and measure the phosphorylation/activation state of the signaling network and thus provide a snapshot of the activity of many of the proteins that are the drug targets of a large number of therapeutics for oncology.

It is now widely known that most cancers are caused by aberrant and hyperactivated kinase-driven signaling pathways that arise from the aggregate genomic alterations. Moreover, posttranslational protein modifications (PTM), mainly phosphorylation, control the kinase-driven signaling networks through SH2, SH3, etc. protein–protein interactions [22–36]. The majority of protein phosphorylation occurs on serine and threonine residues with the remainder (approximately 10%) occurring on tyrosine residues. A large number of receptor tyrosine kinases (RTK) are hyperactivated in cancer and are the targets for clinically used anticancer therapeutics (e.g., EGFR, VEGFR, ROS, HER2 MET, KIT, PDGFR, ALK), and are themselves kinase enzymes. After the receptor binds ligand, or is conformationally altered due to mutation or is overexpressed due to genomic amplification, the receptors hetero- or homodimerize, transphosphorylate, and then form new binding sites for downstream scaffolding and protein kinase interactions [22–36].

The overarching mechanisms and homologous control of these signaling networks are largely unknown and under intense investigation since these mechanisms will undoubtedly help to elucidate better ways to target deranged cellular machinery. New approaches using mathematical modeling of normal and aberrant protein signaling networks is now being explored in order to both reconstruct signaling networks de novo and/or exploit the architecture to identify optimal therapeutic strategies [37–44]. The complexity of the human kinome, comprised of less than a thousand proteins [45], is of low dimensional space compared to the genome or the entire proteome, which ranges from tens of thousands to potentially millions of individual molecular analytes. Indeed, recent full-scale whole genome sequencing of individual human tumor specimens under consortium-based approaches such as the TCGA has shown that each patient's individual tumor is a complex heterogenous portrait of hundreds of independent somatic genetic mutations [11–13] with each tumor being very different from patient to patient. The puzzling aspect of this tremendous heterogeneity is further amplified since it is not known for any individual patient tumor which mutations are the driving mutations and which are the "by-standard" mutations. However, this heterogenous background is resolved at the level of the functional protein pathway networks, which then reveals more clearly what are the functional effects of the mutational load. DNA mutations that ultimately provide a survival advantage to the evolving tumor cell are selected out, and this functional selection is manifest in cell signaling pathway changes that are responsible for altered cell growth, death, motility, differentiation, and metabolism. As the plethora of individualized tumor-by-tumor DNA mutation alterations are realized and condensed down to protein pathway–centered analysis, we start to see that disparate tumor types, defined in the past by organ location and histomorphology, may share common pathway architectural modules. Recent data supports this characterization as a growing cadre of data points to an entirely new categorization of human cancer based on functional protein pathway activation themes and not on mutational status, location, grade, and gene expression. An example of this is the ubiquitous nature of AKT/mTOR pathway derangements, growth factor receptor-mediated signal pathway activation, and ras-raf-ERK network activation in a large number of human cancers, regardless of location and organ microenvironment [46–51].

Indeed, for pancreatic cancer wherein KRAS mutations (as ubiquitous as they are for this tumor) represent a potentially intractable nondruggable target, the focus now is on the downstream targets of KRAS, mainly the AKT-mTOR and MEK-ERK signaling infrastructure [52,53]. These signaling pathways are not pancreatic cancer specific and are central to nearly all tumors. Recent studies have revealed that concurrent targeting of the PI3K and MEK pathways, regardless of KRAS status, could provide a new therapeutic strategy wherein monitoring of the phosphorylation of 4E-BP1 and S6 may serve as a predictive biomarker for response to treatment [53,54]. This is very similar to the recent data that suggest monitoring of these same mTOR markers is of benefit to breast cancer patients [21]. Further evidence of drug "repositioning" is seen as targets such as HER2, EGFR, and STATs (all of which have been extensively exploited in other solid tumors) are now under intense investigation for use in pancreatic cancer [53–55]. Another recent example that demonstrates the profound utility of a protein pathway–centered approach to identify new therapeutic targets and kinase inhibitor drug repositioning for pancreatic cancers is the new initial trial (RECAP:NCT01423604) results whereby an already FDA-approved drug for myelofibrosis (ruxolitinib) that targets JAK kinases 1 and 2 showed exciting response rates [56].

REVERSE PHASE PROTEIN MICROARRAYS AS A TOOL FOR PERSONALIZED CANCER THERAPY

Based on the need to effectively measure the functional activated protein signaling architecture for targeted therapy applications, our laboratory developed a planar array-based technology that can concomitantly quantitatively measure the phosphorylation/activation state of dozens to hundreds of signaling proteins. This technology, the reverse phase protein microarray (RPPA), is proving to be a key enabling technology for the analysis of clinical material [57–65] (Figure 16.1). Unlike a forward phase array format (e.g., antibody array) where the analyte-detecting molecule is immobilized, with the RPPA format, cellular or tissue lysates (or even body fluids) from individual samples are printed directly and immobilized on a planar surface. Depending on the size of the pin used

Reverse phase protein microarray

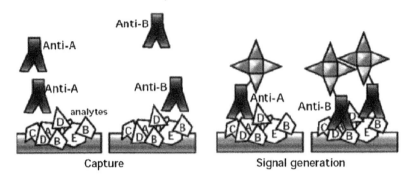

Figure 16.1 *Reverse Phase Protein Microarray Format.* The reverse phase protein microarray is a planar array wherein of denatured or non-denatured cellular lysates, body fluids, culture media, LCM tissue cells, organelles, recombinant proteins, analytes, etc. are immobilized onto a planar substrate. This format allows the direct comparison of hundreds to thousands of individual samples at once since each array is exposed to a single primary antibody. (For color version of this figure, the reader is referred to the online version of this book.)

to print the samples, it is possible to print a few hundred to several thousand spots on each slide. Since each printing deposits as little as 1–5 nl, it is possible to create as many as 100 slides from a lysate of only a few thousand cells. The most widely used substrate is nitrocellulose, which has the aggregate attributes of low cost, high binding capacity, and low relative background. With the RPPA format, each slide is incubated with one specific primary antibody, and a single analyte endpoint is measured and directly compared across multiple samples on each slide. Each array is printed with a series of high and low controls and calibrator samples that contain predetermined and varying amounts of the target analyte that span the expected linear dynamic range of the analyte. The RPPA, when used as a calibrated immunoassay, provides a straightforward means of quantifying any input by interpolation or extrapolation to the printed calibrator. While the RPPA was initially designed for colorimetric detection, florescent detection using near-infrared dye coupled reagents [66] has become popular due to the dramatically increased within spot dynamic range of the assay.

The RPPA is capable of extremely sensitive analyte detection, for example, with reported levels of a few hundred molecules per spot and a CV of less than 10% [64]. Overall analytical sensitivity is ultimately dependent on analyte concentration and antibody affinity and avidity, however, the general sensitivity of detection for the RPPA is such that even extremely low abundance phosphorylated signaling proteins can be measured from a lysate containing less than 10 cell equivalents [64]. The ability to generate a quantitative linear signal from such small amounts of material, and do so in high multiplex, is the unique attribute of the RPPA that distinguishes it from every other proteomic technique. This attribute becomes extremely important for clinical applications where often the starting input material is only a few hundred cells from a needle biopsy or fine needle aspirate specimen. RPPA, like immunohistochemistry, is dependent on the availability of high quality, specific antibodies, particularly those specific for posttranslational modifications or active states of proteins, and is a major limiting factor for the successful implementation of any immunoassay-type platforms. Upfront rigorous validation of each antibody is essential in order to be confident that the signal generated on the array is a result of the specific analyte being detected. Most RPPA work flows include background subtraction from arrays that have been exposed to the secondary antibody alone as well as local intra-array background subtraction. In addition, normalization of the signal itself is usually obtained by measuring the total amount of protein printed on the array, although newer techniques that normalize by DNA content of the lysate can be extremely helpful in instances where the sample is contaminated by exogenous proteins such as blood [67].

Key technological components of the RPPA offer several advantages over other array-based platforms such as tissue arrays [68] or antibody (forward phase) arrays [69] or ex vivo library kinase activity profiling. The RPPA can employ denatured lysates, so that antigen retrieval of sterically hindered phosphorylated epitopes, a significant limitation for tissue arrays, antibody arrays, and immunohistochemistry technologies, is not an issue. Kinase profiling efforts require maintenance of cellular/tissue kinase activity, yet maintaining that activity to reflect only what had occurred in the patient and not influenced by exogenous tissue processing artifact is extremely difficult. RPPAs only require a single class of antibody per analyte protein and do not require direct tagging of the protein as readout for the assay. Other technologies, such as suspension bead array platforms, have significant limitations in the portfolio of analytes that can be measured, even in multiplex, because of the requirement of a two-site assay. Moreover, since the RPPA platform can measure the activation state of so many individual signaling molecules at once, broadscale analysis of the signaling architecture on a pathway basis can provide a detailed understanding of the interconnections within the cellular circuitry even though a single snapshot in time (e.g., biopsy) is the input for analysis.

PRE-ANALYTICAL FACTORS INFLUENCE PHOSPHOPROTEIN PATHWAY ACTIVATION MAPPING

Clinical and preclinical tissues are most often a heterogenous mixture of interacting cell populations, such as fat cells, nerve cells, endothelial vessel cells, muscle cells, fibroblasts, epithelial cells, and immune cells, as well as acellular material such as collagen and serum. Work flows where whole tissue is lysed and analyzed as a whole may generate inaccurate measurements of signaling activation or deactivation since most signaling molecules are ubiquitously expressed in different cell populations. The use of laser capture microdissection (LCM) [70] combined with RPPA provides a facile means of detailed molecular analysis of discreet cell populations within a clinical biopsy specimen [51–65]. The impact of uncontrolled cellular heterogeneity on phosphoprotein measurements was recently described whereby pathway activation mapping was performed on patient-matched undissected and LCM procured colorectal and breast cancer tumor epithelium and revealed significant and numerous differences in pathway activation portraits between the two [60,71], with most patient pairs not revealing any overarching similarity. Moreover, despite the dramatic differences seen between LCM and undissected cells, these past approaches utilized studies wherein many of the cases contained over 50% tumor, which would represent a relatively high upper end of what would normally be seen in a large clinical trial setting (where an average of approximately 20–30% tumor content is seen in a core needle biopsy) [60,71].

Even if the impact of uncontrolled cellular heterogeneity is minimized by cellular enrichment techniques such as LCM, proteins and phosphoproteins are inherently labile and are acutely affected by pre-analytical variables such as post-excision delay, time of the tissue on the pathologist bench prior to fixation, etc. Recent results have found that within 15–30 min after a tissue specimen is removed from the body, many phosphoproteins become both activated and deactivated as the still-living tissue undergoes hypoxic and acidotic changes ex vivo and activate survival signaling [72,73]. Obviously, treatment decisions cannot be based on molecular changes that occur because of how long the tissue sat on the pathologist's table. Since formalin fixation of tissue occurs so slowly (~1 mm/h), simply dropping a piece of tissue into formalin does not solve the issue of preserving the in vivo signaling portraits of a tissue sample. The development of next-generation rapid penetrating fixatives or tissue processing methods that can preserve the labile phosphoprotein signaling architecture while maintaining formalin-equivalent histomorphology is of critical importance, and such reagents and methods are being developed [74,75].

CASE STUDIES IN PATHWAY ACTIVATION MAPPING OF HUMAN CANCER

RPPA technology was first described by our group over a decade ago wherein LCM-RPPA work flow revealed that AKT signaling is activated at the invasion front during prostate cancer progression with a number of those AKT pathway members activated in early stage prostatic intraepithelial neoplasia [51]. Since then, the technology has been used to evaluate the signaling changes in colonic tumor cells undergoing epithelial mesenchymal transition (EMT) [63] whereby LCM-procured tumor, normal epithelium, and matched stromal cells next to each compartment were compared using RPPA analysis. In another study, a phosphoprotein-based signature comprised of multiple members of the AKT-mTOR pathway were found to be systematically activated in rhabdomyosarcoma tumors from children who did not respond to chemotherapy and progressed rapidly [65].

Since cancer is often diagnosed at later stages, many treatments center on management of metastatic disease. Since metastasis is the lethal aspect of the disease, analyzing the signaling profile of the metastatic lesion may be a critical requirement for the correct selection of targeted agents since there is a distinct possibility that the signaling architecture of the metastatic tumor cells will differ significantly from those of the primary tumor cells. In fact, recent analysis of patient-matched primary colorectal cancer lesions and liver metastases suggested that signaling in metastatic hepatic lesions differed considerably from that in the matched primary lesions [76]. These observations are consistent with those in a similar study of six primary ovarian tumors and patient-matched omental metastases taken simultaneously at surgery [77].

Uncovering mechanisms of the development of resistance to targeted agents is another important area where the RPPA technology can have significant impact. In fact, RPPA analysis was to identify protein markers predictive for therapeutic response or resistance in a number of different types of cancers [78]. Studies in ovarian cancer and colon cancer cell lines identified pathway markers involved in nucleotide excision repair that were associated with chemotherapy drug activity [78]. Pathway analysis of melanoma cell lines and patient samples revealed that phosphorylation of 4E-BP1 was increased in melanoma cell lines carrying mutations in BRAF and PTEN compared to cells with wild-type RAS/RAF/PTEN and was associated with worse overall and post-recurrence survival [79]. Analysis of breast cancer cell lines found that distinct patterns of signaling were present in groups representing different molecular subtypes of breast cancer that were not obvious from gene transcription profiling [80]. In another study, the investigators found that treatment of basal-type cells with MEK inhibitors resulted in AKT signaling activation, which could have implications for treatment response to other therapeutic agents [81]. RPPA analysis of the signaling architecture of cells being evaluated for response and resistance to the PI3K inhibitors found that mutations in the genes for PI3K and loss of PTEN activity were potential predictors of sensitivity to these inhibitors [81]. Interestingly, Ras mutations (so prevalent in pancreatic cancers) were a major resistance marker in this study, even in the presence of PI3K mutations and measurements of phosphorylated AKT (S473). Moreover, expression of c-Myc and cyclin B, which are downstream targets of Ras, were upregulated in PI3K inhibitor resistant cell lines in vivo and were also negatively associated with response to the drug in vivo.

Drugs targeting the EGFR and HER family signaling pathway are some of the most intensely studied in the field of molecular-targeted therapies. A recent study by Xia et al. identified an entirely novel mechanism of lapatinib resistance, a small-molecule inhibitor of EGFR and HER2, in breast cancer [82]. Using a series of isogenic lapatinib-sensitive cell lines and those with acquired resistance and broadscale RPPA-based pathway activation mapping of hundreds of key signaling proteins, the investigators found that resistance was due to the "leaky" nature of lapatinib, whereby incomplete inhibition of EGFR phosphorylation by lapatinib supplied effective selective pressure to cause the cells to increase the production of the heregulin ligand and switch from HER2-HER3 signaling to heregulin-driven EGFR-HER3 signaling. Investigators utilized RPPA-based pathway activation mapping to study mechanisms of estrogen resistance in breast cancer, also using matched resistant/sensitive cell lines, and found that several pathways involved in cell proliferation and survival were activated in tamoxifen-resistant lines [83]. The ability to integrate multiplexed RPPA phosphoprotein analysis with multi-omic data (RNA, miRNA, DNA, metabolomic, drug sensitivity data, etc.) was recently described for the NCI-60 cell line series and revealed the distinct nature of the activated protein signaling networks. Interestingly, while a large number of phosphoprotein signaling correlates were found that predicted certain drug sensitivities, little to no correlation was seen between the phosphoprotein/protein signaling architecture and any genomic measurement performed to date [84]. This result emphasizes the need to directly measure the activated protein machinery and the inability to predict this activation from inferential genomic analysis alone.

GENERATION OF A CELLULAR CIRCUIT DIAGRAM FOR PATIENT MANAGEMENT: A SUMMARY

Certainly, RPPAs have become one of the most widely published protein array technologies and perhaps the most dominant technological platform for multiplexed phosphoprotein analysis of clinical biopsy samples. Moreover, recent data indicate that the platform has achieved the necessary analytical fidelity to be used in clinical trial settings. Comparison of HER2 data obtained from RPPA to that generated from the same samples using FDA-approved IHC and FISH measurement technologies revealed excellent concordance (>95%) [85]. The RPPA is a biomarker discovery engine of many cutting edge clinical trials, such as the ISPY-2 TRIAL, where the discovery of rigorously validated CDx markers would be used to accelerate promising molecularly targeted inhibitors to Phase III testing. Techniques such as IHC are a mainstay of many protein-based CDx efforts; however, the use of such methods in a rapidly evolving personalized therapy may become obsolete. Based on the current drug development pipeline, in less than five years there may be >50 targeted therapies cleared for use by the FDA, with as many or more protein CDx markers being offered. Consequently, it will not be possible to measure 50–75 CDx proteins at once from a single biopsy specimen using IHC, ELISA, etc. At this time, the RPPA format is uniquely positioned to produce a quantitative readout of the activation state of dozens to hundreds of drug targets at once. In

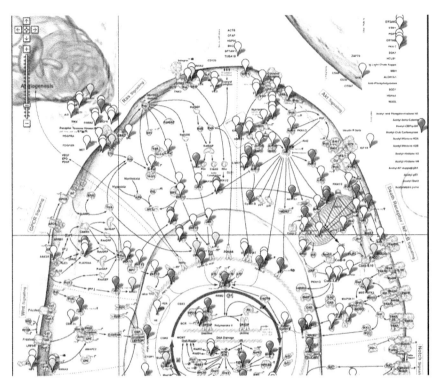

Figure 16.2 A new paradigm for personalized therapy can be envisioned whereby a patient-specific tumor "wiring diagram" of the activated signaling architecture is produced by RPPA data. The "Pathways in Human Cancer" diagram (reproduced courtesy of Cell Signaling, Inc). The Cscape (Cancer Landscape) Program used to map the RPPA data to the image was developed by Eli Lilly, and Company (Kelly Gallagher, Scott McAhren, Loius Stancato) and used collaboratively for RPMA data analysis. Red are high relative levels of drug target activation/phosphorylation and green are low relative levels of drug target activation/phosphorylation. (For color version of this figure, the reader is referred to the online version of this book.)

addition, as combination therapies tailored to each patient's tumor architecture begin to become part of routine pathological workup, the need to effectively measure the activated protein "circuitry" will be central to this effort. Indeed, one can envision a future for pancreatic cancer patients (Figure 16.2) whereby a "wiring diagram" of each patient's tumor biopsy is produced by RPPA technology and provided to the treating oncologist as part of a pathology report, providing a circuit view of the actionable/druggable landscape and a molecular rationale for patient-tailored therapy.

REFERENCES

[1] Lee CK, Brown C, Gralla RJ, Hirsh V, Thongprasert S, Tsai CM, et al. Impact of EGFR inhibitor in non-small cell lung cancer on progression-free and overall survival: a meta-analysis. J Natl Cancer Inst 2013;105(9):595–605.

[2] Rothschild SI, Gautschi O. Crizotinib in the treatment of non–small-cell lung cancer. Clin Lung Cancer 2013;14(5):473–80.

[3] Rexer BN, Arteaga CL. Optimal targeting of HER2-PI3K signaling in breast cancer: mechanistic insights and clinical implications. Cancer Res July 1, 2013;73(13): 3817–20.

[4] Cheng S, Koch WH, Wu L. Co-development of a companion diagnostic for targeted cancer therapy. N Biotechnol 2012;29(6):682–8.

[5] Janku F, Broaddus R, Bakkar R, Hong DS, Stepanek V, et al. PTEN assessment and PI3K/mTOR inhibitors: importance of simultaneous assessment of MAPK pathway aberrations. ASCO Annual Meeting, Abstract 10510. Presented June 5, 2012; 2012.

[6] Ganesan P, Janku F, Naing A, Hong DS, Tsimberidou AM, Falchook GS, et al. Target-based therapeutic matching in early-phase clinical trials in patients with advanced colorectal cancer and PIK3CA mutations. Mol Cancer Ther 2013;12(12):2857–63.

[7] Faivre S, Djelloul S, Raymond E. New paradigms in anticancer therapy: targeting multiple signaling pathways with kinase inhibitors. Semin Oncol 2006;33(4):407–20.

[8] Huang PH, Mukasa A, Bonavia R, Flynn RA, Brewer ZE, Cavenee WK, et al. Quantitative analysis of EGFRvIII cellular signaling networks reveals a combinatorial therapeutic strategy for glioblastoma. Proc Natl Acad Sci USA 2007;104(31): 12867–72.

[9] Engelman JA, Zejnullahu K, Mitsudomi T, Song Y, Hyland C, Park JO, et al. MET amplification leads to gefitinib resistance in lung cancer by activating ERBB3 signaling. Science 2007;316(5827):1039–43.

[10] Sawyers CL. The cancer biomarker problem. Nature April 3, 2008;452(7187):548.

[11] Parsons DW, Jones S, Zhang X, Lin JC, Leary RJ, Angenendt P, et al. An integrated genomic analysis of human glioblastoma multiforme. Science 2008;321(5897): 1807–12.

[12] Jones S, Zhang X, Parsons DW, Lin JC, Leary RJ, Angenendt P, et al. Core signaling pathways in human pancreatic cancers revealed by global genomic analyses. Science 2008;321(5897):1801–6.

[13] Wood LD, Parsons DW, Jones S, Lin J, Sjöblom T, Leary RJ, et al. The genomic landscapes of human breast and colorectal cancers. Science 2007;318(5853):1108–13.

[14] Liotta LA, Kohn EC, Petricoin EF. Clinical proteomics: personalized molecular medicine. JAMA 2001;286(18):2211–4.

[15] Petricoin 3rd EF, Dichsel VE, Calvert VS, Espina V, Winters M, Young L, et al. Mapping molecular networks using proteomics: a vision for patient-tailored combination therapy. J Clin Oncol 2005;23:3614–21.

[16] Wulfkuhle JD, Edmiston KH, Liotta LA, Petricoin EF. Technology insight: pharmacoproteomics for cancer—promises of patient-tailored medicine using protein microarrays. Nat Clin Pract Oncol 2006;3(5):256–68.

[17] Emery IF, Battelli C, Auclair PL, Carrier K, Hayes DM. Response to gefitinib and erlotinib in Non-small cell lung cancer: a retrospective study. BMC Cancer 2009;9:333.

[18] Wang F, Wang S, Wang Z, Duan J, An T, Zhao J, et al. Phosphorylated EGFR expression may predict outcome of EGFR-TKIs therapy for the advanced NSCLC patients with wild-type EGFR. J Exp Clin Cancer Res 2012;31:65.

[19] Anderson L, Seilhamer J. A comparison of selected mRNA and protein abundances in human liver. Electrophoresis 1997;18(3–4):533–7.

[20] Gygi SP, Rochon Y, Franza BR, Aebersold R. Correlation between protein and mRNA abundance in yeast. Mol Cell Biol 1999;19(3):1720–30.

[21] Quaranta V, Tyson DR. What lies beneath: looking beyond tumor genetics shows the complexity of signaling networks underlying drug sensitivity. Sci Signal 2013;6(294): pe32.

[22] Irish JM, Hovland R, Krutzik PO, Perez OD, Bruserud Ø, Gjertsen BT, Bruserud O, et al. Single cell profiling of potentiated phospho-protein networks in cancer cells. Cell 2004;118(2):217–28.

[23] Irish JM, Anensen N, Hovland R, Skavland J, Børresen-Dale AL, Bruserud O, et al. Flt3 Y591 duplication and Bcl-2 overexpression are detected in acute myeloid leukemia cells with high levels of phosphorylated wild-type p53. Blood 2007; 109(6):2589–96.

[24] Stern DF. Phosphoproteomics for oncology discovery and treatment. Expert Opin Ther Targets 2005;9(4):851–60.

[25] Moran MF, Tong J, Taylor P, Ewing RM. Emerging applications for phospho-proteomics in cancer molecular therapeutics. Biochim Biophys Acta 2006;1766(2): 230–41.

[26] Hunter T. Signaling-2000 and beyond. Cell 2000;100:113–27.

[27] Figlin RA. Mechanisms of disease: survival benefit of temsirolimus validates a role for mTOR in the management of advanced RCC. Nat Clin Pract Oncol 2008; 5(10):601–9.

[28] Jin Q, Esteva FJ. Cross-talk between the ErbB/HER family and the type I insulin-like growth factor receptor signaling pathway in breast cancer. J Mammary Gland Biol Neoplasia 2008;13(4):485–98.

[29] Guha U, Chaerkady R, Marimuthu A, Patterson AS, Kashyap MK, Harsha HC, et al. Comparisons of tyrosine phosphorylated proteins in cells expressing lung cancer-specific alleles of EGFR and KRAS. Proc Natl Acad Sci USA 2008;105(37):14112–7.

[30] Cui Q, Ma Y, Jaramillo M, Bari H, Awan A, Yang S, et al. A map of human cancer signaling. Mol Syst Biol 2007;3:152.

[31] Haura EB, Zheng Z, Song L, Cantor A, Bepler G. Activated epidermal growth factor receptor-Stat-3 signaling promotes tumor survival in vivo in non-small cell lung cancer. Clin Cancer Res 2005;11(23):8288–94.

[32] Zandi R, Larsen AB, Andersen P, Stockhausen MT, Poulsen HS. Mechanisms for oncogenic activation of the epidermal growth factor receptor. Cell Signal 2007;19(10):2013–23.

[33] Swanton C, Futreal A, Eisen T. Her2-targeted therapies in non-small cell lung cancer. Clin Cancer Res 2006;12(14 Pt 2):4377s–83s.

[34] Casalini P, Iorio MV, Galmozzi E, Ménard S. Role of HER receptors family in development and differentiation. J Cell Physiol 2004;200(3):343–50.

[35] Wiley HS. Trafficking of the ErbB receptors and its influence on signaling. Exp Cell Res 2003;284(1):78–88.

[36] Arteaga CL. Epidermal growth factor receptor dependence in human tumors: more than just expression? Oncologist 2002;7(Suppl. 4):31–9.

[37] Smock RG, Gierasch LM. Sending signals dynamically. Science 2009;324(5924):198–203.

[38] Ventura AC, Jackson TL, Merajver SD. On the role of cell signaling models in cancer research. Cancer Res 2009;69(2):400–2.

[39] Araujo RP, Liotta LA, Petricoin EF. Proteins, drug targets and the mechanisms they control: the simple truth about complex networks. Nat Rev Drug Discov 2007;6(11):871–80.

[40] Geho DH, Petricoin EF, Liotta LA, Araujo RP. Modeling of protein signaling networks in clinical proteomics. Cold Spring Harb Symp Quant Biol 2005;70:517–24.

[41] Iadevaia S, Lu Y, Morales FC, Mills GB, Ram PT. Identification of optimal drug combinations targeting cellular networks: integrating phospho-proteomics and computational network analysis. Cancer Res 2010;70(17):6704–14.

[42] Araujo RP, Liotta LA. A control theoretic paradigm for cell signaling networks: a simple complexity for a sensitive robustness. Curr Opin Chem Biol 2006;10(1):81–7.

[43] Araujo RP, Petricoin EF, Liotta LA. A mathematical model of combination therapy using the EGFR signaling network. Biosystems 2005;80(1):57–69.

[44] Napoletani D, Sauer T, Struppa DC, Petricoin E, Liotta L. Augmented sparse reconstruction of protein signaling networks. J Theor Biol 2008;255(1):40–52.

[45] Johnson SA, Hunter T. Kinomics: methods for deciphering the kinome. Nat Methods 2005;2(1):17–25.

[46] Hennessy BT, Smith DL, Ram PT, Lu Y, Mills GB. Exploiting the PI3K/AKT pathway for cancer drug discovery. Nat Rev Drug Discov 2005;4(12):988–1004.

[47] O'Reilly KE, Rojo F, She QB, Solit D, Mills GB, Smith D, et al. mTOR inhibition induces upstream receptor tyrosine kinase signaling and activates Akt. Cancer Res 2006;66(3):1500–8.

[48] Grünwald V, Soltau J, Ivanyi P, Rentschler J, Reuter C, Drevs J. Molecular targeted therapies for solid tumors: management of side effects. Onkologie 2009;32(3):129–38.

[49] Huang Z, Brdlik C, Jin P, Shepard HM. A pan-HER approach for cancer therapy: background, current status and future development. Expert Opin Biol Ther 2009;9(1):97–110.

[50] Ramos JW. The regulation of extracellular signal-regulated kinase (ERK) in mammalian cells. Int J Biochem Cell Biol 2008;40(12):2707–19.

[51] Paweletz CP, Charboneau L, Roth MJ, Bichsel VE, Simone NL, Chen T, et al. Reverse phase proteomic microarrays which capture disease progression show activation of pro-survival pathways at the cancer invasion front. Oncogene 2001;20(16):1981–9.

[52] Zhong H, Sanchez C, Spitrzer D, Plambeck-Suess S, Gibbs J, Hawkins WG, et al. Synergistic effects of concurrent blockade of PI3K and MEK pathways in pancreatic cancer preclinical models. PLoS One 2013;8(10):e77243.

[53] Walters DM, Lindberg JM, Adair SJ, Newhook TE, Cowan CR, Stokes JB, et al. Inhibition of the growth of patient-derived pancreatic cancer xenografts with the MEK inhibitor trametinib is augmented by combined treatment with the epidermal growth factor receptor/HER2 inhibitor lapatinib. Neoplasia 2013;15(2):143–55.

[54] Gilmour AM, Abdulkhalek S, Cheng TS, Alghamdi F, Jayanth P, O'Shea LK, et al. A novel epidermal growth factor receptor-signaling platform and its targeted translation in pancreatic cancer. Cell Signal 2013;25(12):2587–603.

[55] Venkatasubbarao K, Peterson L, Zhao S, Hill P, Cao L, Zhou Q, et al. Inhibiting signal transducer and activator of transcription-3 increases response to gemcitabine and delays progression of pancreatic cancer. Mol Cancer 2013;12(1):104.

[56] www.curetoday.com/index.cfm/fuseaction/news.showNewsArticle/id/13/news_id/3785.

[57] Pierobon M, Calvert V, Belluco C, Garaci E, Deng J, Lise M, et al. Multiplexed cell signaling analysis of metastatic and nonmetastatic colorectal cancer reveals COX2-EGFR signaling activation as a potential prognostic pathway biomarker. Clin Colorectal Cancer 2009;8(2):110–7.

[58] Gulmann C, Sheehan KM, Conroy RM, Wulfkuhle JD, Espina V, Mullarkey MJ, et al. Quantitative cell signalling analysis reveals down-regulation of MAPK pathway activation in colorectal cancer. J Pathol 2009;218(4):514–9.

[59] Vanmeter AJ, Rodriguez AS, Bowman ED, Harris CC, Deng J, Calvert VS, et al. LCM and protein microarray analysis of human NSCLC: differential EGPR phosphorylation events associated with mutated EGFR compared to wild type. Mol Cell Proteomics 2008;7(10):1902–24.

[60] Wulfkuhle JD, Speer R, Pierobon M, Laird J, Espina V, Deng J, et al. Multiplexed cell signaling analysis of human breast cancer: applications for personalized therapy. J Proteome Res 2008;7(4):1508–17.

[61] Sanchez-Carbayo M, Socci ND, Richstone L, Corton M, Behrendt N, Wulfkuhle J, et al. Genomic and proteomic profiles reveal the association of gelsolin to TP53 status and bladder cancer progression. Am J Pathol 2007;171(5):1650–8.

[62] Zhou J, Wulfkuhle J, Zhang H, Gu P, Yang Y, Deng J, et al. Activation of the PTEN/mTOR/STAT3 pathway in breast cancer stem-like cells is required for viability and maintenance. Proc Natl Acad Sci USA 2007;104(41):16158–63.

[63] Sheehan KM, Gulmann C, Eichler GS, Weinstein J, Barrett HL, Kay EW, et al. Signal pathway profiling of epithelial and stromal compartments of colonic carcinoma reveals epithelial-mesenchymal transition. Oncogene 2007;27(3):323–31.

[64] Rapkiewicz A, Espina V, Zujewski JA, Lebowitz PF, Filie A, Wulfkuhle J, et al. The needle in the haystack: application of breast fine-needle aspirate samples to quantitative protein microarray technology. Cancer 2007;111(3):173–84.

[65] Petricoin EF, Espina V, Araujo RP, Midura B, Yeung C, Wan X, et al. Phosphoprotein signal pathway mapping: Akt/mTOR pathway activation association with childhood rhabdomyosarcoma survival. Cancer Res 2007;67(7):3431–4.

[66] Calvert VS, Tang Y, Boveia V, Wulfkuhle J, Schutz-Geschwender V, Olive DM, et al. Development of multiplexed protein profiling and detection using near infrared detection of reverse-phase protein microarrays. Clin Proteomics 2004;1(1):81–90.

[67] Chiechi A, Mueller C, Boehm KM, Romano A, Benassi MS, Picci P, et al. Improved data normalization methods for reverse phase protein microarray analysis of complex biological samples. Biotechniques 2012;0(0):1–7.

[68] Avninder S, Ylaya K, Hewitt SM. Tissue microarray: a simple technology that has revolutionized research in pathology. J Postgrad Med 2008;54(2):158–62.

[69] Haab BB. Antibody arrays in cancer research. Mol Cell Proteomics 2005;4(4):377–83.

[70] Emmert-Buck MR, Bonner RF, Smith PD, Chuaqui RF, Zhuang Z, Goldstein SR, et al. Laser capture microdissection. Science 1996;274(5289):998–1001.

[71] Silvestri A, Colombatti A, Calvert VS, Deng J, Mammano E, Liotta L, et al. Protein pathway biomarker analysis of human cancer reveals requirement for upfront cellular-enrichment processing. Lab Invest 2010;90(5):787–96.

[72] Espina V, Edmiston KH, Heiby M, Pierobon M, Sciro M, Merritt B, et al. A portrait of tissue phosphoprotein stability in the clinical tissue procurement process. Mol Cell Proteomics 2008;7(10):1998–2018.

[73] Pinhel IF, Macneill FA, Hills MJ, Salter J, Detre S, A'hern R, et al. Extreme loss of immunoreactive p-Akt and p-Erk1/2 during routine fixation of primary breast cancer. Breast Cancer Res 2010;12(5):R76.

[74] Mueller C, Edmiston KH, Carpenter C, Gaffney E, Ryan C, Ward R, et al. One-step preservation of phosphoproteins and tissue morphology at room temperature for diagnostic and research specimens. PLoS One 2011;6(8):e23780.

[75] Borén M. Methodology and technology for stabilization of specific states of signal transduction proteins. Methods Mol Biol 2011;717:91–100.

[76] Silvestri A, Calvert V, Belluco C, Lipsky M, De Maria R, Deng J, et al. Protein pathway activation mapping of colorectal metastatic progression reveals metastasis-specific network alterations. Clin Exp Metastasis 2013;30(3):309–16.

[77] Sheehan KM, Calvert VS, Kay EW, Lu Y, Fishman D, Espina V, et al. Use of reverse-phase protein microarrays and reference standard development for molecular network analysis of metastatic ovarian carcinoma. Mol Cell Proteomics 2005;4:346–55.

[78] Stevens EV, Nishizuka S, Antony S, Reimers M, Varma S, Young L, et al. Predicting cisplatin and trabectedin drug sensitivity in ovarian and colon cancers. Mol Cancer Ther 2008;7:10–8.

[79] O'Reilly KE, Warycha M, Davies MA, Rodrik V, Zhou XK, Yee H, et al. Phosphory-lated 4E-BP1 is associated with poor survival in melanoma. Clin Cancer Res 2009;15:2872–8.

[80] Boyd ZS, Wu QJ, O'Brien C, Spoerke J, Savage H, Fielder PJ, et al. Proteomic analysis of breast cancer molecular subtypes and biomarkers of response to targeted kinase inhibitors using reverse-phase protein microarrays. Mol Cancer Ther 2008;7:3695–706.

[81] Ihle NT, Lemos R, Wipf P, Yacoub A, Mitchell C, Siwak D, et al. Mutations in the phosphatidylinositol-3-kinase pathway predict for antitumor activity of the inhibitor PX-866 while oncogenic Ras is a dominant predictor for resistance. Cancer Res 2009;69:143–50.

[82] Xia W, Petricoin 3rd EF, Zhao S, Liu L, Osada T, Cheng Q, et al. An heregulin-EGFR-HER3 autocrine signaling axis can mediate acquired lapatinib resistance in HER2+ breast cancer models. Breast Cancer Res 2013;15(5):R85.

[83] van Agthoven T, Godinho MF, Wulfkuhle JD, Petricoin 3rd EF, Dorssers LC. Protein pathway activation mapping reveals molecular networks associated with anti-estrogen resistance in breast cancer cell lines. Int J Cancer 2012;131(9):1998–2007.

[84] Federici G, Gao X, Slawek J, Arodz T, Shitaye A, Wulfkuhle JD, et al. Systems analysis of the NCI-60 cancer cell lines by alignment of protein pathway activation modules with "-OMIC" data fields and therapeutic response signatures. Mol Cancer Res 2013;11(6):676–85.

[85] Wulfkuhle JD, Berg D, Wolff C, Langer R, Tran K, Illi J, et al. Molecular analysis of HER2 signaling in human breast cancer by functional protein pathway activation mapping. Clin Cancer Res 2012;18(23):6426–35.

Computational and Biological Evaluation of Radioiodinated Quinazolinone Prodrug for Targeting Pancreatic Cancer

Pavel Pospisil[1], Amin I. Kassis[2]

[1]Philip Morris International R&D, Philip Morris Products S.A., Neuchâtel, Switzerland, [2]Department of Radiology, Harvard Medical School, Boston, MA, USA

Contents

Introduction to EMCIT Concept 385
Computational Evaluation 387
   Searching for the Target 387
Sequence Alignment of Extracellular Sulfatase 388
   Docking into Sulfatase 389
   Docking into Phosphatases 392
Biological Evaluation 394
   Enzymatic Catalysis 394
   In Vitro Hydrolysis by Human Tumor Cells 396
Discussion 397
   Proof of Concept 399
   Novel Target? 400
Conclusions 401
References 402

INTRODUCTION TO EMCIT CONCEPT

The concept of enzyme-mediated cancer imaging and therapy (EMCIT) [1–5] involves the use of an enzyme specifically overexpressed on the surface of cancer cells. As such, the enzyme can act as a mediator for the hydrolysis of a soluble, radioisotopically labeled prodrug to a water-insoluble drug. This enzyme-dependent and site-specific hydrolysis provides a noninvasive technique for imaging and therapy, based on the rapid in vivo precipitation and entrapment of water-insoluble radioactive molecules within the extracellular spaces of solid tumors and minimal uptake into normal tissues.

The working prototype for the EMCIT approach was first developed and confirmed for alkaline phosphatase (ALP) [1,2,4], a hydrolase with monophosphoesteric activity that is known to be overexpressed on the plasma membranes of many tumor-cell types including breast and ovarian carcinoma [2,6]. In 2008, the EMCIT concept was also successfully established for prostatic acid phosphatase (PAP) in prostate cancer [3]. In both cases, the radiolabeled prodrug, a derivative of quinazolinone, was shown to have very EMCIT-suitable properties. Namely, ammonium 2-(2′-phosphoryloxyphenyl)-6-iodo-4-(3H)-quinazolinone (IQ_{2-P}) was shown to be hydrolyzed by ALP and PAP to the water–insoluble, fluorescent 2-(2′-hydroxyphenyl)-6-iodo-4-(3H)-quinazolinone (IQ_{2-OH}) [1–5]. In vitro incubation of $^{125}IQ_{2-P}/^{127}IQ_{2-P}$ with several human and mouse tumor cell lines (e.g., breast, colon, lung, ovary, and prostate) resulted in the efficient and rapid transformation of the prodrug to the corresponding water–insoluble derivative, which was effectively retained on the surface of cancer cells. The prodrug was minimally hydrolyzed in the presence of normal human mammary epithelial cells (HMEC) and mouse liver, spleen, kidney, and muscle cells [3–5]. Importantly, IQ_{2-P} can be readily radiolabeled with an isotope having decay characteristics suitable for single-photon emission computed tomography (SPECT) or positron emission tomography (PET) imaging (e.g., ^{123}I, ^{124}I) or for therapy (e.g., ^{131}I).

Here we present the application of the EMCIT approach to pancreatic cancer. To a large extent, this chapter is based on the results of our previously published results [7]. In the United States, it is estimated that 45,220 men and women will be diagnosed with pancreatic cancer in 2013, and an estimated 38,460 patients will die from this disease in 2013 (www.cancer. gov/cancertopics/types/pancreatic). Despite the lethal nature of pancreatic tumors, the possibility of early diagnosis is practically nonexistent. Thus, the development of technologies that enable noninvasive sensing of this disease and therapeutic intervention at an early stage is clearly desirable. Therefore, in analogy with our earlier investigations in which the overexpression of ALP was utilized to target such iodoquinazolinone derivatives to various tumors (e.g., colon, lung, ovarian) and PAP in prostate tumors, the intention of our studies is to (1) identify an enzyme that is overexpressed by pancreatic cells and that is able to hydrolyze the quinazolinone prodrug; (2) design, synthesize, and characterize an iodoquinazolinone analog that is a substrate for the extracellular pancreatic cancer–identified hydrolase and with EMCIT-suitable characteristics; and (3) perform in silico as well as in vitro binding assays of such derivatives with the data-mining-identified target prior to in vivo assessment.

In order to investigate a pancreatic target candidate, we have drawn on our recently developed bioinformatics methods of data mining that are based on the combined exploration of scientific literature, gene–protein databases, and knowledge-pathway databases [8,9]. Using this approach, a new target that has been identified is an enzyme overexpressed in human pancreatic cancer called extracellular sulfatase 1 (SULF1). The primary activity of SULF1 is the desulfation of heparan-sulfate-proteoglycan (HSPG) [10]. This sulfatase has also been shown to regulate the growth of pancreatic cancer cells and is overexpressed in pancreatic cancer [11,12]. The enzyme belongs to the arylsulfatase family, whose members have the ability to desulfate molecules with sulfate-attached aromatic rings, e.g., *para*-nitrocatechol sulfate (pNCS) [13]. Because of this activity, and in analogy with the arylphosphatase activity of ALP and PAP, we have modified IQ_{2-P} to its sulfur-derived analog 2-(2′-sulfooxyphenyl)-6-iodo-4-(3H)-quinazolinone (IQ_{2-S}), performed modeling studies, characterized the compound, and determined its hydrolysis in silico and in vitro.

This chapter is mainly based on our published paper [7]. We briefly present how the SULF1 was identified using the combined data mining approaches. We then carried out the in silico molecular docking to predict the potential enzymatic selectivity for the analogs followed by in vitro incubation of the three enzymes (arylsulfatase A (ARSA), ALP, and PAP) with sulfate- and phosphate-quinazolinone derivatives. To further prove that the hydrolysis of these prodrugs occurs on the surface of the cancer cells, T3M4 pancreatic cancer cells (as well as other cancer cell lines: ovarian cancer cells OVCAR-3 and prostate cancer cells LNCaP) were incubated in vitro with the iodoquinazolinone derivatives and showed that their hydrolysis leads to the formation and precipitation of $^{127}IQ_{2-OH}$ fluorescent crystals on the cell surface. These findings were the first to report the targeting of a radioactive substrate to SULF1 and revealed that such structures would be useful in imaging ($^{123}I/^{124}I/^{131}I$) and radiotherapy (^{131}I) of pancreatic cancer.

COMPUTATIONAL EVALUATION
Searching for the Target

The search for hydrolases expressed in the extracellular space of pancreatic cancer cells was completed using our data mining strategy. This approach in a combined manner explores scientific literature, gene and protein databases, and pathway knowledge bases. Our first strategy published in 2006 utilized the text mining software LSGraph and the pathway knowledge bases of Ingenuity Pathways Analysis® (IPA) (version 2.0) [8]. This combined approach of data mining identified 450 proteins related to pan-creatic cancer from which one relevant target, SULF1, was identified (see following) [7].

In 2008, we published the data mining approach based on the knowl-edge base of IPA including the exploration of the cancer microarray platform Oncomine™ (oncomine.org), in order to identify extracellular hydrolases in cancer cells and blood-borne biomarkers for early diagno-sis of cancer [9]. Oncomine™ was chosen because it is a cancer microar-ray platform incorporating over 670 public independent microarray datasets totaling more than 73,000 samples, which span 20 major cancer types (September 2013). It unifies a large compendium of other pub-lished cancer microarray data (Gene Expression Omnibus (GEO; ncbi.nlm.nih.gov/geo)) and Stanford Microarray Database (smd.princeton.edu), and uniquely provides differential expression analyses comparing most major types of cancer with their respective normal tissues. For example, to identify potentially important genes in a particular cancer, users can perform a "cancer vs. normal" analysis for a given cancer type (e.g., pan-creas) and those genes that are upregulated in cancer relative to its nor-mal tissue can be retrieved as a list [9]. Recently, we checked the presence of SULF1 in the oncomine.org database and found that in three out of seven microarray datasets, the gene of this enzyme meets the threshold of being in the top 1% genes of cancer vs. normal datasets. Thus, using this more recent approach, SULF1 would have been identified as the potential target as well.

Extracellular SULF1 is a potential EMCIT target (Figure 17.1). While this enzyme is situated in the endoplasmic reticulum and Golgi stack, it has been shown, by its similarity to homologous proteins, to be secreted outside the cell (UniProt ID: SULF1_HUMAN; Entrez Gene ID: 23213). As indicated in protein and gene databases, its localization in the extracel-lular space infers from direct assays [14,15]. Thus, the combined data min-ing approach used brings together the information on enzyme function, localization, ontology, and known expression in pancreatic cancer micro-array datasets.

SEQUENCE ALIGNMENT OF EXTRACELLULAR SULFATASE

In order to situate the selected enzyme SULF1 with respect to protein family and to determine the closest available structural homologs, sequence align-ments against known protein sequences of the UniProt Knowledgebase 9.2

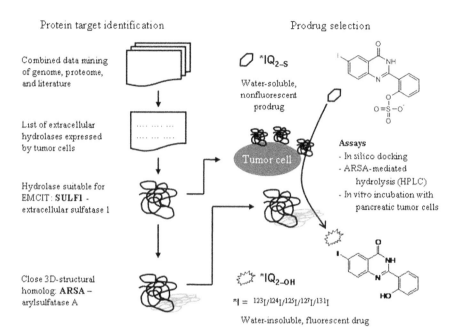

Figure 17.1 *Schematic of Enzyme-Mediated Cancer Imaging and Therapy (EMCIT) Showing Overall Data Mining Approach Used To Identify Hydrolases for Radiolabeled Quinazolinone Derivative Substrates.*

(uniprot.org) were queried using BLAST network service of the Swiss NCBI BLAST program reference (PMID:9254694) [16]. The *blastp* option was set as restricted to mammalian taxon, searched only in UniProt-curated sequences and excluding fragments. The assessment of SULF1 against sequences of proteins with experimentally determined 3-D structures was performed against nonredundant sequences of the Protein Data Bank (PDB, rcsb.org) also using NCBI BLAST2 software (Figure 17.2). Furthermore, sequence alignment of SULF1 against all mammalian proteins in the UniProt database placed SULF1 into the "alkaline-phosphatase-like clan" (Interpro ID: IPRO17849; ebi. ac.uk/interpro/entry/IPR017849). Such findings encouraged us once more to consider SULF1 for the EMCIT concept as this approach was demonstrated to work for the prostatic acid and ALPs [2,3].

Docking into Sulfatase

Since the 3D-resolved structure of SULF1 is not known, we identified in the Protein Data Bank the best aligned structural homolog, arylsulfatase A (ARSA, PDB code 1E2S) (Figure 17.2). As can be seen, the key

(A)

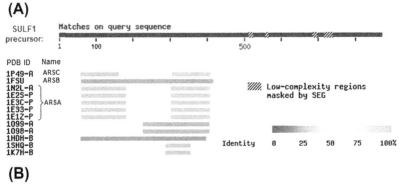

(B)

Common pattern of sulfatases:

$[SAPG]_{85}$-$[LIVMST]_{86}$-$[CS]_{87}$-$[STACG]_{88}$-P_{89}-$[STA]_{90}$-R_{91}-$x(2)_{92,93}$-$[LIVMFW](2)_{94,95}$-$[TAR]_{96}$-G_{97},

where x(2) signifies any residue occurring twice and $[LIVMFW](2)_{94,95}$ denotes that one of the six amino acids is at positions 94 and 95.

ARSA = SLCTPSRAALLTG (in blue: common residues of ARSA and SULF1)

SULF1 = PMCCPSRSSMLTG

Figure 17.2 *SULF1 Sequence Alignment Against Proteins With Resolved 3-D Structures.* (A) SULF1 precursor (blue submission line) is aligned to proteins that are sulfatases with arylsulfatase activities (colored by scale of identities—lowest identity: red; highest identity: green) belonging to alkaline-phosphatase-like family of proteins: 1P49-A – arylsulfatase C (ARSC), 1FSU – arylsulfatase B (ARSB), 1N2L-A through 1E1Z – arylsulfatase A. (B) Sequence shows common pattern of sulfatases that corresponds to active sites. Numbering of residues is consistent with Swiss-Prot original query sequence of SULF1 (1–861). (For interpretation of the references to color in this figure legend, the reader is referred to the online version of this book.)

residues of both sulfatase active sites are identical. When the ARSA crystal structure 1E2S is complexed with pNCS, its sulfate group position showed the expected positioning of sulfate (or phosphate) for the docking of our quinazolinone derivatives (Figure 17.3). Pure ARSA enzyme is available commercially and as such is suitable for in vitro binding assays. Its crystallographically determined structure is the complex ARSA C69A–pNCS that mimics the reaction intermediate during sulfate ester hydrolysis by the active enzyme [17]. The active site of ARSA contains positively charged residues Lys123, Lys302, His229, and Ser150, and divalent Mg^{2+} cation in a small deep pocket capable of coordinating the sulfate moiety (Figure 17.3(B) and (C)). The crystal structure contains one water molecule (WAT57) in close proximity to pNCS. Our docking simulations of all derivatives, which have been performed both keeping and removing water in the active site during the docking process, showed that our derivatives prefer the water-deprived active site.

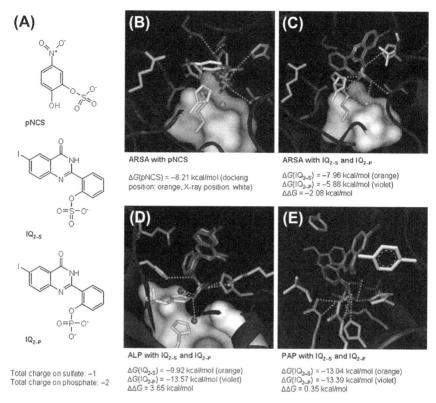

Figure 17.3 *Docking Positions of pNCS, IQ$_{2-S}$, and IQ$_{2-P}$ in Active Sites of ARSA, ALP, and PAP.* Compounds are docked charged as depicted (A). Original crystallographic position of pNCS and its docked position in ARSA are shown with C atoms in white and orange, respectively (B). IQ$_{2-S}$ and IQ$_{2-P}$, depicted with C atoms colored in orange and violet, respectively, are docked in energetically most favorable positions in ARSA (C), ALP (D), and PAP (E). Positively charged residues are green, histidines cyan, and negatively charged residues are red. H-bond interactions to sulfuric group of docked pNCS (B), IQ$_{2-S}$ (C–E), or phosphatidic group of IQ$_{2-P}$ (C–E) are shown as green dotted lines. White surface (B–D) represents amino acid residues complexing Mg^{2+} (green ball) or Zn^{2+} (magenta ball) cations. Ionic groups (sulfate, phosphate) are ideally positioned for nucleophilic attack on sulfur/phosphorus atom. (For interpretation of the references to color in this figure legend, the reader is referred to the online version of this book.)

pNCS is docked deeply in the pocket within 1.5 Å RMSD of distances of docked vs. crystal ligand atoms, in close proximity to the Mg^{2+} cation and Ala69 (Figure 17.3(B)).

Three-dimensional conformers of all sulfate and phosphate derivatives studied were prepared and docked fully flexible into rigid proteins as described previously [3,13]. The protein active sites were defined as amino acid residues 7 Å from the sulfurous or phosphorous atoms of their respective crystal structure substrates. All ligands were docked in the active site of the arylsulfatase ARSA (PDB ID: 1E2S, monomer A) in their charged form. The sulfate group of IQ_{2-S} and pNCS, as well as the phosphate group of IQ_{2-P}, were dehydrogenated in order to simulate the intermediate state of these compounds [3,13]. To test the accuracy of docking to ARSA, modeling was run first with complexed ligand pNCS, then for IQ_{2-S} and IQ_{2-P}. The best docking poses were estimated in terms of docking energy and closest position of sulfur (for IQ_{2-S} and pNCS) or phosphorus (for IQ_{2-P}) atom to the Mg^{2+} cation and the $C\beta$ of Ala69.

Docking into Phosphatases

In order to compare the ability of the arylsulfatase to accommodate IQ_{2-S} with the ability of phosphatases to accommodate IQ_{2-P}, both quinazolinone derivatives have been docked to ARSA, ALP, and PAP. Docking poses of IQ_{2-S} and IQ_{2-P} in the sulfatase were compared to those done to alkaline and acid phosphatases, keeping in account particular differences between the protein active sites [2,3]. For docking into ALP, the structure of human placental ALP (PDB ID: 1EW2) was used. The metal ions Zn and Mg at the active binding site were retained with +2.0 charges, whereas all bound waters except the five involved in interactions with the substrates were discarded. Water hydrogen atoms were added by the PDB2PQR program [18], and then the hydrogen-bonding network was optimized while keeping the heavy atoms rigid. Binding free energy (ΔG) and inhibition constant (K_i) values were calculated and estimated within the AutoDock scoring function. The obtained complexes were utilized for interpretation of the bioactivity potential of the ligands.

Comparison of docking poses and energies can be seen for all compounds in Figure 17.3. The iodine atom of the quinazolinone derivatives point outward from the active site, and the quinazolinone moiety itself does not hinder the binding to studied enzymes (Figure 17.3(C–E)). IQ_{2-P} docks successfully into all three enzymes ARSA, ALP, and PAP. The favorable binding selectivity of IQ_{2-S} and IQ_{2-P} is, therefore, given in terms of the difference of their respective free energies of binding to the enzyme, $\Delta\Delta G$. Thus, IQ_{2-P} binds more tightly than IQ_{2-S} to ALP ($\Delta\Delta G = 3.65\,kcal/mol$) and at similar energies to PAP ($\Delta\Delta G = 0.35\,kcal/mol$) (Figure 17.3, Table 17.1). Similarly to ARSA, docking orientations are almost identical, with the phosphate placed closer to the anchoring residues then sulfate (Figure 17.3(D) and (E)).

Table 17.1 Hydrolysis of IQ_{2-S} and IQ_{2-P} by Arylsulfatase A (ARSA), Alkaline Phosphatase (ALP), and Prostatic Acid Phosphatase (PAP)

Experiment	Target	IQ_{2-S} Hydrolysis	IQ_{2-P} Hydrolysis			Note
In silico docking binding in terms of ΔG (kcal/mol)	ARSA	−7.96	−5.88			ARSA is closest 3-D-structure available homolog to SULF1. IQ_{2-S} docks successfully and more favorably than IQ_{2-P} ($\Delta\Delta G = \Delta G(IQ_{2-S}) - \Delta G(IQ_{2-P}) = -2.08\,\text{kcal/mol}$)
	ALP	−9.92	−13.57			IQ_{2-S} docks successfully but less favorably than IQ_{2-P} ($\Delta\Delta G = 3.65\,\text{kcal/mol}$)
	PAP	−13.04	−13.39			Both IQ_{2-S} and IQ_{2-P} dock at favorable energies to PAP ($\Delta\Delta G = 0.35\,\text{kcal/mol}$)
Phosphatase inhibitors[a]						
In vitro incubations		No	Yes			
In solution (HPLC)	ARSA	98%	ND	7%	12%	Arylsulfatase from Helix pomatia
	ALP	44%	ND	98%	18%	Human placental alkaline phosphatase
	PAP	45%	ND	98%	17%	Human semen prostatic acid phosphatase
Tumor cells (microscopy)[b]	Pancreatic cancer (T3M4)	++	++			Data mining identified SULF1 and PPAP2A (phosphatidic acid phosphatase 2A) related to pancreatic cancer
	Ovarian cancer (OVCAR-3)	++	−			ALP and PAP are known to be expressed in ovarian cancer[c]
	Prostate cancer (LNCaP)	++	−			PAP is known to be expressed in prostate cancer cell LNCaP cells shown to overexpress PAP[c]

[a]Inhibition determined by HPLC with 5% inhibitor (20× dilution); enzyme concentration 0.01 unit/μl.
[b]Density of crystals: −, no fluorescent crystals; +, few scattered fluorescent crystals; ++, cells covered with crystals.
[c]Reference [3].

BIOLOGICAL EVALUATION

Enzymatic Catalysis

We have designed, characterized, and synthesized IQ_{2-S} using organic synthetic methods that are analogous to those used with phosphate-containing IQ_{2-P} [2]. Syntheses of 2-(2'-phosphoryloxyphenyl)-6-[$^{125}I/^{127}I$]iodo-4-(3H)-quinazolinone (IQ_{2-P}), its hydroxylated analog 2-(2'-hydroxyphenyl)-6-iodo-4-(3H)-quinazolinone (IQ_{2-OH}), and the stannylated analog 2-(2'-hydroxyphenyl)-6-tributylstannyl-4-(3H)-quinazolinone (SnQ_{2-OH}) were published in [3,4]. IQ_{2-OH} and SnQ_{2-OH} are starting materials for the synthesis of IQ_{2-S} and $^{125}IQ_{2-S}$, respectively. Synthesis of pure (>96%) compounds 2-(2'-sulfooxyphenyl)-6-[^{127}I]iodo-4-(3H)-quinazolinone (IQ_{2-S}), 2-(2'-sulfooxyphenyl)-6-tributylstannyl-4-(3H)-quinazolinone (SnQ_{2-S}), and 2-(2'-sulfooxyphenyl)-6-[^{125}I]iodo-4-(3H)-quinazolinone ($^{125}IQ_{2-S}$) is shown in [7].

In analogy with the in silico docking simulations, we have performed comparable experiments in vitro. The hydrolysis of compounds was assessed by measuring the formation of radioactive ^{125}I-labeled products with HPLC [1–5]. The retention times of each sample were determined and compared with those obtained prior to the addition of enzymes. In essence, $^{125}IQ_{2-S}$ and $^{125}IQ_{2-P}$ were incubated with (1) 1 unit of ARSA from *Helix pomatia*; (2) 1 unit of ALP from human placenta; or (3) 1 unit of PAP from human semen. The enzymes were examined at three concentrations (0.1, 0.01, and 0.001 units/μl). Figure 17.4 shows HPLC profiles and retention times of the radiolabeled prodrugs $^{125}IQ_{2-S}$ and $^{125}IQ_{2-P}$ in solution in the absence and presence of the enzymes. All three enzymes mediate the hydrolysis of $^{125}IQ_{2-S}$ and $^{125}IQ_{2-P}$, but, at different rates (Table 17.1). Arylsulfatase (0.01 unit/μl) cleaves sulfate very efficiently from $^{125}IQ_{2-S}$, completely transforming this molecule to $^{125}IQ_{2-OH}$ within 10 min. At the same concentration, this sulfatase is quite inefficient at the hydrolysis of $^{125}IQ_{2-P}$ (~7%). When the concentration of the enzyme was 10-fold higher, only partial hydrolysis (37%) was observed (Figure 17.4(B)). These results indicate that arylsulfatase exhibits partial phosphatidic activity. Hydrolysis of both compounds with alkaline and acid phosphatases demonstrates the reverse pattern. With both phosphatases (0.01 unit/μl), there is partial hydrolysis of $^{125}IQ_{2-S}$ (~45%), as seen previously [3–5]. Complete hydrolysis of $^{125}IQ_{2-P}$ occurs in the presence of either enzyme (Figure 17.4, Table 17.1). Therefore, it seems that besides the enzymes' prime activities, both ALP and PAP also have sulfatidic activity, while ARSA has phosphatidic activity.

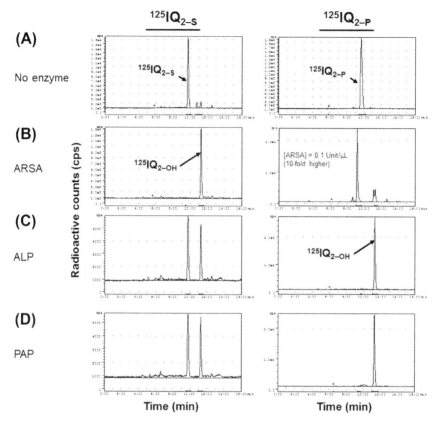

Figure 17.4 ARSA-, ALP-, and PAP-Mediated Hydrolysis of $^{125}IQ_{2-S}$ and $^{125}IQ_{2-P}$ HPLC profiles of $^{125}IQ_{2-S}$ (left column) and $^{125}IQ_{2-P}$ (right column) are shown for pure compounds in solution (A), and after 10-min incubation (Trizma® buffer, pH 7.4, 37°C) of derivatives with ARSA (B), ALP (C), and PAP (D). All profiles are performed with 0.01 unit/μl enzyme with exception of ARSA assay with $^{125}IQ_{2-P}$ which is done at 10-fold-higher concentration of enzyme (0.1 unit/μl).

Enzymatic hydrolysis in solution of $^{125}IQ_{2-P}$ by ARSA, ALP, and PAP was also determined in the presence of phosphatase inhibitors. A mixture of compounds, "Phosphatase Inhibitor Cocktail 2" known to inhibit acid and ALPs (10 μl), was used in a total volume of 20 μl solution (two-fold dilution of purchased inhibitor concentration) containing $^{125}IQ_{2-P}$ (200 μCi in 5 μl), Tris buffer (0.1 M, pH 7.4), and selected enzyme concentrations (0.1, 0.01, or 0.001 units/μl). The hydrolysis of IQ_{2-P} is completely inhibited in the presence of the phosphatase inhibitors. When IQ_{2-S} was incubated with these tumor cells, efficient hydrolysis and formation of crystals occurred (Figure 17.5). The addition of phosphatase inhibitors led to an absence of fluorescent crystals only with the LNCaP and OVCAR-3 cells and not the T3M4 cells.

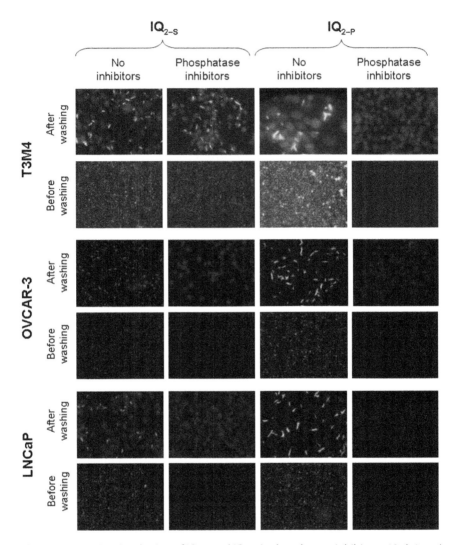

Figure 17.5 In vitro incubation of IQ_{2-S} and IQ_{2-P} (±phosphatase inhibitors; 10 μl, 1 mg/ ml) with viable human pancreatic, ovarian, and prostatic cancer cells showing hydrolysis of compounds and precipitation of IQ_{2-OH} (green crystals) before washing cells (low power) and after washing cells (high power). Cell nuclei (blue) are counterstained with DAPI. (For interpretation of the references to color in this figure legend, the reader is referred to the online version of this book.)

In Vitro Hydrolysis by Human Tumor Cells

The in vitro hydrolysis of IQ_{2-S} and IQ_{2-P} with pancreatic T3M4, ovarian OVCAR-3, and prostate LNCaP cancer cells was assessed by fluorescence microscopy examined under the same conditions (pH 7.4, 37 °C) as published [3,7]. Briefly, logarithmically growing cells were trypsinized, suspended in medium, and allowed to adhere by an overnight incubation at 37 °C. The chambers were then washed, the medium removed, and the slides reincubated for up to 24 h with IQ_{2-S} or IQ_{2-P} (30 μg/ml). The slides were incubated an additional 24 h, the cells were observed under a fluorescence microscope, and the density of the green crystals formed was semiquantitatively recorded (− (minus): no fluorescent crystals; ++: cells covered with crystals, (Table 17.1)). The slides were then washed 3× in PBS and then fixed in ice-cold acetone. The washed fixed cells were counterstained with diamidino-2-phenylindole (DAPI), a nuclear stain, and the distribution and intensity of fluorescent crystals were observed and compared with those prior to washing of the cell monolayer. The inhibition of IQ_{2-S} or IQ_{2-P} (10 μg/ml) hydrolysis was assessed in the presence of the phosphatase inhibitors by the simultaneous addition of the aqueous solution of inhibitor mixture (30 μl, Phosphatase Inhibitor Cocktail 2, 1 mg/ml). When the three cell lines are incubated with IQ_{2-P}, fluorescent crystals, i.e., the corresponding product of hydrolysis IQ_{2-OH}, are formed and retained (before and after cell washing) on the cell surface (Figure 17.5). No hydrolysis and formation of fluorescent IQ_{2-OH} crystals are observed when HMEC are incubated with IQ_{2-S} or IQ_{2-P} or when both compounds are incubated in medium in the absence of cells.

DISCUSSION

The computational data mining approach utilized in our studies, which uses a combination of searches through scientific literature, gene and protein databases, and pathway knowledge bases, identified 450 entities hits (gene/protein). This number is much larger than that obtained using the classic search exploring the protein database only. Interestingly, most of these proteins (390 of 450, >86%) are expressed in the extracellular space of the pancreatic cancer cell or are integral to its plasma membrane, which is a considerable number of cell-surface entities. As we are interested in finding an EMCIT-suitable hydrolase, we identified five phosphatases and one sulfatase—extracellular sulfatase 1 that we predicted would be an excellent target suitable for EMCIT (Figure 17.1). SULF1 has been shown to have high specific endoglucosamine-6-sulfatase activity [14] and to exhibit arylsulfatase activity, described as the cleavage of sulfate from the aromatic phenyl ring. Thus, arylsulfatase activity can be compared to the arylphosphatase activity known for ALP and PAP that has been successfully applied to the hydrolysis of IQ_{2-P} in our previous EMCIT studies [1–5]. Interestingly,

SULF1 sequence alignment to all mammalian proteins (Figure 17.2) demonstrated its "alkaline-phosphatase-like" properties, which provided us an additional argument for using SULF1 as the target for enzyme-mediated imaging.

Therefore, we have modified IQ_{2-P} to its sulfate-derived analog IQ_{2-S} and docked it into the closest homologous 3-D structure of SULF1, ARSA. The accurate docking pose of pNCS into its ARSA binding pocket (1.5 Å RMSD) shows the right selection of the docking procedure. Docking of both derivatives IQ_{2-S} and IQ_{2-P} into ARSA, ALP, and PAP (Figure 17.3) showed that besides the common classification of the three enzymes in the alkaline-phosphatase-like family, they are known to bind *para*-nitrophenyl sulfates or phosphates and have both partial sulfatidic and phosphatidic activities [19,20]. From the point of view of the ligand structures alone, pNCS and IQ_{2-S} and IQ_{2-P} share some chemical–structural similarities that make quinazolinones promising scaffolds. Particularly, IQ_{2-S} contains a sulfate group that is attached to the phenyl ring as in pNCS that can be hydrolyzed. Actually, this characteristic is successfully predicted by the docking of IQ_{2-S}, which embeds the sulfate in its pocket of ARSA (Figure 17.3(B)). Additionally, we gain new aromatic hydrophobic interactions between the quinazolinone phenyl moiety and Val91 residue. The phenyl portion of the quinazolinone moiety of IQ_{2-S} lies parallel to the phenyl portion of pNCS in the crystal complex. It seems that the sulfate drives the binding. Comparison of pNCS and IQ_{2-S} energies indicates that the resulting free-energy binding value of IQ_{2-S} (-7.96 kcal/mol) is similar to that of pNCS (-8.21 kcal/mol). The slight difference of 0.25 kcal/mol indicates that iodoquinazolinone does not prohibit the sulfate ion from being anchored into the sulfate pocket.

IQ_{2-P} docks into the active site of ARSA exactly as IQ_{2-S}, placing the phosphate moiety into the sulfate-binding pocket (Figure 17.3(C)). The H-bonding system between phosphate and Mg^{2+} cation is somewhat weaker (fewer bonds and longer interactions, $\Delta G = -5.88$ kcal/mol) and 2 kcal/mol less favorable than that for IQ_{2-S}. Despite the number of H-bonds and the difference in docking pose, the program shows a distinct preference toward a sulfate rather than a phosphate moiety. Even with the -2 charge of phosphate compared with the -1 charge of sulfate, the sulfate derivative binding energy (-7.96 kcal/mol) is more favorable than that of the phosphate derivative (-5.88 kcal/mol) (Figure 17.3(C)). Overall, docking predicts that replacing phosphate by sulfate on the iodoquinazolinone scaffold would permit shifting the EMCIT concept from phosphatases to sulfatases and suggests a novel prodrug target system. Particularly with respect to pancreatic cancer, the sulfate-derived IQ_{2-S} is a potential prodrug for ARSA and subsequently its closest analog SULF1 (due to its high sequence homology and identical key active site interacting residues).

The successful docking of IQ_{2-S} and IQ_{2-P} into sulfatase (though with different binding energies) led us to carry out the reciprocal tests of docking into alkaline and PAPs [2,3]. The favorable binding selectivity of IQ_{2-S} and IQ_{2-P} is given in terms of $\Delta\Delta G$ (Table 17.1). Similarly to ARSA, docking orientations are almost identical (Figure 17.3(D) and (E)) and the preference of the enzymes for their respective substrates is given in binding energies predicted by docking. In analogy with the in silico docking simulations, we have performed comparable experiments in vitro, and it can be seen that all three enzymes mediate the hydrolysis of $^{125}IQ_{2-S}$ and $^{125}IQ_{2-P}$. The binding determinants here are the % rates (Table 17.1). The results indicate that arylsulfatase exhibits partial phosphatidic activity, while phosphatases show partial sulfatidic activities. These findings are in agreement with previous studies showing enzymatic promiscuity of ALP toward hydrolysis of sulfate derivatives and vice versa [19,20]. Furthermore, based on the difference in the observed percentage of hydrolysis in solution, it is possible to conclude that this sulfatase is very effective at the hydrolysis of IQ_{2-S} while being quite ineffective at hydrolyzing IQ_{2-P}. On the other hand, both phosphatases, which very efficiently hydrolyze IQ_{2-P}, seem to exhibit stronger sulfatidic activities with IQ_{2-S} (~45% hydrolysis at 0.01 unit/μl enzyme).

Proof of Concept

In order to confirm that the hydrolysis of IQ_{2-S} is mediated by sulfatase, both quinazolinone derivatives were also incubated with each hydrolase in the presence of the phosphatase inhibitors. As expected, the presence of inhibitors reduced the ALP and PAP-mediated hydrolyses of IQ_{2-P} approximately five times to 18% and 17%, respectively (Table 17.1). Since ARSA poorly hydrolyzes this quinazolinone derivative (~7%), it was difficult to ascertain the effect of these inhibitors (similar hydrolysis was seen, ~12%). These data confirm the poor ability of this sulfatase to hydrolyze the phosphorylated quinazolinone derivative.

Recently, we demonstrated that in vitro incubation of water-soluble nonfluorescent IQ_{2-P} with various viable ALP-expressing human and mouse tumor cell lines (breast, colorectal, lung, ovarian, rhabdomyosarcoma, and teratocarcinoma) leads to its hydrolysis and the formation of large fluorescent water-insoluble crystals of IQ_{2-OH} [1,2,4], and no hydrolysis occurs when the tumor cells are in the presence of levamisole, a specific inhibitor of ALP [2,4]. In an analogous study [3], we determined that three human prostatic cancer cell lines (LNCaP, PC-3, and 22Rv1) hydrolyze IQ_{2-P} or its radiolabeled analog $^{125}IQ_{2-P}$ to IQ_{2-OH} or $^{125}IQ_{2-OH}$, respectively, with time-dependent formation of very large (up to 20-μm long) fluorescent crystals, many of which were irreversibly bound at the surface of the tumor cells.

The in vitro hydrolysis assay of IQ_{2-S} and IQ_{2-P} with the three cancer cells (T3M4, OVCAR-3, and LNCAP) showed in all cases clear formation of crystals of the corresponding product IQ_{2-OH} (Figure 17.4). However, the addition of phosphatase inhibitors inhibited the formation of fluorescent crystals only with the LNCaP (PAP positive) and OVCAR-3 (ALP positive) cells, and not the T3M4 (pancreatic) cells. Taken together, these findings indicate the presence of (1) phosphatase hydrolytic activity on all three cell lines, and (2) sulfatase activity on the extracellular surface of pancreatic tumor cells only. Based on the results obtained from the combined data-mining approach, docking, and in vitro HPLC assay, it can be suggested that the observed hydrolysis-dependent fluorescence is due to a presence of an arylsulfatase (the group of which SULF1 is a member). From the lack of formation of crystals when both compounds are incubated with ovarian and prostatic cancer cell lines in the presence of phosphatase inhibitors, it can be further concluded that the above-mentioned sulfatase, potentially responsible for the hydrolysis of IQ_{2-S} in T3M4 cells, is not expressed by OVCAR-3 and LNCaP cells. This is in agreement with our data mining, which has identified phosphatases (ALP, PAP)—whose activity here is successfully inhibited—but not sulfatases, overexpressed in the extracellular space of ovarian and prostatic cancer cells.

Novel Target?

As mentioned previously, when we assess the hydrolysis of IQ_{2-P} without inhibitors in pancreatic cancer cells, the substrate is hydrolyzed on the cell surface. Interestingly, this in turn could be explained by the activity of a phosphatase specifically expressed by pancreatic cells of which we are unaware. The observations that in vitro HPLC profiles show weak phosphatidic activity of arylsulfatase and that neither ALP nor PAP is known to be excreted in the outer space of pancreatic cancer cells suggest that there is a phosphatase specifically expressed in the extracellular space of these cells. Retrospectively, we have checked the results of our data mining and have identified a phosphatidic acid phosphatase type 2A (PPAP2A) (see open access additional file in reference [8]). PPAP2A is an integral membrane glycoprotein that hydrolyzes a number of structurally related lipid phosphate substrates and plays an active role in the hydrolysis and uptake of lipids [21]. Two human isoforms of membrane-associated phosphatidic acid phosphatase have been described (PPAP-2A and PPAP-2B), and both enzymes have been shown to have broad substrate specificity and wide tissue distribution [21,22]. The isoform 2A is predominantly present in heart and pancreas and also expressed in prostate, and it belongs to the same family of proteins as PAP [23]. For example, PPAP2A is known to dephosphorylate phosphatidic acid (PA) and its activity (as PAP) is Mg^{2+} independent [22]. Several of these indications point to a possible PPAP-2A arylphosphatase activity hydrolyzing IQ_{2-P} on the surface of T3M4 pancreatic cells. In the recent characterization of the pancreatic juice proteome in patients with pancreatic adenocarcinoma, PPAP2A was identified and described as a potential biomarker of pancreatic cancer suitable for early diagnosis [24]. It suggests one new direction where the EMCIT efforts could be focused in the future.

CONCLUSIONS

Using advanced computational data mining and modeling methods, we have identified human extracellular SULF1 as a suitable target for the enzyme-mediated cancer imaging and therapy technology in pancreatic cancer. Based on previously published work, we have synthesized, radiolabeled, and characterized a sulfate derivative, IQ_{2-S}. In vitro incubation of $^{125}IQ_{2-S}$ with a SULF1-homologous arylsulfatase leads to its hydrolysis and the formation of fluorescent crystals of its product IQ_{2-OH}. Similarly, its incubation with pancreatic cancer cells leads to fluorescent crystals of product IQ_{2-OH} irreversibly attached to the extracellular membranes of these cells. Furthermore, we have unveiled the possible role of PPAP2A phosphatase in the hydrolysis and have suggested this protein too as a potential EMCIT target.

It is our hope that these quinazolinone-based radiopharmaceuticals will eventually lead to the development of a novel noninvasive approach for imaging (^{123}I-SPECT; ^{124}I-PET) and treating (^{131}I) pancreatic cancer. We believe that the EMCIT concept works for sulfatase, as well as phosphatase-mediated hydrolysis of quinazolinone derivatives, providing an active insoluble drug, IQ_{2-OH}, that can move meaningful intervention to a much earlier point in the path of progression of pancreatic cancer before the disease becomes untreatable.

REFERENCES

[1] Ho NH, Harapanhalli RS, Dahman BA, Chen K, Wang K, Adelstein SJ, et al. Synthesis and biologic evaluation of a radioiodinated quinazolinone derivative for enzyme-mediated insolubilization therapy. Bioconjug Chem 2002;13:357–64.

[2] Chen K, Wang K, Kirichian AM, Al Aowad AF, Iyer LK, Adelstein SJ, et al. In silico design, synthesis, and biological evaluation of radioiodinated quinazolinone derivatives for alkaline phosphatase-mediated cancer diagnosis and therapy. Mol Cancer Ther 2006;5:3001–13.

[3] Pospisil P, Wang K, Al Aowad AF, Iyer LK, Adelstein SJ, Kassis AI. Computational modeling and experimental evaluation of a novel prodrug for targeting the extracellular space of prostate tumors. Cancer Res 2007;67:2197–205.

[4] Wang K, Kirichian AM, Aowad AF, Adelstein SJ, Kassis AI. Evaluation of chemical, physical, and biologic properties of tumor-targeting radioiodinated quinazolinone derivative. Bioconjug Chem 2007;18:754–64.

[5] Kassis AI, Korideck H, Wang K, Pospisil P, Adelstein SJ. Novel prodrugs for targeting diagnostic and therapeutic radionuclides to solid tumors. Molecules 2008;13:391–404.

[6] Benham FJ, Fogh J, Harris H. Alkaline phosphatase expression in human cell lines derived from various malignancies. Int J Cancer 1981;27:637–44.

[7] Pospisil P, Korideck H, Wang K, Yang Y, Iyer LK, Kassis AI. Computational and biological evaluation of quinazolinone prodrug for targeting pancreatic cancer. Chem Biol Drug Des 2012;79:926–34.

[8] Pospisil P, Iyer LK, Adelstein SJ, Kassis AI. A combined approach to data mining of textual and structured data to identify cancer-related targets. BMC Bioinf 2006;7.

[9] Yang Y, Pospisil P, Iyer LK, Adelstein SJ, Kassis AI. Integrative genomic data mining for discovery of potential blood-borne biomarkers for early diagnosis of cancer. Plos One 2008;3:e3661.

[10] Lai J, Chien J, Staub J, Avula R, Greene EL, Matthews TA, et al. Loss of HSulf-1 up-regulates heparin-binding growth factor signaling in cancer. J Biol Chem 2003;278:23107–17.

[11] Abiatari I, Kleeff J, Li J, Felix K, Buchler MW, Friess H. Hsulf-1 regulates growth and invasion of pancreatic cancer cells. J Clin Pathol 2006;59:1052–8.

[12] Li J, Kleeff J, Abiatari I, Kayed H, Giese NA, Felix K, et al. Enhanced levels of Hsulf-1 interfere with heparin-binding growth factor signaling in pancreatic cancer. Mol Cancer 2005;4:14.

[13] von Bulow R, Schmidt B, Dierks T, von Figura K, Uson I. Crystal structure of an enzyme-substrate complex provides insight into the interaction between human aryl-sulfatase A and its substrates during catalysis. J Mol Biol 2001;305:269–77.

[14] Morimoto-Tomita M, Uchimura K, Werb Z, Hemmerich S, Rosen SD. Cloning and characterization of two extracellular heparin-degrading endosulfatases in mice and humans. J Biol Chem 2002;277:49175–85.

[15] Frese MA, Milz F, Dick M, Lamanna WC, Dierks T. Characterization of the human sulfatase Sulf1 and its high affinity heparin/heparan sulfate interaction domain. J Biol Chem 2009;284:28033–44.

[16] Altschul SF, Madden TL, Schaffer AA, Zhang J, Zhang Z, Miller W, et al. Gapped BLAST and PSI-BLAST: a new generation of protein database search programs. Nucleic Acids Res 1997;25:3389–402.

[17] Lukatela G, Krauss N, Theis K, Selmer T, Gieselmann V, von Figura K, et al. Crystal structure of human arylsulfatase A: the aldehyde function and the metal ion at the active site suggest a novel mechanism for sulfate ester hydrolysis. Biochemistry 1998;37:3654–64.

[18] Dolinsky TJ, Nielsen JE, McCammon JA, Baker NA. PDB2PQR: an automated pipeline for the setup of Poisson-Boltzmann electrostatics calculations. Nucleic Acids Res 2004;32:W665–7.

[19] Catrina I, O'Brien PJ, Purcell J, Nikolic-Hughes I, Zalatan JG, Hengge AC, et al. Probing the origin of the compromised catalysis of *E. coli* alkaline phosphatase in its promiscuous sulfatase reaction. J Am Chem Soc 2007;129:5760–5.

[20] O'Brien PJ, Herschlag D. Catalytic promiscuity and the evolution of new enzymatic activities. Chem Biol 1999;6:R91–105.

[21] Roberts R, Sciorra VA, Morris AJ. Human type 2 phosphatidic acid phosphohydrolases. Substrate specificity of the type 2a, 2b, and 2c enzymes and cell surface activity of the 2a isoform. J Biol Chem 1998;273:22059–67.

[22] Kai M, Wada I, Imai S, Sakane F, Kanoh H. Cloning and characterization of two human isozymes of Mg2+-independent phosphatidic acid phosphatase. J Biol Chem 1997;272:24572–8.

[23] Ulrix W, Swinnen JV, Heyns W, Verhoeven G. Identification of the phosphatidic acid phosphatase type 2a isozyme as an androgen-regulated gene in the human prostatic adenocarcinoma cell line LNCaP. J Biol Chem 1998;273:4660–5.

[24] Gronborg M, Bunkenborg J, Kristiansen TZ, Jensen ON, Yeo CJ, Hruban RH, et al. Comprehensive proteomic analysis of human pancreatic juice. J Proteome Res 2004;3:1042–55.

CHAPTER 18

Systems and Network Pharmacology Strategies for Pancreatic Ductal Adenocarcinoma Therapy: A Resource Review

Irfana Muqbil[1], Asfar S. Azmi[2], Ramzi M. Mohammad[3,4]

[1]Department of Biochemistry, Faculty of Life Sciences, AMU, Aligarh, UP, India, [2]Department of Pathology, Wayne State University, Detroit, MI, USA, [3]Department of Oncology, Karmanos Cancer Institute, Wayne State University, Detroit, MI, USA, [4]Hamad Medical Corporation, Doha, Qatar

Contents

Introduction   405
Need for Revisiting the Progression Model of PDAC: Departure from Genes to Network 407
Defining Biological Networks   408
   Local Network Topology (Hubs, Motifs, and Graphlets)   409
   Broader Network Topology: Modules, Bridges, Bottlenecks, and Choke Points 410
     Applications on Network Pharmacology   411
     Network-Based PDAC Biomarker Identification   412
   Optimal Intervention Strategies in PDAC Networks Using Network Pharmacology 413
Network Pharmacology to Unwind PDAC microRNA Complexity   414
Network Pharmacology in Drug Repositioning for PDAC   416
Networks in Polypharmacology Strategies against PDAC   418
Conclusions and Future Perspectives   420
References   421

INTRODUCTION

According to the World Cancer Research Fund (WCRF) there were 279,000 cases of pancreatic cancer diagnosed worldwide in 2008 (http://www.wcrf.org/cancer_statistics/). The estimated five-year prevalence of people living with pancreatic cancer is projected at 3.5% per 100,000 and it is the 13th most common cancer in the world. Pancreatic cancer is almost always fatal and is the eighth leading cause of cancer-related deaths in the world. The most common form of pancreatic cancer is the pancreatic ductal adenocarcinoma (PDAC). In the United States it is the fourth leading cause of cancer-related deaths [1]. PDAC kills ~39,000 patients each year [1], which translates to two American deaths every 30 min. The disease is presented at a very late stage and the symptoms are very complex, oftentimes overlapping with that of other disorders, leading to misdiagnoses. Aggressive and therapy resistant PDAC is refractory to any of the currently available treatment modalities. Gemcitabine and its combination with platinum-based compounds have minimal impact and improve the survival by a mere few weeks. Recently, gemcitabine-nab-paclitaxel (Abraxane) has been investigated, and that too has shown very nominal benefits. These morbid statistics and lack of effective drugs indicate that modern approaches to understanding the disease as well as novel molecularly targeted therapies are urgently needed in order to advance the current state of PDAC therapy.

The genetics of therapy resistant PDAC is highly complex [2]. The refractory tumors harbor multiple aberrations in oncogenic and tumor suppressor signaling pathways [3]. PDAC signaling networks are highly intertwined and robust, meaning that they resist changes such as that induced by targeted therapies. According to the most accepted PDAC progression model, normal duct epithelium progresses to infiltrating cancer through a series of histologically defined precursors (PanINs). The overexpression of HER-2/*neu* and point mutations in the K-*ras* gene occur early, inactivation of the *p16* gene at an intermediate stage, while the inactivation of *p53*, *DPC4*, and *BRCA2* occur relatively late [4]. It has previously been proposed that PDAC robustness stems from "passing of the baton" between genes responsible for driving the various stages of the tumor, and therefore an effective therapy should likely target an entire set of genes across a succession of stages to break such robustness [5]. It is interesting to note that to date the moderately successful agents against PDAC have been the nucleoside analogs such as gemcitabine, 5FU, platinum drugs such as cisplatin or oxaliplatin, and recently nab-paclitaxel. While nucleoside analogs and platinum are considered DNA intercalators [6] and nab-paclitaxel was originally discovered as an antimicrotubule agent [7], studies have shown that most of these agents have multiple network pharmacology type of effects on cancer cells [8]. For example, the nucleoside analog gemcitabine has been shown to interact with a wide range of proteins such as P8 [9], and oxaliplatin (a component of FULFIRNOX) was shown to form 10 times more protein adducts than its originally designated DNA adduct forming anticancer mechanisms [10]. Similarly the permutations and combinations of targets of individual components in FULFIRINOX have not been fully elucidated. Although stagnated at six to eight months overall survival benefit for the past 40 years, the multitargeted therapeutics mentioned previously have remained the most widely used agents for the treatment of PDAC. There is no doubt that these chemotherapeutic drugs work through network pharmacology principles. In this chapter, we present the case for using systems and network biology sciences to better understand PDAC complexity and provide examples of how network pharmacology strategies can be used to design superior network targeted single agent and combination strategies against PDAC leading to better treatment outcome.

NEED FOR REVISITING THE PROGRESSION MODEL OF PDAC: DEPARTURE FROM GENES TO NETWORK

There is general consensus over the heterogenous nature of PDAC. Advances in genomic assessment tools have highlighted the intricate signaling network complexity that emanates from the interactions between the different components in PDAC tumor microenvironment. Differential gene expression (DE) analysis has been the traditionally adopted model to identify driver genes. This is the criteria used in the Hruban's progression model where a set of driver gene mutations have been attributed to each specific stage in PDAC development. While these analyses manage to capture several major genes that show noticeable changes in expression/mutation, there are many more important genes that often do not display such drastic changes (do not fall under the DE criteria or cutoff values). These genes are not identifiable through their own behavior, rather, their changes are only quantifiable when evaluated in conjunction with other genes within their vicinity (i.e., through their role in the networks) [5]. However, traditional molecular biology cannot sieve through this complexity, and systems and network level investigations that take a holistic view are needed [11]. In this direction, Srihari and colleagues have utilized PDAC expression datasets comparing 39 paired normal vs. tumor samples to track the progression based on protein–protein (PPI) and gene interactions. Their analysis utilized a novel algorithm, MIN FLIP (FLIP are genes that are flipped in response to stage transition or perturbations). Their analysis shows that serine/threonine kinase are the major genes that act as ON/OFF switches regulating cell cycle progression during the PDAC differentiation process [5]. The MIN FLIP resulted in the discovery of genes that were not marked in the traditional DE system.

Table 18.1 Network Visualization Resources

Network Visualization Resources (2012)	Website Resource
Arena3D	http://arena3d.org
BiologicalNetworks	http://biologicalnetworks.net
BioTapestry	http://www.biotapestry.org
Hive Plots	http://www.hiveplot.com
Hybridlayout	http://www.cadlive.jp/hybridlayout/hybridlayout.html
Hyperdraw	http://www.bioconductor.org/packages/release/bioc/html/hyperdraw.html
ModuLand	www.linkgroup.hu/modules.php
Multilevel Layout	http://code.google.com/p/multilevellayout
MAVisto	http://mavisto.ipk-gatersleben.de
Multilevel Layout	http://code.google.com/p/multilevellayout
RedeR	http://bioconductor.org/packages/release/bioc/html/RedeR.html
VANTED	http://vanted.ipk-gatersleben.de

Logically, the approaches that could break down the PDAC signaling complexity into smaller easily decipherable fragments should make rational design of drugs or their combination easier. There are a number of different network visualizing tools available that can be used to evaluate PDAC expression datasets to obtain sub network information both for diagnostic and therapeutic purposes. With the advent of high-throughput analyses systems, diseases such as PDAC are routinely investigated at multiple levels such as genomics, transcriptomics, and interactomics (metabolomics) levels. These large-scale analyses systems can further be benefited by applying network interaction visualization tools that are readily and publicly available. Table 18.1 lists some of the major network visualization tools that are freely available to evaluate expression datasets such as that derived from PDAC cell line, animal models, human primary tumors, and patient samples. These network visualization tools give a fairly good amount of insight into the interactions between the defined set of differentially identified genes (for example, differentially expressed genes) within a given expression dataset.

DEFINING BIOLOGICAL NETWORKS

The selection of important network positions as drug targets faces major hurdles. An ideal target in cancer network has to be important enough to influence the disease, however, such network position must not be so critical for normal cell physiology that targeting it leads to outward toxicity.

The answer to this problem can come from detailed knowledge on the structure and dynamics of complex cancer related networks that are presented in the following discussion. A biological network is composed of nodes and edges [12]. Nodes can be either amino acids, genes, microRNAs, or proteins, and edges are the interactions between two nodes. Depending on the threshold of detection limits, the edges can connect more than two nodes. Even though these simplistic definitions hold true, there are exceptions, such as in case the node is a protein that is secretory in nature, and then definitions of nodes become diffused. There are a number of excellent reviews that detail the network identification methods and dilemmas associated with defining certain molecular networks [13]. This chapter will not rereview the existing knowledge but will instead focus on how these existing resources will be applied for PDAC biomarker identification and drug discovery.

Local Network Topology (Hubs, Motifs, and Graphlets)

When a node in a biological network has an unusually higher number of neighbors, it is termed as a hub. It is imperative that if a hub is disturbed then the information is rapidly distributed across all the partnering neighbors. Cancer hubs have more interacting partners compared to noncancer proteins, thereby making them good targets in network-based drug design [14,15]. Nevertheless, if the hubs are critical/essential proteins (such as transcription factors that are needed for normal cell function as well), their targeting becomes problematic. At the next level, there have been attempts to define amino acid hubs as intraprotein information distributors, thereby making them targets for drug intervention [16,17]. In this direction, Laonnis and colleagues using mass spectrometry–based quantitative proteomics and stable isotope labeling of amino acids in cell culture coupled with bioinformatics gave indirect evidence identifying interferons as the major hub in cardiac glycoside (e.g., digoxin, digitoxin) mediated PDAC cell death [18]. On the other hand *motifs* are circuits of 3–6 nodes in directed networks that are highly overrepresented as compared to randomized networks [19]. Graphlets are similar to motifs, but are unidirected [20,21]. Nevertheless, targeting local network topology has its limitations, and network robustness overcomes the specific attacks against hubs, motifs, or graphlets. For example, Schramm and colleagues demonstrated that in many different malignancies including PDAC the signaling networks were more diverse (average number of nodes in the networks of tumor > normal tissue nodes), shorter path length (average path length for cancer < normal), less centralized (average clustering coefficient of cancer < normal tissue), and less dependent on hubs (average increase of network diameter after hub removal, for cancer < normal tissue) [22]. They concluded that cancer (PDAC) networks demonstrated signaling maintenance and increased error tolerance to punctual attacks even at hubs, making the design of highly specific drugs (targeted therapies) extremely challenging. These challenges have forced researchers to define and identify opportunities in the broader network topology as presented below.

Broader Network Topology: Modules, Bridges, Bottlenecks, and Choke Points

The broader network topology definitions became necessary once it was realized that the impact of targeting hubs alone may not lead to desirable therapeutic outcome. Modules represent the networking nodes that are linked to a particular group and classified for a single function (readers are referred to our comprehensive review on network pharmacology for details on network topology and illustrations that can be found at Azmi et al., [12]). Modules in the networks are responsible for giving a cellular/molecular function. Modules arise when nodes are more densely connected with one another as compared to their neighborhood. In cancer the modules of disease-related genes in PPI networks have been suggested as attractive network drug targets. On the other hand, bridges connect two neighboring modules and they are independently regulated from the nodes belonging to both modules, which they interconnect. Such module interconnecting properties makes them attractive as drug targets. An agent against a bridge can impact numerous modules at the same time, resulting in synergistic effects. By definition, a bottleneck is a phenomenon where the performance or capacity of an entire system is limited by a single component. Bottlenecks are in fact key connector proteins with key functional and dynamic properties. In the past a number of computational strategies have been applied to identify bottleneck proteins in cancer. In particular, they are more likely to be essential proteins such as transcription factors. Choke defines a point of attack that requires a lesser degree of effort to achieve the desired outcome on the entire network. Therefore, choke points in a network serve as excellent points for drug intervention. Ideally a choke point would allow an inferior drug or its combination to successfully prevent the entire network of major protein functions even though the latter may be comprised of highly resistant components. For example, the nuclear export protein Exportin1/ Xpo1/CRM1 is a recognized exporter of most of the tumor suppressor proteins (TSPs) and fits the bill of a choke point (Figure 18.1). High expression of CRM1, as observed in most cancers including PDAC, results

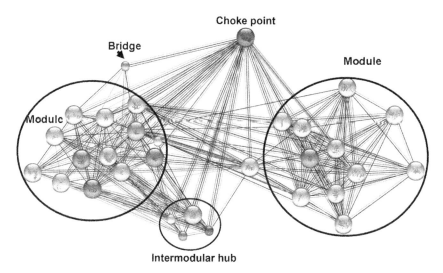

Figure 18.1 *Network Topology. Modules, Bridges, Intermodular Hubs, and Bottle-necks.* Showing module in a protein network that represents the networking nodes related to a particular group and classified, for example, for a single function. Bridges connect two neighboring modules. Intermodular hubs are key connector proteins between two modules. Choke points are critical entities in the network attacking that require lesser degree of effort to achieve the optimal outcome on the entire network. (For color version of this figure, the reader is referred to the online version of this book.)

in constant nuclear expulsion (cytoplasmic retention/mislocalization) of major TSPs. Inhibition of CRM1 should result in blocking of the nuclear export of most of the target TSPs. As demonstrated by our group, the targeted inhibition of CRM1 results in nuclear retention of different TSPs in PDAC cell nuclei leading to inhibition of proliferation and suppression of tumor growth in subcutaneous and orthotopic mice tumor models [23]. Older examples of the importance of choke points came from pathogens such as bacteria for enzymes that either uniquely produce or consume a given metabolite leading to their survival. Once verified, inhibition of these enzymes was proven to result in either lethal inability to produce an essential metabolite or toxic accumulation of another metabolite.

Applications on Network Pharmacology

Network-based approaches are increasingly being applied in different areas of cancer research. A number of different network methodologies presented in the last decade have allowed superior understanding of cancer heterogeneity, biomarker identification, microRNA stratification, drug design, drug repurposing, and even clinical trial design. In the following section, we elaborate on some of the uses of network-based approaches in cancer, particularly PDAC.

Network-Based PDAC Biomarker Identification

The concept of utilizing networks in identifying PDAC-related biomarkers has been presented by many different groups [24]. The last several years have witnessed the emergence of several network-based methods that have been developed to help in the identification of specific genes and proteins related to a particular disease. Most of these methods couple protein microarrays with bioinformatics and computational analyses such as principal component analysis and hierarchical clustering [25,26]. Table 18.2 lists the network-based methods that are being used to identify novel disease-associated genes as biomarkers. These network-based methods show marked improvements over their predecessor that utilized sequence-based methods in the classification of novel, disease-associated genes. The methods, including nonlocal information of network topology, usually perform better than methods based on local network properties. As a general trend, the more information the method includes, the better prediction it may achieve. However, with the multiplication of datasets, biases may also be introduced, which will lead to an overestimation of the performance of the test system.

Table 18.2 Web Resources to Evaluate Disease, Drug, MicroRNA, and Environment Interactions

Types of Network Investigated	Alternative Names and Website
Disease and disease-related genes	Human disease network (Cytoscape plug-in DisGeNET: http://ibi.imim.es/DisGeNET/DisGeNETweb.html)
Disease, drug associations, tissue, interactome	iCTNet: a Cytoscape plug-in to construct an integrative network of diseases, associated genes, drugs, and tissues (http://www.cs.queensu.ca/ictnet)
Disease, gene ontology	Biomine: an integrated bio-entity network with more than a million entities and 8 million edges (http://biomine.cs.helsinki.fi)
Expression patterns, microRNAs	PAGED: an integrated bio-entity network with more than a million entities from 20 organisms (http://bio.informatics.iupui.edu/PAGED)
Disease and environment-related factors, patients' response	Etiome: a database + clustering analysis of environmental + genetic (=etiological) factors of human diseases

Moreover, it is difficult to dissect the performance contribution of the datasets and the prediction method itself. Additionally, each type of dataset may require a different method for optimal analysis. Therefore, the separate analysis of each data source has been suggested with a subsequent combination of the ranking lists using rank aggregation algorithms. This procedure also facilitates backtracking the origin of the most relevant information. The functional gene ontology term annotations usually bring crucially important information to the analyses. The inclusion of interactome edge-based disease perturbations may improve the performance of these methods even further in the future. Aside from disease-associated genes, there has been a recent spurt in evaluating metabolic networks, microRNAs networks, drugs association networks, environment associated networks, and many more.

Optimal Intervention Strategies in PDAC Networks Using Network Pharmacology

A number of research groups have presented PDAC network–targeted strategies using network pharmacology and other systems methodologies. Recently, Jing Tang and colleagues used maximization and minimization averaging (TIMMA) approaches to selectively target PDAC survival pathways [27]. Their focus was to evaluate combinatorial effects of kinase inhibition by utilizing the results from a kinome-wide drug sensitization screen, in which the kinase siRNA silencing was combined with the treatment of Aurora kinase inhibitors in BxPC-3 PDAC cell line. As the Aurora kinases (A–C) are frequently overexpressed in many tumors (such as PDAC), they have been proposed to be potential cancer therapeutics that can interfere with cancer cell division. The purpose of their TIMMA study was to identify a specific set of kinases that when silenced would sensitize PDAC cells to the Aurora kinase inhibitors. The RNAi screen was done using the Human Validated Kinase Set (HVKS) siRNA library. Their study identified a total of 17 kinases and confirmed in a validation screen to have at least two out of four siRNA sequences showing greater than 1.5-fold decreases in EC50 or EC30 values of the Aurora kinase inhibitor AKI-1. Their group further evaluated whether the TIMMA model could help in predicting the kinases that would sensitize the pancreatic cancer cells to the AKI-1. Their TIMMA analysis identified 19 kinases that showed stronger synthetic lethality interactions with Aurora B than with itself. Two (MET, PDGFRA) out of the three targets (MET, PDGFRA, and PYK2) were experimentally validated as sensitizing targets of AKI-1 in the pancreatic cancer, representing a highly significant enrichment (that was hypergeometric).

Table 18.3 Drug Interactions, Target Visualization, and Prioritization Tools
Drug Target Prioritization,

Validation	Website
Pubchem	http://pubchem.ncbi.nlm.nih.gov
chEMBLdb	https://www.ebi.ac.uk/chembldb
DailyMed	http://dailymed.nim.nih.gov
DrugBank	http://drugbank.ca
MATADOR	http://matador.embl.de
Supertarget	http://insilico.charite.de/supertarget
KEGG drug	http://genome.jp/kegg/drug
TDR	http://tdrtargets.org
PROMISCUOUS	http://bioinformatics.charite.de/promiscuous
MANTRA	http://mantra.tigem.it
CDA	http://cda.i-pharm.org

Working in this direction, our group had earlier presented p53 reactivation optimizing strategies using network identified combinations of MDM2 inhibitors in PDAC [28]. Considering p53 as a network object, its direct and indirect activators were analyzed using network-based predictions leading to the identification of MDM2 inhibitor–oxaliplatin combination [29]. Through these approaches synergy unique genes were mapped and modeled using pathway analyses that demonstrated the role of important hubs such as CDH1, CARF, EGR, RelA, and CREBP in promoting optimal p53 reactivation [30]. When investigated in resistant PDAC animal tumor models, the combination resulted in synergistically enhanced tumor growth inhibition and 50% cure [31]. These are examples where systems and network pharmacology can be applied in the design of optimal intervention strategies to desirable therapeutic outcome in PDAC.

A number of resources are available for the identification of network targeted drugs (Table 18.3). However, at present, there are not many groups working on utilizing these resources for PDAC. We anticipate that in the coming years, researchers will put more emphasis on network-based drug strategies that could positively impact modern PDAC therapy.

NETWORK PHARMACOLOGY TO UNWIND PDAC microRNA COMPLEXITY

MicroRNAs are key players in the gene regulatory networks that can influence the expression of numerous genes by binding to complementary sequences on target mRNAs leading to the repression of their translation

[32]. This inherent multigene modulating property indicates that microRNAs should have a major regulatory role on gene networks. This is especially important when earlier studies have demonstrated that the hubs, bottlenecks, and their targets such as TFs are more frequently regulated by microRNAs than other nodes in the biological networks [33]. These findings indicate that microRNAs have a systems function and, therefore, their targeting should also be approached using systems and network sciences. The complexity of microRNAs can be appreciated from the fact that although occupying <15% of the genome, they can influence more than 30% of the genes in the entire genome [34]. The weak and promiscuous nature of the interactions of microRNAs with the 3′ UTRs of their many target genes can result in an exponential number of interaction possibilities. As the microRNA targets include a diverse set of signaling proteins, enzymes, and TFs [35], their targets appear to form complex regulatory networks that are intertwined with other cellular networks. It is still not clear how microRNAs might orchestrate the regulation of different cellular signaling networks and how this may contribute to the myriad biological functions of microRNAs. As with other cancers, there is published evidence that in PDAC, the microRNAs either regulate or are themselves under epigenetic control [36]. In recent years tumor suppressor miRNA mimics and oligonucleotide inhibitors complementary to oncogenic miRNA have been shown to restore normal cell programming [37]. The most important question is whether in cancer a set of microRNA target genes regulated by an individual miRNA generally constitute a functionally associated network or simply reflect a random set of unrelated entities. Key questions remain such as what kind of biological networks does the human microRNAome most actively regulate? Answering such questions may allow clinical progress in the direction of incorporating microRNA into mainstream PDAC medicine.

Network biology has shown that the microRNA network is arranged in hierarchical layers that harbor hundreds of "target hubs" and each is potentially subject to massive regulation by scores of additional secondary microRNAs [38]. Most importantly, striking differences between cancer cells (including PDAC) and normal cell microRNA networks have been noted with microRNA-regulated drug targets closely interacting with each other and tending to form hub bottlenecks in the human interactome [39]. However, the history of microRNA-based drug development strategies has shown that there are many important challenges in this area [40]. As one microRNA can regulate many genes, it is still not clear whether targeting a single microRNA would result in a restricted set of gene modulations with minimal desired effect or whether it may cause multigene changes leading to undesirable or toxic side effects. Therefore, true understanding of microRNA regulatory network is integral to the successful design of microRNA-based targeted therapy. Despite several technical advances, there are still many challenges, such as determining the ideal design of antimicroRNA sequence, bypassing the activation of the immune system, off-target effects, and competition with endogenous microRNAs for cellular miRNA-processing machinery. Additionally, one must first identify the correct and relevant target microRNA that is critical in the disease of choice prior to designing anti- or premicroRNA therapy. Therefore, the translation of microRNA-targeted technology into the clinic depends on resolving these important systems level challenges.

Expression profiles of microRNAs could be highly informative in discriminating malignant from the normal pancreas in view of the different patterns of expression of microRNAs in PDAC tumors. In tumors from K-ras–driven transgenic pancreas mice model (KCI), we observed overexpression of *miR-21*, *miR-221*, *miR-27a*, *miR-27b*, and *miR-155*, and downregulation of *miR-216a*, *miR-216b*, *miR-217*, and *miR-146a*. These findings were replicated in KCI-derived RInk-1 cells. Most interestingly, biological validation experiments revealed a significant induction of aberrant micro RNA-driven overexpression of EGFR, K-Ras, and MT1-MMP protein expression in tissues from tumorigenic mice models. Again, tumor tissue analysis was comparable to RInk-1 cells and MIAPaCa-2 cells indicating the involvement of common networks [41,42]. Ingenuity modeling extracted key microRNAs that were targeted using different strategies (RNAi and chemical) to induce cell killing in these transgenic mice–derived Rink-1 cells. As a proof of concept, instead of targeting all deregulated miRNAs, we focused on key microRNAs (miR-21, miR-155, miR-220, miR-143, and miR-217) in the entire network. Knocking down miR-155 in RInk-1 cells inhibited PDAC growth, colony formation, and was consistent with suppression of K-ras signaling expression. On the contrary, forced expression of Ras targeting *miR-216b* inhibited PDAC cell proliferation and colony formation with consequent reduction of Ras and related signaling. These findings clearly suggest that network-based approaches would be useful for preclinical evaluation of novel microRNA-targeted agents for designing personalized therapy for PDAC.

NETWORK PHARMACOLOGY IN DRUG REPOSITIONING FOR PDAC

The cost of bringing one drug from the researcher's lab bench to the patient's bedside ranges from 3 to 5 billion dollars. Even if a drug passes through all the stringent preclinical screening procedures, there is no guarantee that the agent may prove efficacious in patients. While the cost of developing new drugs has witnessed a continuous upward trend, drug attrition has risen considerably as well. Therefore, strategies that can cut the cost of drug development are being aggressively pursued by the pharmaceutical industry worldwide. Drug repositioning or drug repurposing aims to find a new therapeutic modality for an existing or established drug, and thus provides a cost-efficient way to enhance the repertoire of available drugs and also the druggable space. Drug repurposing uses a compound having a well-established safety profile, such as the IND-approved drugs from the FDA that have passed the strict criteria of having proven good lab practice (GLP) formulation procedures and clinically acceptable pharmacokinetic parameters. It is through these efforts that the utility of multikinase HIV treatment drugs [43] and the diabetes drug metformin [44] have been realized in cancer. Drug target networks are highly useful in drug repositioning. It has been proposed that modularization/edge prediction of drug target networks may reveal novel applications of existing drugs [45]. Novel drug indications can be revealed from central drugs of drug therapy networks in which two drugs are connected, if they share a common therapeutic application. For example, intermodular drugs that connect two distant therapies oftentimes reveal novel drug indications. Tightly interacting modules of drug–drug interaction networks have been shown to also reveal unexpected therapeutic applications [46]. Perhaps the biggest advantage of utilizing network approaches to drug discovery is that the technology allows us to make sense of side effects of drugs. Such analysis, in many instances, reveals novel therapeutic areas and offers a number of options for network-based drug repositioning [47]. Our group has earlier shown that the diabetes drug metformin can induce PDAC cell growth inhibition and apoptosis in multiple cellular models including highly resistant pancreatic cancer stem cells (CSC) and their corresponding xenograft tumor models [48]. Mechanistically, it is still not clear how this agent can eliminate PDAC cells as our preliminary studies demonstrated a highly promiscuous behavior involving metformin-induced suppression of CSC, microRNAs, and notch signaling. Nevertheless, based on the work done from our laboratory and those of others (in different tumor models), metformin is in 23 different clinical trials (clinicaltrial.gov). These studies not only support the network theory in drug action but also lend support to drug reposition principles in PDAC. Although this is one successful example, drug repositioning nevertheless has more challenges than one would expect, such as validation of the drug candidate from incomplete and outdated data (oftentimes discontinued drugs). However, most network-based methods helping drug repositioning may also be used to predict multitarget drugs.

Most of the drug repositioning efforts utilize large-scale screens of FDA-approved drugs against a multitude of novel targets [49]. From literature data mining–driven network-based method modularization, edge prediction, or machine learning methods, researchers have unexpectedly found links between remote drug targets highlighting possible cross-reactivity of known drugs with novel targets [50,51]. Network-based comparison of drug-induced changes in gene expression profiles that is combined with disease-induced gene expression changes, disease drug associations, interactomes, or signaling networks have been used to identify unexpected or previously understudied uses of existing drugs [52]. Further, genome-wide association studies (GWAS) have been used to construct drug-related networks, helping drug repositioning even in a personalized manner [53]. Ongoing studies include the comparison of phosphoproteome and metabolome datasets to reveal additional drug repositioning options. These approaches are expected to aid the design of personalized drug application protocols.

NETWORKS IN POLYPHARMACOLOGY STRATEGIES AGAINST PDAC

Rewiring of cancer related signaling networks to that of healthy cells is the primary aim of drugs that work on signal transduction pathways [54]. As most cellular proteins belong to multiple network modules in the human interactome, efficient targeting of a single protein may influence multiple cellular functions at the same time. In contrast, efficient restoration of a particular cellular function to that of the healthy state can often be accomplished only by a simultaneous attack on multiple proteins. The targeting efficiency on each protein may only be partial since these target sets preferentially contain proteins with an intermediate number of neighbors having an intermediate level of influence of their own. The above systems-level considerations explain the success of polypharmacology, i.e., the development and use of multitarget drugs. The goal of polypharmacology is to identify a multitargeted compound with a desired biological profile across multiple targets whose combined modulation reverses disease state to normal. Multiple targeting is a well-established strategy as more than 20% of approved agents are multitarget drugs [55]. Most treatments against deadly diseases such as AIDS and cancer have a multicomponent attached to it.

Multitarget drugs possess a number of beneficial network-related properties: (1) they can be designed to act on a carefully selected set of primary targets influencing a set of key, therapeutically relevant secondary targets; (2) they may need a compromise in binding affinity, however, even low-affinity binding multitarget drugs are efficient; (3) indirect targeting via their low-affinity binding multitarget drugs has been shown to overcome the dual trap of drug resistance and toxicity; and (4) low-affinity binding multitarget drugs may often stabilize diseased cells, which may be sometimes at least be as beneficial as their primary therapeutic effect [56].

A number of natural compounds from dietary sources, especially from fruits and vegetables, have been investigated for their cancer preventive benefits [57,58]. Researchers have tried to identify the exact mechanism behind their cancer preventive activities and also their cancer cell selectivity. Such work has led to the identification of multitargeted and promiscuous mechanism of action of agents such as grape polyphenol resveratrol (Stilbene), curcumin, Catechins, and compounds such as Delphinidin and Anthocynadins that are found in pomegranate [59]. However, the promiscuous behavior of most of these natural agents is a heatedly debated topic [60]. As identified by network pharmacological analysis, the vast majority (>80%) of the cellular protein, signaling, and transcriptional networks are in a low-affinity, or transient, "weak linkage" with each other, i.e., forming a complex network. Therefore, natural compounds are a perfect fit where network pharmacology can be applied to predict their scope of action against cancer.

Difluorinated-Curcumin (CDF) is a difluoro synthetic analog chemopreventive agent curcumin (difluoro curcumin) [61,62]. It has pleiotropic activity with proven anticancer effects in vitro and in vivo [63,64]. Like other natural agents, CDF has lower target binding affinity to different proteins than a targeted SMI. Using pathway network modeling, we previously showed that CDF can modulate a unique set of microRNAs resulting in the activation of a c-Myc hub, and these perturbations orchestrated a unique set of events that eventually led to the induction of apoptosis [65]. Fitting into the model of a multitargeted agent, CDF has also been reported to influence epithelial-to-mesenchymal transition (EMT), inhibit bottleneck transcription factors such as NF-kB, and also inhibit different cancer-promoting microRNAs in PDAC. It is highly possible that there may be other potential targets of CDF that are context driven and tumor dependent and yet to be discovered.

Two other agents, Diindolylmethane (DIM) and its more bioavailable form BR-DIM, have been extensively investigated for their anticancer effects. They primarily work through downregulation of the TF NF-kB. Nevertheless, numerous other mechanisms have also been proposed such as through activation of pro-death protein prostate apoptosis response 4 (Par-4) [66], suppression of androgen receptor (AR) [67], MMP9 [68], uPA [69,70], FOXO3 [71], and mTOR pathway [72]. They act as potent chemosensitizers and are now under clinical investigation for treating patients with prostate cancer undergoing radical prostatectomy. We proposed that such multitargeted effects of DIM/BR-DIM may be through rewiring of cancer cell networks that lead to resensitization to chemotherapeutic agents. In order to explore this hypothesis, our group recently utilized network analysis to identify the set of target genes of BR-DIM. Ingenuity analysis showed both isoflavone- and BR-DIM–induced changes in multiple signaling pathways such as AR/PSA, NKX3-1/Akt/p27, MITF, etc. [42,73]. These studies proved that BR-DIM with their multitargeted effects could be useful for the prevention of progression, especially by attenuating bone metastasis in a prostate model. Other promising anticancer activities of BR-DIM include the modulation of noncoding RNAs. These proof-of-concept investigations showed that network-based studies could be useful in designing promiscuous strategies incorporating such multitargeted therapeutic agents, which would likely aid in designing optimized therapy for cancer in future.

CONCLUSIONS AND FUTURE PERSPECTIVES

PDAC remains a deadly and by far incurable disease. The last 40 years have not seen any major advancement in the area of PDAC diagnostics and therapeutics. Targeted therapies have largely failed to deliver expected promise. On the other hand, promiscuous chemotherapeutics and their combinations show some efficacy, but these too do not prolong the life of patients beyond a few additional weeks. The incidence and death rates closely mirror each other, and such poor overall statistics indicate that the field of PDAC research needs a major revamp in its approach in order to impact the disease. Systems and network biology have allowed researchers to dwell much deeper into the complexity of PDAC and sieve through the heterogeneity in more meaningful ways. Such approaches have emerged to identify key points in the highly robust and resistant PDAC network attacking that can lead to superior outcomes in patients. However, selection of key network positions in PDAC as drug target options has a major dilemma. On the one hand, the network position has to be important enough to influence the PDAC tumor; conversely, the selected network position must not be so important that its attack would lead to toxicity to normal tissue. The successful solution of this dilemma requires a detailed knowledge on the structure and dynamics of the complex PDAC sustaining networks. Incorporation of personalized information, such as mutations, singalome or metabolome profiles to the molecular networks is expected to enhance patient and disease stage–specific drug targeting in the future. The current boom in network methods (listed in the three tables in this chapter) can help in discovering the truly surprising, novel actors of the cellular community, which are the hidden masterminds responsible for initiation, sustenance, and resistance of PDAC. Nevertheless, proponents of this technology must be proactive in presenting convincing evidence that promotes these emerging tools and rapidly merge them into mainstream PDAC biomarker identification and cancer drug discovery. These strategies may help revive some shelved drugs and could also reduce the cost of new drugs entering the PDAC treatment pipeline. It is predicted that within the next 10 years, newer technological advances plus methodologies better developed to make analysis software economical, easy to use, and more acceptable to molecular biologists and pharma researchers will, no doubt, result in the use of network analyses as a priority tool in PDAC-related research. In conclusion, systems biology in general and network pharmacology in particular certainly have the potential to change our view of PDAC complexity as well as aid in the successful design of drugs for better treatment outcome of therapies against this important disease. If used correctly, network pharmacology is predicted to significantly de-risk PDAC drug discovery.

REFERENCES

[1] Siegel R, Naishadham D, Jemal A. Cancer statistics, 2013. CA Cancer J Clin 2013;63: 11–30.
[2] Wolfgang CL, Herman JM, Laheru DA, Klein AP, Erdek MA, Fishman EK, et al. Recent progress in pancreatic cancer. CA Cancer J Clin 2013;63(5):318–48.
[3] Iacobuzio-Donahue CA, Velculescu VE, Wolfgang CL, Hruban RH. Genetic basis of pancreas cancer development and progression: insights from whole-exome and whole-genome sequencing. Clin Cancer Res 2012;18:4257–65.
[4] Hruban RH, Goggins M, Parsons J, Kern SE. Progression model for pancreatic cancer. Clin Cancer Res 2000;6:2969–72.
[5] Srihari S, Ragan MA. Systematic tracking of dysregulated modules identifies novel genes in cancer. Bioinformatics 2013;29:1553–61.
[6] Kostova I. Platinum complexes as anticancer agents. Recent Pat Anticancer Drug Discov 2006;1:1–22.
[7] Mecucci C, La SR, Negrini M, Sabbioni S, Crescenzi B, Leoni P, et al. t(4;11)(q21;p15) translocation involving NUP98 and RAP1GDS1 genes: characterization of a new subset of T acute lymphoblastic leukaemia. Br J Haematol 2000;109:788–93.

[8] Lee KH,Yim EK, Kim CJ, Namkoong SE, Um SJ, Park JS. Proteomic analysis of anti-cancer effects by paclitaxel treatment in cervical cancer cells. Gynecol Oncol 2005;98:45–53.

[9] Giroux V, Malicet C, Barthet M, Gironella M, Archange C, Dagorn JC, et al. p8 is a new target of gemcitabine in pancreatic cancer cells. Clin Cancer Res 2006;12:235–41.

[10] Alian OM, Azmi AS, Mohammad RM. Network insights on oxaliplatin anti-cancer mechanisms. Clin Transl Med 2012;1:26.

[11] Alian OM, Philip PA, Sarkar FH, Azmi AS. Systems biology approaches to pancreatic cancer detection, prevention, and treatment. Curr Pharm Des 2013.

[12] Azmi AS. Adopting network pharmacology for cancer drug discovery. Curr Drug Discov Technol 2013;10:95–105.

[13] Csermely P, Korcsmaros T, Kiss HJ, London G, Nussinov R. Structure and dynamics of molecular networks: a novel paradigm of drug discovery: a comprehensive review. Pharmacol Ther 2013;138:333–408.

[14] Jonsson PF, Bates PA. Global topological features of cancer proteins in the human interactome. Bioinformatics 2006;22:2291–7.

[15] Jonsson PF, Cavanna T, Zicha D, Bates PA. Cluster analysis of networks generated through homology: automatic identification of important protein communities involved in cancer metastasis. BMC Bioinformatics 2006;7:2.

[16] Pandini A, Fornili A, Fraternali F, Kleinjung J. Detection of allosteric signal transmission by information-theoretic analysis of protein dynamics. FASEB J 2012;26:868–81.

[17] Pandini A, Fornili A, Fraternali F, Kleinjung J. GSATools: analysis of allosteric communication and functional local motions using a structural alphabet. Bioinformatics 2013;29:2053–5.

[18] Prassas I, Karagiannis GS, Batruch I, Dimitromanolakis A, Datti A, Diamandis EP. Digitoxin-induced cytotoxicity in cancer cells is mediated through distinct kinase and interferon signaling networks. Mol Cancer Ther 2011;10:2083–93.

[19] Kashtan N, Itzkovitz S, Milo R, Alon U. Topological generalizations of network motifs. Phys Rev E Stat Nonlin Soft Matter Phys 2004;70:031909.

[20] Przulj N, Wigle DA, Jurisica I. Functional topology in a network of protein interactions. Bioinformatics 2004;20:340–8.

[21] Przulj N. Biological network comparison using graphlet degree distribution. Bioinformatics 2007;23:e177–83.

[22] Schramm G, Kannabiran N, Konig R. Regulation patterns in signaling networks of cancer. BMC Syst Biol 2010;4:162.

[23] Azmi AS, Aboukameel A, Bao B, Sarkar FH, Philip PA, Kauffman M, et al. Selective inhibitors of nuclear export block pancreatic cancer cell proliferation and reduce tumor growth in mice. Gastroenterology 2013;144:447–56.

[24] Krauthammer M, Kaufmann CA, Gilliam TC, Rzhetsky A. Molecular triangulation: bridging linkage and molecular-network information for identifying candidate genes in Alzheimer's disease. Proc Natl Acad Sci USA 2004;101:15148–53.

[25] Zhao J, Patwa TH, Lubman DM, Simeone DM. Protein biomarkers in cancer: natural glycoprotein microarray approaches. Curr Opin Mol Ther 2008;10:602–10.

[26] Zhao J, Patwa TH, Qiu W, Shedden K, Hinderer R, Misek DE, et al. Glycoprotein microarrays with multi-lectin detection: unique lectin binding patterns as a tool for classifying normal, chronic pancreatitis and pancreatic cancer sera. J Proteome Res 2007;6:1864–74.

[27] Tang J, Karhinen L, Xu T, Szwajda A, Yadav B, Wennerberg K, et al. Target inhibition networks: predicting selective combinations of druggable targets to block cancer survival pathways. PLoS Comput Biol 2013;9:e1003226.

[28] Azmi AS, Beck FW, Sarkar FH, Mohammad RM. Network perspectives on HDM2 inhibitor chemotherapy combinations. Curr Pharm Des 2011;17:640–52.

[29] Azmi AS, Wang Z, Philip PA, Mohammad RM, Sarkar FH. Proof of concept: network and systems biology approaches aid in the discovery of potent anticancer drug combinations. Mol Cancer Ther 2010;9:3137–44.

[30] Azmi AS, Banerjee S, Ali S, Wang Z, Bao B, Beck FW, et al. Network modeling of MDM2 inhibitor-oxaliplatin combination reveals biological synergy in wt-p53 solid tumors. Oncotarget 2011;2:378–92.

[31] Azmi AS, Aboukameel A, Banerjee S, Wang Z, Mohammad M, Wu J, et al. MDM2 inhibitor MI-319 in combination with cisplatin is an effective treatment for pancreatic cancer independent of p53 function. Eur J Cancer 2010;46:1122–31.

[32] Doench JG, Sharp PA. Specificity of microRNA target selection in translational repression. Genes Dev 2004;18:504–11.

[33] Hsu CW, Juan HF, Huang HC. Characterization of microRNA-regulated protein-protein interaction network. Proteomics 2008;8:1975–9.

[34] Axtell MJ. Evolution of microRNAs and their targets: are all microRNAs biologically relevant? Biochim Biophys Acta 2008;1779:725–34.

[35] Hieronymus H, Silver PA. A systems view of mRNP biology. Genes Dev 2004;18: 2845–60.

[36] Azmi AS, Beck FW, Bao B, Mohammad RM, Sarkar FH. Aberrant epigenetic grooming of miRNAs in pancreatic cancer: a systems biology perspective. Epigenomics 2011;3:747–59.

[37] Medina PP, Slack FJ. Inhibiting microRNA function in vivo. Nat Methods 2009; 6:37–8.

[38] Shalgi R, Lieber D, Oren M, Pilpel Y. Global and local architecture of the mammalian microRNA-transcription factor regulatory network. PLoS Comput Biol 2007;3:e131.

[39] Wang J, Haubrock M, Cao KM, Hua X, Zhang CY, Wingender E, et al. Regulatory coordination of clustered microRNAs based on microRNA-transcription factor regulatory network. BMC Syst Biol 2011;5:199.

[40] Rupaimoole R, Han HD, Lopez-Berestein G, Sood AK. MicroRNA therapeutics: principles, expectations, and challenges. Chin J Cancer 2011;30:368–70.

[41] Ali S, Ahmad A, Aboukameel A, Bao B, Padhye S, Philip PA, et al. Increased Ras GTPase activity is regulated by miRNAs that can be attenuated by CDF treatment in pancreatic cancer cells. Cancer Lett 2012;319(2):173–81.

[42] Li Y, Kong D, Ahmad A, Bao B, Sarkar FH. Targeting bone remodeling by isoflavone and 3,3′-diindolylmethane in the context of prostate cancer bone metastasis. PLoS One 2012;7:e33011.

[43] Xie L, Evangelidis T, Xie L, Bourne PE. Drug discovery using chemical systems biology: weak inhibition of multiple kinases may contribute to the anti-cancer effect of nelfinavir. PLoS Comput Biol 2011;7:e1002037.

[44] Bednar F, Simeone DM. Metformin and cancer stem cells: old drug, new targets. Cancer Prev Res (Phila) 2012;5:351–4.

[45] Nacher JC, Schwartz JM. Modularity in protein complex and drug interactions reveals new polypharmacological properties. PLoS One 2012;7:e30028.

[46] Lehar J, Zimmermann GR, Krueger AS, Molnar RA, Ledell JT, Heilbut AM, et al. Chemical combination effects predict connectivity in biological systems. Mol Syst Biol 2007;3:80.

[47] Campillos M, Kuhn M, Gavin AC, Jensen LJ, Bork P. Drug target identification using side-effect similarity. Science 2008;321:263–6.

[48] Bao B, Wang Z, Ali S, Ahmad A, Azmi AS, Sarkar SH, et al. Metformin inhibits cell proliferation, migration and invasion by attenuating CSC function mediated by deregulating miRNAs in pancreatic cancer cells. Cancer Prev Res (Phila) 2012;5: 355–64.

[49] Chong CR, Sullivan Jr DJ. New uses for old drugs. Nature 2007;448:645–6.

[50] Achenbach J, Tiikkainen P, Franke L, Proschak E. Computational tools for polypharmacology and repurposing. Future Med Chem 2011;3:961–8.

[51] Deftereos SN, Andronis C, Friedla EJ, Persidis A, Persidis A. Drug repurposing and adverse event prediction using high-throughput literature analysis. Wiley Interdiscip Rev Syst Biol Med 2011;3:323–34.

[52] Hu G, Agarwal P. Human disease-drug network based on genomic expression profiles. PLoS One 2009;4:e6536.

[53] Sanseau P, Agarwal P, Barnes MR, Pastinen T, Richards JB, Cardon LR, et al. Use of genome-wide association studies for drug repositioning. Nat Biotechnol 2012;30:317–20.

[54] Papatsoris AG, Karamouzis MV, Papavassiliou AG. The power and promise of "rewiring" the mitogen-activated protein kinase network in prostate cancer therapeutics. Mol Cancer Ther 2007;6:811–9.

[55] Ma'ayan A, Jenkins SL, Goldfarb J, Iyengar R. Network analysis of FDA approved drugs and their targets. Mt Sinai J Med 2007;74:27–32.

[56] Farkas IJ, Korcsmaros T, Kovacs IA, Mihalik A, Palotai R, Simko GI, et al. Network-based tools for the identification of novel drug targets. Sci Signal 2011;4:t3.

[57] Sarkar FH. Current trends in the chemoprevention of cancer. Pharm Res 2010;27:945–9.

[58] Sarkar FH, Li Y, Wang Z, Padhye S. Lesson learned from nature for the development of novel anti-cancer agents: implication of isoflavone, curcumin, and their synthetic analogs. Curr Pharm Des 2010;16:1801–12.

[59] Lewandowski C, Pezzuto JM. Pharmaceutical biology: a retrospective. Pharm Biol 2012;50:1–5.

[60] Azmi AS, Mohammad RM, Sarkar FH. Can network pharmacology rescue neutraceutical cancer research? Drug Discov Today 2012;17:807–9.

[61] Padhye S, Banerjee S, Chavan D, Pandye S, Swamy KV, Ali S, et al. Fluorocurcumins as cyclooxygenase-2 inhibitor: molecular docking, pharmacokinetics and tissue distribution in mice. Pharm Res 2009;26:2438–45.

[62] Padhye S, Yang H, Jamadar A, Cui QC, Chavan D, Dominiak K, et al. New difluoro Knoevenagel condensates of curcumin, their Schiff bases and copper complexes as proteasome inhibitors and apoptosis inducers in cancer cells. Pharm Res 2009;26:1874–80.

[63] Dandawate PR, Vyas A, Ahmad A, Banerjee S, Deshpande J, Swamy KV, et al. Inclusion complex of novel curcumin analogue CDF and beta-cyclodextrin (1:2) and its enhanced in vivo anticancer activity against pancreatic cancer. Pharm Res 2012;29(7):1775–86.

[64] Bao B, Ali S, Banerjee S, Wang Z, Logna F, Azmi AS, et al. Curcumin analogue CDF inhibits pancreatic tumor growth by switching on suppressor microRNAs and attenuating EZH2 expression. Cancer Res 2012;72:335–45.

[65] Azmi AS, Ali S, Banerjee S, Bao B, Maitah MN, Padhye S, et al. Network modeling of CDF treated pancreatic cancer cells reveals a novel c-myc-p73 dependent apoptotic mechanism. Am J Transl Res 2011;3:374–82.

[66] Azmi AS, Ahmad A, Banerjee S, Rangnekar VM, Mohammad RM, Sarkar FH. Chemoprevention of pancreatic cancer: characterization of Par-4 and its modulation by 3,3′ diindolylmethane (DIM). Pharm Res 2008;25:2117–24.

[67] Singh-Gupta V, Banerjee S, Yunker CK, Rakowski JT, Joiner MC, Konski AA, et al. B-DIM impairs radiation-induced survival pathways independently of androgen receptor expression and augments radiation efficacy in prostate cancer. Cancer Lett 2012;318:86–92.

[68] Kong D, Li Y, Wang Z, Banerjee S, Sarkar FH. Inhibition of angiogenesis and invasion by 3,3′-diindolylmethane is mediated by the nuclear factor-kappaB downstream target genes MMP-9 and uPA that regulated bioavailability of vascular endothelial growth factor in prostate cancer. Cancer Res 2007;67:3310–9.

[69] Ahmad A, Kong D, Sarkar SH, Wang Z, Banerjee S, Sarkar FH. Inactivation of uPA and its receptor uPAR by 3,3′-diindolylmethane (DIM) leads to the inhibition of prostate cancer cell growth and migration. J Cell Biochem 2009;107:516–27.

[70] Ahmad A, Kong D, Wang Z, Sarkar SH, Banerjee S, Sarkar FH. Down-regulation of uPA and uPAR by 3,3′-diindolylmethane contributes to the inhibition of cell growth and migration of breast cancer cells. J Cell Biochem 2009;108:916–25.

[71] Li Y, Wang Z, Kong D, Murthy S, Dou QP, Sheng S, et al. Regulation of FOXO3a/ beta-catenin/GSK-3beta signaling by 3,3′-diindolylmethane contributes to inhibition of cell proliferation and induction of apoptosis in prostate cancer cells. J Biol Chem 2007;282:21542–50.

[72] Kong D, Banerjee S, Huang W, Li Y, Wang Z, Kim HR, et al. Mammalian target of rapamycin repression by 3,3′-diindolylmethane inhibits invasion and angiogenesis in platelet-derived growth factor-D-overexpressing PC3 cells. Cancer Res 2008;68: 1927–34.

[73] Li Y, Wang Z, Kong D, Li R, Sarkar SH, Sarkar FH. Regulation of Akt/FOXO3a/ GSK-3beta/AR signaling network by isoflavone in prostate cancer cells. J Biol Chem 2008;283:27707–16.

INDEX

Note: Page numbers with "*f*" denote figures; "*t*" tables.

A

A1BG. *See* Alpha-1B-glycoprotein
ABC. *See* Antibody binding capacity
Aberrant Notch pathway activation, 78
ABO gene, 176–177
Abraxane. *See* Gemcitabine-nab-paclitaxel
Acetonitrile (ACN), 223–224
ACOSOG. *See* American College of
    Surgeons Oncology Group
Actinin-4 (ACTN4), 203
Activity-based proteomics approach, 210
Adaptive rank truncated product (ARTP),
    183
Adenocarcinoma, 3–4
Adenomatous polyposis coli (APC), 15
Affymetrix platform, 156–157
Ago-2 enzyme. *See* Argonaute-2 enzyme
AGR2. *See* Anterior gradient-2
AIO. *See* Arbeitsgemeinschaft Internistische
    Onkologie
Akt kinase, 286–287
Aldehyde dehydrogenase (ALDH), 81–82
ALDH. *See* Aldehyde dehydrogenase
Alkaline phosphatase (ALP), 386
    $^{125}IQ_{2-P}$ and $^{125}IQ_{2-S}$ mediated hydrolysis,
        395f
Alpha-1B-glycoprotein (A1BG), 207–208
α-smooth muscle actin (SMA), 80–81
American College of Surgeons Oncology
    Group (ACOSOG), 44–45
American Society of Clinical Oncology
    (ASCO), 60
Ankyrin (ANK), 76
Annexin II (ANXA2), 202–203
Anterior gradient-2 (AGR2), 207–208,
    225–230
Antibody binding capacity (ABC), 264
ANXA2. *See* Annexin II
APC. *See* Adenomatous polyposis coli
Arbeitsgemeinschaft Internistische
    Onkologie (AIO), 57

Area under the receiver operating curve
    (AUROC), 335
Area-under-curve (AUC), 206–207
Argonaute-2 enzyme (Ago-2 enzyme),
    266–267
Array-Express, 117
ARTP. *See* Adaptive rank truncated
    product
Arylsulfatase A (ARSA), 387
    docking positions of pNCS, IQ_{2-S}, and
        IQ_{2-P}, 391f
    enzyme, 389–391
    hydrolysis of $^{125}IQ_{2-P}$ and $^{125}IQ_{2-S}$, 395f
    IQ_{2-S}, and IQ_{2-P} hydrolysis, 393t
ASCO. *See* American Society of Clinical
    Oncology
Ataxia telangiectasia mutated (ATM), 114
AUC. *See* Area-under-curve
AUROC. *See* Area under the receiver
    operating curve

B

Bead arrays, 158
Bevacizumab, 58–59
BFAST. *See* BLAT-Like Fast Accurate
    Search Tool
Bioinformatic analysis
    in microarrays
        DGE, 97–98
        genotyping, 98
        GWAS, 98–99
        housekeeping genes, 97
        normalization, 96–97
        unit of analysis, 98
        unsupervised methods, 98
    in NGS
        alignment strategies, 103
        data visualization, 103
        dozens of peak callers, 103
        IgG antibodies, 103–104
        motif databases, 104–105

Bioinformatic analysis (*Continued*)
   peak detection algorithm, 104
   raw sequenced reads, 103
  in RNA-seq
   DGE, 109–110
   raw sequence, 108–109
   splice junctions, 109
   statistical distribution, 110
Biological networks, 408–409. *See also*
   Proteomic analysis
  analysis, 230, 230f
   comparative pathway maps, 233, 233f
   cytoskeleton_intermediate filaments
    network, 231–232
   drug-resistance and metastasis group,
    231
   functional ontologies, 232, 232f
   pathway analysis tools, 230–231
  broader network topology, 410–413
  local network topology, 409–410
  network-based methods, 412t
Biomarkers, 333–334
  CDx, 368
  metabolomic, 330–331
  network-based PDAC, 412–413
  Notch-3 and Hey-1 as, 80
  pancreatic juice as, 247–249
  proteomics for identification, 247
  RPPA and, 377–378
  vimentin, 241
BLAT-Like Fast Accurate Search Tool
   (BFAST), 103
Blood biomarker discovery
  global profiling, 205
   functional proteins, 205–206
   in plasma or serum, 205
  protein biomarker detection, proteomics
   for, 206–207
Body mass index (BMI), 174–175
BORA gene, 179
BRCA2 tumor suppressor gene, 15. *See also*
   Dpc4 tumor suppressor gene
Broader network topology, 410–411
  applications on network pharmacology,
   411–412
  PDAC biomarker identification,
   411–412
Burrows-Wheeler Aligner (BWA), 103

C

c-Myc protein, 326, 336–337
C14ORF1. *See* Chromosome 14 open-
   reading frame 1
Cabozantinib, 61
CAM-DR. *See* Cell adhesion mediated
   drug resistance
Cancer and Leukemia Group B (CALGB),
   49–50
Cancer Cell Line Encyclopedia (CCLE), 125
Cancer genome sequencing. *See also*
   Genome–exome sequencing studies
  alignment quality, 111
  bioinformatics, 113
  clonal evolution characterization, 113
  DNA fragmentation, 111
  genome discovery cohorts, 112
  GSEA method, 112–113
  IGV, 111
  kataegis, 113
  mutations and statistical accumulation, 112
  single-nucleotide variants, 112
  somatic mutational signatures, 111
  tumor and normal samples, 111–112
  variant calling algorithms, 111
Cancer stem cells (CSC), 61–62, 75–76,
   81–82, 307–308, 349, 416–418
  microRNA network, 314–316
   differentially expressed, 316t
   microarrays in, 315f
  pancreatic cancer
   isolation and biological
    characterization, 308–309, 309f
   molecular analysis, 310f
   therapy resistance and role, 307–308
   triple-positive PC CSC cells, 309–310
  systems and pathway analysis, 310–311,
   312f
   FoxQ1 expression, 311–314
   mRNA microarray assay use, 311–314
   top-ranked differentially expressed
    genes, 314
Cancer-associated cell invasiveness
   investigation, 210
Canonical pathway analysis
  cell adhesion and endothelial cell
   contacts, 236f
  chemoresistance of cancer cell, 235–236

cytoplasmic proteins, 236–237
cytoskeleton remodeling, 234f, 235
keratin family proteins, 236
mesenchymal-type movement, 237–238
using MetaCore™, 233, 238
TGF-β-dependent induction, 235f
vimentin overexpression, 237
Capecitabine-based clinical trials, 50
Carcinoembryonic antigen (CEA),
247–249, 334
Carcinoembryonic antigen-related cell
adhesion molecule (CEACAM),
208–209
Catalogue of Somatic Mutations in Cancer
(COSMIC), 122–123
cBioPortal for Cancer Genomics, 123–124
CCLE. *See* Cancer Cell Line Encyclopedia
CD298. *See* Na+/K+ ATPase Beta 3
Cdk4. *See* Cyclin-dependent kinase 4
cDNA microarrays, 157–158
CDx. *See* Companion diagnostic tests
CEA. *See* Carcinoembryonic antigen
CEACAM. *See* Carcinoembryonic antigen-
related cell adhesion molecule
Cell adhesion mediated drug resistance
(CAM-DR), 34
Cell culture
cell lines, 16
characterization, 26
origin tissue *vs.*, 27
of PDAC, 16
primary cell cultures, 17
3-D, 34
Cell lines, 16
Cell signaling, 368–369
Cell surface glycoproteins, 253
cellular viability, 254–255
isolation process, 254f
Cell surface proteins, 246
Cellular growth, 28–29
Censoring, 135–136
Cetuximab, 58
CF. *See* Cystic fibrosis
CFL1. *See* Cofilin
Chemical derivatization, 200–201
Chemoradiotherapy (CHRT), 50–51
Chemoresistance, 221–222
Chinese scan (ChinaPC), 180

ChIP-seq, 101. *See also* RNA sequencing
(RNA-seq)
applications, 105–110
encyclopedia of DNA elements, 102
of pancreatic cancer, 107
Chromosome 14 open-reading frame 1
(C14ORF1), 212–213
Chromothripsis, 113
Chronic pancreatitis
isolated cell analysis, 204–205
PDAC, 204
CHRT. *See* Chemoradiotherapy
CID. *See* Collision-induced dissociation
Cleft lip and palate-associated transmembrane
1-like protein (*CLPTM1L*), 178
Clinical tumor volume (CTV), 58
Clonal evolution characterization, 113
CLPTM1L. *See* Cleft lip and palate-associated
transmembrane 1-like protein
cnLOH. *See* Copy-neutral regions of loss
of heterogeneity
CNV. *See* Copy number variation
Cofilin (CFL1), 202–203
Collision-induced dissociation (CID),
200–201
Companion diagnostic tests (CDx), 368
ISPY-2 TRIAL, 377–378
phosphoproteins as, 368–369
homologous control, 370–371
kinase-driven signaling pathways,
369–370
KRAS mutations, 371
Computed tomography (CT), 5–6, 40–41,
335–336
Connective tissue growth factor (CTGF),
59–60
Coordinate descent algorithm, 136
cyclic, 138
for DrCox regression model, 141–143
Copy number variation (CNV), 112
Copy-neutral regions of loss of
heterogeneity (cnLOH), 112
COSMIC. *See* Catalogue of Somatic
Mutations in Cancer
Cox proportional hazards model, 135, 137
COX-2. *See* Cyclooxygenase-2
CSC. *See* Cancer stem cells
CT. *See* Computed tomography

Ct. *See* Cycle threshold
CTGF. *See* Connective tissue growth factor
CTV. *See* Clinical tumor volume
Cycle threshold (Ct), 155–156
Cyclic coordinate descent algorithms, 136
Cyclin-dependent kinase 4 (Cdk4), 14–15
Cyclooxygenase-2 (COX-2), 55, 76–77
Cystic fibrosis (CF), 171
Cytokeratin expression, 237–238
Cytoskeleton remodeling, 234f, 235

D

DAPI. *See* Diamidino-2-phenylindole
Data compiling, 224
dbSNP. *See* Single-Nucleotide
        Polymorphism Database
DCC. *See* Deleted in colorectal cancer
DCN. *See* Decorin
DDR. *See* DNA damage response
2-DE. *See* Two-dimensional electrophoresis
Decorin (DCN), 203
Deleted in colorectal cancer (DCC), 15
Desmoplasia, 59–60
DGE. *See* Differential gene expression
2-DGE. *See* Two-dimensional gel
        electrophoresis
Diabetes, 328
    development of, 5
    of pancreatic cancer, 328–329
Diabetes mellitus (DM), 328
Diamidino-2-phenylindole (DAPI),
        396–397
Difference gel electrophoresis (DIGE),
        207–208
Differential gene expression (DGE), 97–98,
        407
Differential stable isotopic labeling,
        200–201
Diindolylmethane (DIM), 419–420
Disease priming, 346–347
    drivers of human cancer, 347f
    key regulatory pathways components, 349
    MAPK/ERK signaling pathway,
        348–349
DM. *See* Diabetes mellitus
DNA damage response (DDR), 288
DNase I hypersensitive sites sequencing
        (DNase-seq), 106

Dose-limiting toxicity (DTL), 49–50
Doubling time (DT), 28
    calculation, 29
    cellular division, 28, 29f
    function, 28
    speed of growth, 28
Doubly regularized Cox regression model
        (DrCox regression model), 136
    coordinate descent algorithm, 141–143
    for non-overlap case, 140–141
    for overlap cases, 143–144
    for pancreatic cancer survival analysis, 140
Downstream signaling, 56
Dpc4 tumor suppressor gene, 15. *See also*
        p16 tumor suppressor gene
DrCox regression model. *See* Doubly
        regularized Cox regression model
DT. *See* Doubling time
DTL. *See* Dose-limiting toxicity

E

Eastern Cooperative Oncology Group
        (ECOG), 49
EBRT. *See* External beam radiotherapy
ECM. *See* Extracellular matrix
ECOG. *See* Eastern Cooperative Oncology
        Group
ECSA. *See* Epithelial cell surface antigen
EGF. *See* Epidermal growth factor
EGFR. *See* Epidermal growth factor
        receptor; Epithelial growth factor
        receptor
ELISA. *See* Enzyme-linked immunosorbent
        assay
EMCIT. *See* Enzyme-mediated cancer
        imaging and therapy
EMT. *See* Epithelial-to-mesenchymal
        transition
ENA. *See* European Nucleotide Archive
ENCODE project, 116–117
    data type in, 119t–121t
    pancreas cell lines, 118t
Endoscopic retrograde
        cholangiopancreatography (ERCP),
        5–6
Endoscopic ultrasonography, 5–6
Enzyme-linked immunosorbent assay
        (ELISA), 205–206

Enzyme-mediated cancer imaging and therapy (EMCIT), 385
  data mining approach, 389f
  extracellular SULF1, 388
  working prototype, 386
EORTC. *See* European Organization for Research and Treatment of Cancer
Epidermal growth factor (EGF), 76
Epidermal growth factor receptor (EGFR), 57, 185–186
Epithelial cell population selection, 25
Epithelial cell surface antigen (ECSA), 251–252
Epithelial growth factor receptor (EGFR), 26–27
Epithelial-specific antigen (ESA), 61–62, 81–82
Epithelial-to-mesenchymal transition (EMT), 75–76, 80–81, 221–222, 297–298, 348–349, 375, 419
ERCP. *See* Endoscopic retrograde cholangiopancreatography
ERK. *See* Extracellular signal-regulated kinase
ES. *See* Exome sequencing
ESA. *See* Epithelial-specific antigen
ESPAC-1. *See* European Study Group for Pancreatic Cancer
EST. *See* Expressed sequence tag
European Nucleotide Archive (ENA), 116
European Organization for Research and Treatment of Cancer (EORTC), 43–44
European Study Group for Pancreatic Cancer (ESPAC-1), 43–44
Exome sequencing (ES), 174
Expressed sequence tag (EST), 109, 157
Expression microarrays, 99–100. *See also* Genotyping microarrays
Expression validation methods, 260, 261f
  tissue factor
    by IHC, 263f
    by Q-FACS, 265f
  validation expression, 260
    in membrane, 263–266
    in tumor cells, 261–266
External beam radiotherapy (EBRT), 41–43
Extracellular matrix (ECM), 59–60, 133–134, 204, 235–236

Extracellular signal-regulated kinase (ERK), 76–77, 348–349
Extracellular Sulfatase 1 (Extracellular SULF1), 388
  docking
    into phosphatases, 392
    positions, 391f
    into sulfatase, 389–392
  hydrolysis of IQ_{2-S} and IQ_{2-P}, 393t
  SULF1 sequence alignment, 390f

F

FAIRE-seq. *See* Formaldehyde-Assisted Isolation of Regulatory Elements sequencing
FAK. *See* Focal adhesion kinase
False discovery rate (FDR), 97–98
Familial adenomatous polyposis (FAP), 173
Familial Atypical Multiple Mole Melanoma (FAMMM), 171
Familial pancreatic cancer (FPC), 171
Farnesyl protein transferase (FPT), 56
FBS. *See* Fetal bovine serum
FDR. *See* False discovery rate
Feature extraction approach, 134
Feature selection approach, 134
Fédération Francophone de Cancérologie Digestive (FFCD), 50–51
Fetal bovine serum (FBS), 25
FFPE tissue. *See* Formalin-fixed paraffin-embedded tissue
Fine-needle aspirate (FNA), 352
[18]F-fluorodeoxyglucose positron emission tomography (^{18}F-FDG-PET), 324–325
5-fluorouracil (5-FU), 41–43
  chemotherapy, 43–44
  clinical studies, 49
FNA. *See* Fine-needle aspirate
Focal adhesion kinase (FAK), 236–237
FOLFIRINOX, 7–8, 245–246
  clinical benefit of, 53
  treatment activity, 53–54
  treatment establishment, 52
Forkhead box Q1 (FoxQ1), 311–314
Formaldehyde-Assisted Isolation of Regulatory Elements sequencing (FAIRE-seq), 106

Formalin-fixed paraffin-embedded tissue
    (FFPE tissue), 163–164
FoxQ1. *See* Forkhead box Q1
FPC. *See* Familial pancreatic cancer
FPT. *See* Farnesyl protein transferase
5-FU. *See* 5-fluorouracil
Functional analysis, 98
Functional and hypothesis-driven proteomic
    studies. *See also* Proteomics
  cell invasiveness investigation, 210
  KRAS proteins
    protein receptor identification, 210
    targeted interrogation, 209
  protein activities, 210

G

Gain of function, 26–27
γ-secretase inhibitor (GSI), 83–84
GAPs. *See* GTPase-activating proteins
Gas chromatography–mass spectrometry
    (GC–MS), 330
Gastro-Intestinal Tumor Study Group
    (GITSG), 41–43
Gastroduodenal artery (GDA), 47
Gastrointestinal malignancies (GI
    malignancies), 41
GC. *See* Guanine–cytosine
GC–MS. *See* Gas chromatography–mass
    spectrometry
GDA. *See* Gastroduodenal artery
GDP. *See* Guanosine diphosphate
GEF. *See* Guanine nucleotide exchange
    factor
Gelsolin (GSN), 202–203
GemCap. *See* Gemcitabine and
    capecitabine
Gemcitabine (GEM), 221–222
  and FU, 50–51
  gemcitabine-clinical trials, 49–50
  gemcitabine-nab-paclitaxel, 54, 405–406
Gemcitabine and capecitabine (GemCap), 51
Gemcitabine-based
  clinical trials, 49–50
  combination chemotherapy
    GemCap, 51–52
    gemcitabine and FU, 50–51
Gene Expression Barcode, 122
Gene Expression Omnibus (GEO), 117, 388

Gene expression profiling
  affymetrix microarrays, 156–157, 161
  agilent bioanalyzer 2100 assay, 154f
  biological information, 162
  cDNA microarrays, 157–158
  data collection, 162
  data repositories, 158
  using DNA sequencing, 160
  lack of reproducibility, 163–164
  microarray technologies, 157
  oligonucleotide and bead arrays, 158
  pancreatic cancer expression, 152
  protein kinases in PDAC, 163f
  qRT-PCR, 155
  RIN, 153–154
  RNA
    molecules, 151
    preparation, 154–155
    RNA-seq, 160–161
  solid tumor samples, 152–153
  tissue banks, 152
  tissue sampling, 151–152
  Web links for databases and software, 159t
Gene set ridge regression in association
    studies (GRASS), 185
Gene transfer format (GTF), 105
Gene-Set Enrichment Analysis (GSEA), 98
Genome–exome sequencing studies
  genetic heterogeneity in metastases, 115
  neoplastic pancreatic cysts, 115
  PALB2, 114
  in pancreas, 114
  pancreatic cancer cases, 114
Genomewide association studies (GWAS),
    98–99, 170, 418
Genotype-Tissue Expression (GTEx), 116
Genotyping microarrays, 100–101
GEO. *See* Gene Expression Omnibus
GERCOR. *See* Groupe Coopérateur
    Multidisciplinaire en Oncologie
GI malignancies. *See* Gastrointestinal
    malignancies
GITSG. *See* Gastro-Intestinal Tumor Study
    Group
Global profiling, 205
  functional proteins, 205–206
  in plasma or serum, 205
  protein profiling methods, 200–201

GLP. *See* Good lab practice
GLS. *See* Glutaminase
Glucose transporter-1 (GLUT1), 326
Glutaminase (GLS), 326
Glycoprotein (GP2), 207–208, 212
Glycosylation, 212–213. *See also*
        Phosphorylation
Good lab practice (GLP), 416–418
GP2. *See* Glycoprotein
GRASS. *See* Gene set ridge regression in
        association studies
Gross tumor volume (GTV), 58
Groupe Coopérateur Multidisciplinaire en
        Oncologie (GERCOR), 50–51
GSEA. *See* Gene-Set Enrichment Analysis
GSI. *See* γ-secretase inhibitor
GSN. *See* Gelsolin
GTEx. *See* Genotype-Tissue Expression
GTF. *See* Gene transfer format
GTPase-activating proteins (GAPs), 283
GTV. *See* Gross tumor volume
Guanine nucleotide exchange factor (GEF),
        56, 283
Guanine–cytosine (GC), 97
Guanosine diphosphate (GDP), 56, 283
GWAS. *See* Genomewide association
        studies

H
Haplotype analysis, 178
HBOC. *See* Hereditary breast and ovarian
        cancer
Heat shock protein 27 (Hsp27), 211
Helicobacter pylori (*H. pylori*), 177
Heparan-sulfate-proteoglycan (HSPG), 387
Hepatocarcinoma-intestinepancreas (HIP),
        247–249
Hepatocyte growth factor (HGF), 59–61
Hereditary breast and ovarian cancer
        (HBOC), 173–174
Hereditary pancreatitis (HP), 171
HGF. *See* Hepatocyte growth factor
High-dimensional data, 136
    censoring, 135–136
    cyclic coordinate descent algorithms, 136
    DrCox regression model, 140–144
    feature extraction and selection, 134
    features and predictors, 136

genetic signatures and signaling pathways,
        135
    LASSO penalized regression method,
        137–140
    pancreatic cancer survival analysis,
        144–146
    PDAC, 133–134
    statistical models and methods, 134–135
    truncation, 135–136
HIP. *See* Hepatocarcinoma-
        intestinepancreas
HMEC. *See* Human mammary epithelial
        cells
Housekeeping genes, 97
HP. *See* Hereditary pancreatitis
Hsp27. *See* Heat shock protein 27
HSPG. *See* Heparan-sulfate-proteoglycan
Human Genome Project, 94
Human mammary epithelial cells (HMEC),
        386
Human Validated Kinase Set (HVKS), 413
HVKS. *See* Human Validated Kinase Set
2-(2′-hydroxyphenyl)-6-iodo-4-(3H)-
        quinazolinone (IQ$_{2-OH}$), 386
2-(2′-hydroxyphenyl)-6-tributylstannyl-4-
        (3H)-quinazolinone (SnQ$_{2-OH}$), 394
Hypoxia inducing factor-1 (HIF-1),
        225–230
    HIF-1α protein, 326
    transcription factor, 326

I
ICAT. *See* Isotope coded affinity tag
ICGC. *See* International Cancer Genome
        Consortium
IF. *See* Intermediate filament
IGF-1R. *See* Insulin-like growth factor
        receptor
IGFBP2. *See* Insulin-like growth factor
        binding protein 2
IgG antibodies. *See* Immunoglobulin G
        antibodies
IGV. *See* Integrative Genomics Viewer
IHC. *See* Immunohistochemistry
ILGF. *See* Insulin-like growth factor
ILK. *See* Integrin-linked kinase
Immunoglobulin G antibodies (IgG
        antibodies), 103–104

Immunohistochemistry (IHC), 260
IMRT. *See* Intensity-modulated radiation
    therapy
In vivo models, 34–35
Ingenuity Pathway Analysis (IPA), 230–231,
    298–299, 387–388
Ink4a protein, 287
    against microRNAs, 289–290
    nFBL *vs.* pFBL with Kras, 288–289, 289f
Institutional review boards (IRB), 151–152
Insulin-like growth factor (ILGF), 247–249
Insulin-like growth factor binding protein
    2 (IGFBP2), 204
Insulin-like growth factor receptor
    (IGF-1R), 59
Integrative Genomics Viewer (IGV), 111
Integrin Beta 6, 258
    peptide intensity plots, 259f
Integrin-linked kinase (ILK), 236–237
Integrin-signaling system, 235–236
Integrins, 235–236
Intensity-modulated radiation therapy
    (IMRT), 58
Intermediate filament (IF), 237–238
International Cancer Genome Consortium
    (ICGC), 114, 124, 160
International Protein Index (IPI), 224
IntOGen, 122
Intraductal papillary mucinous neoplasm
    (IPMN), 4, 115, 207–208
Intraoperative radiation therapy (IORT), 46
IPA. *See* Ingenuity Pathway Analysis
IPI. *See* International Protein Index
IPMN. *See* Intraductal papillary mucinous
    neoplasm
IRB. *See* Institutional review boards
Isotope coded affinity tag (ICAT), 256

K

Kallikrein 1 (KLK1), 207–208
Kataegis, 113
KEGG. *See* Kyoto Encyclopedia of Genes
    and Genomes
Keratin family proteins, 236
Knowledge-based pathway analysis
    biological network analysis, 230f
        comparative pathway maps, 233,
            233f

cytoskeleton_intermediate filaments
    network, 231–232
drug-resistance and metastasis group, 231
functional ontologies, 232, 232f
pathway analysis tools, 230–231
PLGEM data, 230
canonical pathway analysis, 233–238
comparative analysis
    PLGEM analysis, 225
    vimentin, 225–230
using comparative data sets, 222
data compiling, 224
growth behavior, 221–222
PC, 221
protein identification, 224
proteomic analysis
    cell lines, 222–223
    metastatic cell lines, 223
    pathway analysis work flow, 223f
    peptide samples, 224
    trypsinized cells, 223–224
vimentin expression and
    chemoresistance, 238–241
Kras gene, 282, 328
    activation threshold, 282–283
        GTP-bound Ras, 283
        Kras GTPase cycle, 284–285, 284f
        property of a Ras, 283
        total Ras protein, 285, 285f
    effector pathways in PDAC development,
        285–288, 286f
    Ink4a
        against microRNAs in, 289–290
        nFBL *vs.* pFBL with, 288–289, 289f
    K-ras mutations, 14
    Kras-miR-21 pFBL, 290
    proteins
        protein receptor identification, 210
        targeted interrogation, 209
    proto-oncogene, 56
Kyoto Encyclopedia of Genes and
    Genomes (KEGG), 183

L

Laminin beta 1 (LAMB1), 203
Laparoscopic distal pancreatectomy (LDP), 41
Laparoscopic pancreaticoduodenectomy
    (LPD), 41

LAPC. *See* Locally advanced unresectable
    pancreatic cancer
Laser capture microdissection (LCM), 250,
    374
Laser microdissection (LMD), 16, 29–30
    goal, 31–34
    on primary cell cultures, 29–30
        advantages, 30
        of PDAC, 31f
        PET membrane, 32f–33f
        preparation, 31f
LASSO. *See* Least absolute shrinkage and
    selection operator
LASSO penalized regression method, 137
    cyclic coordinate descent
        coordinate descent algorithms, 138
        directional derivatives calculation, 139
        Newton's method, 139–140
        number of selected predictors, 140
    variable selection
        Cox proportional hazards regression
            model, 137
        via LASSO regularized partial
            likelihood, 137
        penalty function, 138
LC. *See* Liquid chromatography
LC-MS/MS analysis, 254–255
LCM. *See* Laser capture microdissection
LDP. *See* Laparoscopic distal
    pancreatectomy
Least absolute shrinkage and selection
    operator (LASSO), 134
Left pancreatectomy (LP), 17
LET. *See* Linear energy transfer
Leucine-rich alpha-2-glycoprotein (LRG),
    205–206
Li–Fraumeni syndrome, 173
Linear energy transfer (LET), 62
Lipolysis, 329
Liquid chromatography (LC), 199–200
LMD. *See* Laser microdissection
Local network topology, 409–410, 411f
Locally advanced unresectable pancreatic
    cancer (LAPC), 48
    clinical trials
        capecitabine-based, 50
        gemcitabine-based, 49–50
        5-FU–based clinical studies, 49

gemcitabine-based combination
        chemotherapy
    GemCap, 51–52
    gemcitabine and FU, 50–51
    randomized trials of therapy, 48t
Loss of heterozygosity (LOH), 98–99
LP. *See* Left pancreatectomy
LPD. *See* Laparoscopic
        pancreaticoduodenectomy
LRG. *See* Leucine-rich alpha-2-glycoprotein
Lumican (LUM), 202–203
Lynch syndrome, 172–173

M
Magnetic resonance
        cholangiopancreatography
        (MRCP), 5–6
Magnetic resonance imaging (MRI), 40–41
MALDI. *See* Matrix-assisted laser
        desorption/ionization
Malignant tumors (TNM), 22
Mammalian target of rapamycin (mTOR),
        76–77
MAPK/ERK. *See* Mitogen-activated protein
        kinase/extracellular regulated kinase
Mass spectrometer, 201
Mass spectrometry (MS), 201, 329–330
Matrix metalloproteinase-9 (MMP-9),
        76–77, 207–208
Matrix-assisted laser desorption/ionization
        (MALDI), 201
Maturity onset diabetes of the young
        (MODY), 183–185
Maximum tolerated dose (MTD), 49–50
MCN. *See* Mucinous neoplasms
MD Anderson Cancer Center (MDACC), 47
MEK1/2. *See* Mitogen-activated protein
        kinases 1/2
Metabiomarker, 330–331
Metabolomic effect characterization, 329
    advantages, 330–331
    biological insights, 332–333
    contains genetic aberrations, 323
    metabolic derangements, 324
        alterations by pathogenic process, 328
        in host tissues, 328–329
        reprogrammed energy metabolism
            features, 327f

Metabolomic effect characterization
    (*Continued*)
    tissues contributing representation, 325f
    in tumor cells, 324–326
    metabolomics-based diagnostic testing,
        333–334
        ¹H-NMR spectroscopy, 335–336
        malignant pancreatic, 335
        serum tumor markers, 334
    ¹H-NMR spectroscopy, 330
    therapeutics development, 336–337
    urine metabolome, 331–332
Metabolomics, 329–331
Metabolomics-based diagnostic testing
        development, 333–334
    ¹H-NMR spectroscopy, 335–336
    malignant pancreatic, 335
    serum tumor markers, 334
MetaCore™, 231
Metastasis, 221–222
Metastatic disease, 52
    FOLFIRINOX treatment establishment,
        52
    gemcitabine, 52
    nab-paclitaxel, 54
    PFS, 52–53
Microarrays
    bioinformatic analysis
        DGE, 97–98
        genotyping, 98
        GWAS, 98–99
        housekeeping genes, 97
        normalization, 96–97
        unit of analysis, 98
        unsupervised methods, 98
    in pancreas
        expression microarrays, 99–100
        genotyping microarrays, 100–101
    technique, 96
Micrococcal Nuclease sequencing
        (MNase-seq), 106
Microdissection, 152–153
MicroRNAs (miRNAs), 82, 107–108,
        298–299, 303–304, 345–346,
        414–415
    in cellular systems, 346
    clinical targeting, 352–354
        discovering of miRNAs, 354–355

mirDREM method, 355–356
        miRNA placements, 356–357
        miRNAs paradigm, 355
    diagnostic, prognostic, and therapeutic
        value, 349
        CSCs bolstering, 349–350
        miR-21identification, 352
        PDAC analysis, 350–351
    disease priming and progression,
        346–347
        interrelated drivers of human cancer,
            347f
        key regulatory pathways components,
            349
        MAPK/ERK signaling pathway,
            348–349
    implications, 357–359
    prioritizing pancreatic, 352
    prioritizing PDAC, 353f
    selected candidate miRNAs, 358t
mirDREM. *See* MIRna Dynamic
        Regulatory Events Miner
MIRna Dynamic Regulatory Events Miner
        (mirDREM), 355–356
miRNAs. *See* MicroRNAs
Mismatch repair genes (MMR genes),
        172–173
Mitogen-activated protein kinase (MAPK),
        348–349
Mitogen-activated protein kinase/
        extracellular regulated kinase
        (MAPK/ERK), 236–237
Mitogen-activated protein kinases 1/2
        (MEK1/2), 56
MMP-9. *See* Matrix metalloproteinase-9
MMR genes. *See* Mismatch repair genes
MNase-seq. *See* Micrococcal Nuclease
        sequencing
Modular enrichment analysis, 98
MODY. *See* Maturity onset diabetes of the
        young
Moesin (MSN), 202–203
Molecular targeted therapies
    activity of TGFβ, 61
    bevacizumab, 58–59
    cellular and molecular mechanisms,
        54–55
    cetuximab, 58

CSC, 61–62
CTGF, 60
downstream signaling, 56
EGFR, 57
using FG-3019, 60
FPT, 56
HGF, 61
hyaluronic acid, 59
IGF-1R, 59
K-Ras proto-oncogene, 56
K-Ras signaling, 56
for pancreas cancer, 55f
PI3K/Akt/mTOR pathway, 57
prostaglandin synthase, 55
Ras synthesis, 56
targeting pancreas tumor stroma, 59–60
VEGFR, 58
Motif Elicitation Suite, 104–105
MRCP. *See* Magnetic resonance
    cholangiopancreatography
MRI. *See* Magnetic resonance imaging
MS. *See* Mass spectrometry
MSN. *See* Moesin
MTD. *See* Maximum tolerated dose
mTOR. *See* Mammalian target of
    rapamycin
Mucin-5AC (MUC5AC), 212–213
Mucinous neoplasms (MCN), 208–209
Mucins (MUC), 212, 247–249
Multimodal therapies
    molecular targeted therapies, 54–62
    next generation radiation oncology,
        62–63
    pancreatic cancer, 40
        borderline resectable, 47
        current therapy options in, 40f
        LAPC, 48–52
        metastatic disease, 52–54
        resectable, 40–46
Myc gene, 281
    Myc-p53 interaction, 282, 288–289
    overexpression, 292, 326
MZT1 gene, 179

N

Na+/K+ ATPase, 258
Na+/K+ ATPase Beta 3, 258
    peptide intensity plots, 259f

Nab-paclitaxel, 54
National Cancer Institute (NCI), 47
National Comprehensive Cancer Network
    (NCCN), 47
National Human Genome Research
    Institute (NHGRI), 185
Negative feedback loop (nFBL), 281
Neoadjuvant therapy, preoperative, 45–46
Network pharmacology, 302
    in drug repositioning for PDAC,
        416–418
    to unwind PDAC miRNA complexity,
        414–416
Neuroendocrine tumors (NET), 208–209
Next generation radiation oncology
    dose escalation, 63
    pancreas cells, 62–63
    particle therapy, 62
    in vitro experimentation, 62
Next-generation sequencing (NGS), 94, 101.
        See also RNA sequencing (RNA-seq)
    bioinformatic analysis workflow, 102,
        102f
        alignment strategies, 103
        data visualization, 103
        dozens of peak callers, 103
        IgG antibodies, 103–104
        motif databases, 104–105
        peak detection algorithm, 104
        raw sequenced reads, 103
    ChIP-seq, 101
        applications, 105–110
        encyclopedia of DNA elements, 102
        of pancreatic cancer, 107
    technique, 101
NF-κB. *See* Nuclear factor-kappa B
nFBL. *See* Negative feedback loop
NGS. *See* Next-generation sequencing
NHGRI. *See* National Human Genome
    Research Institute
NICD. *See* Notch intracellular domain
NLS. *See* Nuclear localization signals
¹H-NMR spectroscopy, 330–331
Non-small cell lung cancer (NSCLC), 367
Normalization, 96–97
Normalized spectral abundance factor
    (NSAF), 225
Notch intracellular domain (NICD), 76–77

Notch signaling pathway, 76
  development and progression of cancer, 86f
  notch inhibition, 83–84
  notch receptors and ligands structure, 77f
  notch-ligand binding, 76–77
  in PC
    cell apoptosis, 79
    cell cycle, 79
    cell growth, 78
    crosstalks with miRNA, 82
    CSC regulation, 81–82
    drug resistance, 83
    EMT, 80–81
    overexpression, 78
    poor prognosis, 80
    tumor angiogenesis, 80
    tumor cell invasion, 79–80
  role in CSC, 82
  through systems biology, 84–85
NSAF. *See* Normalized spectral abundance
    factor
NSCLC. *See* Non-small cell lung cancer
Nuclear factor-kappa B (NF-κB), 76–77
Nuclear localization signals (NLS), 76
Nucleosome positioning, 106

O

Octamer-binding protein 4 (Oct-4), 177
Odds ratio (OR), 170
Oligonucleotide arrays, 158
Omics technologies, 151
Oncomine, 118
Overall survival (OS), 44, 52–53
Oxythiamine (OT), 211

P

p16 tumor suppressor gene, 14–15
p53 gene, 14, 281
  DDR pathway, 288
  Myc-p53 interaction, 282, 288–289
Paclitaxel, 54
Pair-end sequencing, 107–108
PALB2. *See* Partner and localizer of *BRCA2*
Palladin (PALLD), 210
PALLD. *See* Palladin
Panc-1 cells, 239
PanC4. *See* Pancreatic Cancer Case
    Control Consortium

Pancreas
  cell lines in ENCODE Project, 118t
  cells, 62–63
  genome–exome sequencing studies,
    114–115
  magnification of head, 18f
  microarrays
    expression, 99–100
    genotyping, 100–101
  RNA-seq in, 110
  surgical resection, 18f, 20f
Pancreas cancer genome
  databases and resources, 115
    1000 Genomes Project, 124
    Array-Express, 117
    cBioPortal for cancer genomics,
      123–124
    CCLE, 125
    COSMIC, 122–123
    data visualization in, 123f
    dbSNP, 122
    ENA, 116
    ENCODE project, 116–117
    GenBank, 116
    Gene Expression Barcode, 122
    GEO, 117
    ICGC, 124
    IntOGen, 122
    Oncomine, 118
    PED, 125
    SRA, 116
    TCGA, 124
  high-throughput genomic technologies
    bioinformatics approaches, 95–96
    heterogeneity and quality of samples, 95
    pancreatic tumors, 95
  microarrays
    bioinformatic analysis, 96–99
    in pancreas, 99–101
    technique, 96
  NGS, 101–110
  RNA-seq, 107–110
Pancreas stellate cells (PSC), 59–60
Pancreas–duodenum homeobox protein 1
    (*PDX1*), 177–178
Pancreatic cancer (PC), 3, 12, 221, 297–298,
    323, 349, 405–406
  applications, 35

biological models, 29–34
CF, 171–172
characterization of cell cultures, 26
chronic inflammatory conditions, 171
clinical presentation, 5
complexity, 298–299
    IPA, 298–299, 300f
    pathways identification, 301
CSCs role, 307–308
    differentially expressed miRNAs, 316t
    isolation and biological
        characterization, 308–310, 309f
    microRNA network, 314–316
    miRNA microarrays in, 315f
    molecular analysis, 310f
    systems and pathway analysis,
        310–314
diagnosis, 5–6
epidemiology, 3–4, 12–13
familial risk, 170
FAMMM syndrome, 172
FAP, 173
FPC cases, 174
genotyping, 26–27
GWAS and gene mapping approaches,
    186–188
HBOC, 173–174
HP, 171
in vivo models, 34–35
isolation
    of epithelial component, 16
    and establishment procedure, 17–25
kras activation threshold, 282
    GTP-bound Ras, 283
    Kras GTPase cycle, 284–285, 284f
    property of a Ras, 283
    total Ras protein, 285, 285f
Kras effector pathways in PDAC,
    285–288, 286f
Li–Fraumeni syndrome, 173
low-risk
    ABO gene, 176–177
    BORA gene, 179
    CLPTM1L, 178
    GWAS, 174–175
    H. pylori, 177
    haplotype analysis, 178
    linkage approach, 174

    NR5A2 gene, 177–178
    PanC4, 175–176
    PDX1, 177–178
Lynch syndrome, 172–173
miRNAs diagnostic, prognostic, and
    therapeutic value, 349
    CSCs bolstering, 349–350
    miR-21 identification, 352
    PDAC analysis, 350–351
morphology, 26
neoadjuvant therapy, 7
in non-European populations
    ChinaPC, 180
    inherited susceptibility variants,
        180–181, 181f
    Japanese GWAS, 180
    PANDoRA, 180
    PanScan GWAS, 179
pathway analyses, 181–182, 184t
    dense module searching, 185–186
    GRASS, 185
    GWAS, 181–182
    high-throughput data sets, 185
    mapping SNPs from GWAS, 186
    using *P*-values, 182–183
    SNP, 183
PDAC
    cell culture, 16–17
    molecular genetics, 13–15
    pathway view, 300f
phenotyping, 27–29
PJS, 172
potentially curative, 6–7
prognosis, 3, 8
significance of Kras-Ink4a nFBL, 282
systems biology, 302
    assessment of toxicity, 306–307
    curation methodologies using, 303
    miRNAs role, 303–304
    network pharmacology, 302
    network-based analyses, 307
    neutraceutical use, 304–305
    systems science, 304
3-D cell cultures, 34
treatment, 6
    adjuvant, 7
    palliative, 7–8
types, 4, 4t

Pancreatic Cancer Case Control
    Consortium (PanC4), 175–176
Pancreatic cancer GWAS data sets
  dense module searching, 185–186
  GRASS, 185
  high-throughput data sets, 185
  mapping SNPs from GWAS, 186
  using *P*-values, 182–183
  pathway analyses, 181–182, 184t
  SNP, 183
Pancreatic cancer stem cells, 308
  miRNA microarrays in, 315f
  systems analysis, 312f
  systems biology, 302
    assessment of toxicity, 306–307
    curation methodologies using, 303
    miRNAs role, 303–304
    network pharmacology, 302
    network-based analyses, 307
    neutraceutical use, 304–305
    systems science, 304
Pancreatic cancer survival analysis
  data analysis
    with DrCox regression, 145–146
    with LASSO penalized cox
      regression, 145
  microarray data, 144
  signaling pathways, 144–145
Pancreatic cyst fluid, 208–209
PANcreatic Disease ReseArch
    (PANDoRA), 180
Pancreatic ductal adenocarcinoma (PDAC),
    4t, 16, 39, 99–100, 133–134,
    202–203, 281, 350–351, 405–406
  applications, 35
  biological networks, 408–409
    broader network topology, 410–413
    local network topology, 409–410
    network-based methods, 412t
  cell culture
    cell lines, 16
    characterization, 26
    primary cell cultures, 17
  cellular growth, 28–29
  culturing and storage, 25
  desmoplastic reaction, 19f
  diagnosis, 17
    autopsy case studies, 17–19
    hemorrhage and necrosis, 19–20

epithelial and fibroblast cells, 24f
epithelial cell population selection, 25
genotyping, 26–27
histological diagnosis, 22–23
identification of network targeted drugs,
    414t
in vivo models, 34–35
Kras effector pathways, 285–288
microscopic features, 20–21
  grading of exocrine pancreatic tumor,
    22t
  moderately differentiated, 21f
  poorly differentiated, 21–22, 22f
  well-differentiated, 21f
molecular genetics, 13
  Dpc4 tumor suppressor gene, 15
  general considerations, 15–16
  K-ras mutations, 14
  other genes, 15
  p16 tumor suppressor gene, 14–15
  p53 tumor suppressor gene, 14
morphology, 26, 27f
need for progression model revisiting, 407
  DE analysis, 407
  network visualization resources, 408t
network pharmacology
  in drug repositioning for PDAC,
    416–418
  to unwind PDAC microRNA
    COMPLEXITY, 414–416
networks in polypharmacology strategies,
    418–419
  BR-DIM, 419–420
  CDF, 419
  DIM, 419–420
  multiple targeting, 418–419
  natural compound investigation, 419
optimal intervention strategies in,
    413–414
pancreatic resections for, 17
phenotyping, 27–29
primary cell culture, 26f
protein kinases in, 163f
second level of biological models, 29–34
sorting by surgical resection type, 23t
staging and TNM relationship, 23t
at surgical pathology unit, 24f
3-D cell cultures, 34
tumor tissue isolation, 23–24

Pancreatic duodenectomy (PD), 17
Pancreatic Expression Database (PED),
    99–100, 125
Pancreatic intraepithelial neoplasias
    (PanINs), 4
Pancreatic juice, 207–208
Pancreatitis-associated protein (PAP),
    207–208, 247–249
Pancreative intraepithelial neoplasia
    (PanIN), 203
PANDoRA. *See* PANcreatic Disease
    ReseArch
PanIN. *See* Pancreative intraepithelial
    neoplasia
PanINs. *See* Pancreatic intraepithelial
    neoplasias
Panther Classification System, 230–231
PAP. *See* Pancreatitis-associated protein;
    Prostatic acid phosphatase
Para-nitrocatechol sulfate (pNCS), 387
    $^{125}IQ_{2-p}$ and $^{125}IQ_{2-S}$ mediated hydrolysis,
    395f
  docking positions, 391f
Partner and localizer of *BRCA2* (PALB2),
    114
PBS. *See* Phosphate-buffered saline
PC. *See* Pancreatic cancer; Pseudo-cyst
PCA. *See* Principal component analysis
PCR. *See* Polymerase chain reaction
PD. *See* Pancreatic duodenectomy
PDAC. *See* Pancreatic ductal
    adenocarcinoma
PDB. *See* Protein Data Bank
*PDX*1. *See* Pancreas–duodenum homeobox
    protein 1
PED. *See* Pancreatic Expression Database
Pegylated hyaluronidase (PEGPH20), 59
Peripherin, 225–230
Personalized therapy, 367. *See also* Protein
    network activation mapping
    technology
  molecularly targeted agents, 368
  "Pathways in Human Cancer" diagram,
    377–378, 378f
  RPPA as tool for, 371–374
PEST residues. *See* Proline, glutamine,
    serine, and threonine residues
PET. *See* Positron emission tomography
Peutz–Jeghers syndrome (PJS), 171

pFBL. *See* Positive feedback loop
PFS. *See* Progression-free survivals
Phosphate-buffered saline (PBS),
    223–224
Phosphatidic acid phosphatase type 2A
    (PPAP2A), 400–401
Phosphatidylinositol-3 kinase (PI3K),
    236–237
Phosphoprotein
  as CDx markers, 368–369
    homologous control, 370–371
    kinase-driven signaling pathways,
    369–370
    KRAS mutations, 371
  pathway activation mapping
    case studies in, 375–377
    pre-analytical factors influence,
    374–375
Phosphorylation, 211
2-(2′-phosphoryloxyphenyl)-6-[^{127}I]
    iodo-4-(3H)-quinazolinone
    ($^{127}IQ_{2-p}$), 394
2-(2′-phosphoryloxyphenyl)-6-iodo-4-
    (3H)-quinazolinone (IQ_{2-p}), 386
  docking positions, 391f
  hydrolysis, 393t
PI3K. *See* Phosphatidylinositol-3 kinase
Piwi-interacting RNAs (piRNAs),
    107–108
PJS. *See* Peutz–Jeghers syndrome
PK. *See* Pyruvate kinase
Plectin-1 (PLEC), 202–203, 237–238
Pleiotropy scan method, 185
PLGEM. *See* Power law global error
    model
pNCS. *See* Para-nitrocatechol sulfate
Polymerase chain reaction (PCR), 102,
    155–156
Polypharmacology, networks in, 418–420
Portal vein (PV), 47
Positive feedback loop (pFBL), 282
Positron emission tomography (PET),
    386
Post-translational modification (PTM),
    198, 211. *See also* Functional and
    hypothesis-driven proteomic
    studies
  glycosylation, 212–213
  phosphorylation, 211

Postoperative adjuvant therapy
  beneficial effects, 44
  chemoradiation phase II trial, 44–45
  EORTC, 43–44
  ESPAC-3 trial, 45
  GI malignancies, 41
  randomized trials of, 41–43, 42t
  RTOG, 44
Posttranslational protein modifications
        (PTM), 369–370
Power law global error model (PLGEM), 225
PPAP2A. *See* Phosphatidic acid phosphatase
        type 2A
PPI. *See* Protein–protein interaction
Primary cell cultures, 17, 33f
  gain of function, 26–27
  LMD on, 29–30
    advantages, 30
    of PDAC, 31f
    PET membrane, 32f–33f
    primary cell culture preparation, 31f
    stained with hematoxylin, 32f
  of pancreatic adenocarcinoma, 23–24
  PDAC, 17, 26f
  pure population, 27f
Principal component analysis (PCA), 134
Prognostic biomarkers, 350–354
Progression-free survivals (PFS), 52–53
Proline, glutamine, serine, and threonine
        residues (PEST residues), 76
Prostaglandin synthase, 55
Prostatic acid phosphatase (PAP), 386
Protein activities determination, 210
Protein Data Bank (PDB), 388–389
Protein network activation mapping
        technology
  CDx, 368
  cellular circuit diagram generation,
        377–378, 378f
  defective protein signaling networks
    phosphoproteins as CDx markers,
        368–371
  phosphoprotein pathway activation
        mapping
    case studies in, 375–377
    pre-analytical factors influence,
        374–375
  Prottein receptor identification, 210

Protein–peptide analysis
  bioinformatics for, 201–202
  targeted proteomics, 202
Protein–protein interaction (PPI), 185–186,
        407
Proteomics, 246–247
  blood biomarker discovery, 205–207
  global protein profiling
    quantitative methods for, 200–201
  using ICAT technology, 255–256
    2-DE, 255–256
    decoupled ICAT process, 257f
    multiplex analysis, 257
    peptide intensity plots, 259f
    tissue factor, 258
  mass spectrometry, 201
  in pancreatic cancer studies, 199f
  pancreatic cyst fluid, 208–209
  pancreatic juice, 207–208
  of pancreatic tissue
    chronic pancreatitis, 204
    PanIN, 203
    PDAC, 202–203
  pipeline, 198–199
  plasma membrane proteins identification
    biological samples for analysis,
        247–253
    enrichment for cell surface
        glycoproteins, 253–255, 254f
    epithelial cell enrichment, 251f
    for overexpressed tumor antigens, 248f
    pancreatic cell line models, 252f
  post-translational modifications, 211
    glycosylation, 212–213
    phosphorylation, 211
  protein–peptide analysis
    bioinformatics for, 201–202
    targeted proteomics, 202
  proteins and peptides separation,
        199–200
PSC. *See* Pancreas stellate cells
Pseudo-cyst (PC), 208–209
Pten gene, 287
PTM. *See* Post-translational modification;
        Posttranslational protein modifications
PubMed literature search, 158
PV. *See* Portal vein
Pyruvate kinase (PK), 326

Q

Quantitative flow cytometry (Q-FACS), 263–264

Quantitative real-time polymerase chain reaction (qRT-PCR), 155–156

R

Radiation Therapy Oncology Group (RTOG), 44

Radiofrequency (RF), 330

Radioiodinated quinazolinone prodrug biological evaluation

ARSA, ALP, and PAP-mediated hydrolysis, 395f

enzymatic catalysis, 394–395

in vitro hydrolysis, 396–397

in vitro incubation of IQ_{2-S} and IQ_{2-P}, 396f

data mining approach, 397–398

docking of IQ_{2-S} and IQ_{2-P}, 399

docking pose of pNCS, 398

EMCIT, 385, 389f

extracellular SULF1 sequence alignment, 388–389

docking into phosphatases, 392

docking into sulfatase, 389–392

docking positions, 391f

hydrolysis of IQ_{2-S} and IQ_{2-P}, 393t

SULF1 sequence alignment, 390f

PAP, 386

searching for target, 387–388

SULF1, 387

Ras protein, 283

GTP-bound Ras, 283

Ras synthesis, 56

total Ras protein, 285

Ras-GTPase activating proteins (Ras-GAP), 56

RBBP9. *See* Retinoblastoma-binding protein 9

Reads/fragments per kilobase per million (RPKM/FPKM), 109

Receptor tyrosine kinases (RTK), 369–370

Resectable pancreatic cancer, 40–41

borderline, 47

LDP and LPD, 41

postoperative adjuvant therapy beneficial effects, 44

chemoradiation phase II trial, 44–45

EORTC, 43–44

ESPAC-3 trial, 45

GI malignancies, 41

randomized trials of, 41–43, 42t

RTOG, 44

preoperative neoadjuvant therapy, 45–46

Retention time (RT), 256

Retinoblastoma-binding protein 9 (RBBP9), 210

Reverse phase protein microarray (RPPA), 371–372, 372f

analysis protein marker identification, 376

for multiplexed phosphoprotein analysis, 377–378

tool for personalized cancer therapy, 371–372

advantages of technological components, 373–374

for sensitive analyte detection, 372–373

RF. *See* Radiofrequency

Ribonuclease (RNASE1), 207–208

Ribonucleic acid (RNA), 94

Right censoring, 135–136

RIN. *See* RNA integrity number

RISC. *See* RNA-induced silencing complex

RNA. *See* Ribonucleic acid

RNA integrity number (RIN), 95, 153–154

RNA interference (RNAi), 266–267

cell surface proteins, 246

challenging disease, 245

expression validation methods, 260

in membrane, 263–266

for proteomically identified candidates, 260, 261f

tissue factor by IHC, 263f

tissue factor by Q-FACS, 265f

in tumor cells, 261–266

functional validation, 266

high-throughput target validation, 266–267

MPANC96 cells, 272

processes in cancer, 269–270

RNAi knockdown results, 270–271, 271f

RNA interference (RNAi) (*Continued*)
    RNAi mechanism, 266–267
    RNAi mediated gene knockdown,
        267–268
    siRNA transfections, 269
    mediated gene knockdown, 267–268
    platform, 270
    program, 268
    proteomics, 246–247
        biological samples for analysis, 247–253
        decoupled ICAT process, 257f
        enrichment for cell surface
            glycoproteins, 253–255, 254f
        epithelial cell enrichment, 251f
        pancreatic cell line models, 252f
        peptide intensity plots, 259f
        quantitative proteomics, 255–260
        for tumor antigens identification, 248f
RNA sequencing (RNA-seq), 94
    bioinformatic analysis
        DGE, 109–110
        raw sequence, 108–109
        splice junctions, 109
        statistical distribution, 110
    cancer genome sequencing, 111–115
    ENCODE guidelines, 108
    expression microarrays, 107
    genome–exome sequencing studies,
        114–115
    in pancreas, 110
    technique, 107–108
RNA-induced silencing complex (RISC),
    266–267
RNA-seq. *See* RNA sequencing
RNAi. *See* RNA interference
RNASE1. *See* Ribonuclease
RPKM/FPKM. *See* Reads/fragments per
    kilobase per million
RPPA. *See* Reverse phase protein microarray
RT. *See* Retention time
RTK. *See* Receptor tyrosine kinases
RTOG. *See* Radiation Therapy Oncology
    Group

S

SAM. *See* Significance analysis of microarray
SDS-PAGE. *See* Sodium dodecyl sulfate
    polyacrylamide gel electrophoresis

SEA. *See* Singular enrichment analysis
Sequence Read Archive (SRA), 116
SFRO. *See* Société Francophone de
    Radiothérapie Oncologique
sh. *See* Short hairpin
Shh. *See* Sonic hedgehog
SHH. *See* Sonic hedgehog signaling
    pathway
Short hairpin (sh), 267–268
Signal-to-noise (STN), 222
Significance analysis of microarray (SAM),
    135
Single-end sequencing, 107–108
Single-nucleotide polymorphism (SNP),
    98, 174–175
Single-Nucleotide Polymorphism Database
    (dbSNP), 122
Single-photon emission computed
    tomography (SPECT), 386
Singular enrichment analysis (SEA), 98
siRNA. *See* Small interfering RNA
SMA. *See* Superior mesenteric artery;
    α-smooth muscle actin
Smad4 tumor suppressor gene. *See* Dpc4
    tumor suppressor gene
Small interfering RNA (siRNA), 266–267
SMF. *See* Streptozocin, mitomycin, and 5-FU
SMPV. *See* Superior mesenteric-portal vein
SMV. *See* Superior mesenteric vein
SNP. *See* Single-nucleotide polymorphism
Société Francophone de Radiothérapie
    Oncologique (SFRO), 50–51
Sodium dodecyl sulfate polyacrylamide gel
    electrophoresis (SDS-PAGE),
    223–224
Sonic hedgehog (Shh), 61–62
Sonic hedgehog signaling pathway (SHH),
    298–299
SOP. *See* Standard operating procedures
Southwest Oncology Group–directed
    intergroup Phase III trial
    (SWOG-S0205), 58
SPECT. *See* Single-photon emission
    computed tomography
Splice junctions, 109
SRA. *See* Sequence Read Archive
Standard operating procedures (SOP),
    151–152

STN. *See* Signal-to-noise
Streptozocin, mitomycin, and 5-FU (SMF), 49
Stromal cells, 204–205
Sulfatase 1 (SULF1), 387
2-(2′-sulfooxyphenyl)-6-[^{125}I]iodo-4-(3H)-quinazolinone (^{125}IQ$_{2-S}$), 394
ARSA, ALP, and PAP-mediated hydrolysis, 395f
2-(2′-sulfooxyphenyl)-6-[^{127}I]iodo-4-(3H)-quinazolinone (^{127}IQ$_{2-S}$), 394
2-(2′-sulfooxyphenyl)-6-iodo-4-(3H)-quinazolinone (IQ$_{2-S}$), 387
docking positions, 391f
hydrolysis, 393t
2-(2′-sulfooxyphenyl)-6-tributylstannyl-4-(3H)-quinazolinone (SnQ$_{2-S}$), 394
Superior mesenteric artery (SMA), 40–41, 47
Superior mesenteric vein (SMV), 47
Superior mesenteric-portal vein (SMPV), 40–41
Surgical resection, 6
SWOG-S0205. *See* Southwest Oncology Group–directed intergroup Phase III trial
SYBR green assay, 155–156
Systems biology, 302
    assessment of toxicity, 306–307
    curation methodologies using, 303
    miRNAs role, 303–304
    network pharmacology, 302
    network-based analyses, 307
    neutraceutical use, 304–305
    patient-specific molecular signature, 304

T

T-cell receptor beta chain (TCRB), 207–208
TAD. *See* Transactivation domain
TaqMan assay, 155–156
TAR-RNA–binding protein (TRBP), 266–267
Target validation, 267–268
Taxol®. *See* Paclitaxel
TCA. *See* Tricarboxylic acid
TCGA. *See* The Cancer Genome Atlas
TCRB. *See* T-cell receptor beta chain
TF. *See* Tissue factor; Transcription factor

TGF-β. *See* Transforming growth factor-β; Tumor growth factor-β
TGM2. *See* Transglutaminase 2
The Cancer Genome Atlas (TCGA), 122–124, 160
Therapeutics targeting disordered metabolism, 336–337
1000 Genomes Project, 124
Three-dimensional cell cultures (3-D cell cultures), 34
Time-of-flight (TOF), 201
TIMP1. *See* Tissue inhibitor of metalloproteinase 1
Tissue banks, 152
Tissue factor (TF), 212–213, 246–247, 258
    expression validation, 262–263, 263f, 265f
    peptide intensity plots, 259f
    RNAi
        functional validation, 271f
        knockdown results, 270–271
Tissue inhibitor of metalloproteinase 1 (TIMP1), 205–206
Tissue microarray analysis (TMA), 163–164
Tissue plasminogen activator (tPA), 202–203, 210
TMA. *See* Tissue microarray analysis
TNF. *See* Tumor necrosis factor
TNM. *See* Malignant tumors
TOF. *See* Time-of-flight
tPA. *See* Tissue plasminogen activator
Transactivation domain (TAD), 76
Transcription factor (TF), 103
Transcription start site (TSS), 105
Transcription termination site (TTS), 105
Transforming growth factor-β (TGF-β), 59–60, 311–314
Transglutaminase 2 (TGM2), 206–207
TRBP. *See* TAR-RNA–binding protein
Tricarboxylic acid (TCA), 332
Truncation, 135–136
Trypsinized cells, 223–224
TSP. *See* Tumor suppressor protein
TSS. *See* Transcription start site
TTS. *See* Transcription termination site
Tumor growth factor-β (TGF-β), 225–230
Tumor necrosis factor (TNF), 328

Tumor suppressor protein (TSP), 410–411
Tumor tissue isolation, 23–24
Tumor-associated syndrome, 329
Two-dimensional electrophoresis (2-DE),
    199–200
Two-dimensional gel electrophoresis
    (2-DGE), 249–250, 255

U

Ultrasonography (US), 5–6
Union for International Cancer Control
    (UICC), 22
University of California, Santa Cruz
    (UCSC), 103
Untranslated region (UTR), 105

V

Variant calling algorithms, 111

Vascular endothelial growth factor (VEGF),
    76–77
Vascular endothelial growth factor receptor
    (VEGFR), 58
Vimentin (VIM), 203, 225–230, 238, 239f
    knockdown in Panc-1 cells, 239, 240f
    overexpression and role, 238
    sensitivity on GEM treatment, 241

W

Whole genome sequencing (WGS), 174
World Cancer Research Fund (WCRF),
    405–406
World Health Organization (WHO), 22

Z

Zinc-finger E-box binding homeobox
    (ZEB), 80–81

Printed and bound by CPI Group (UK) Ltd, Croydon, CR0 4YY

03/10/2024

01040425-0015